HEALERS IN THE NIGHT

Eric de Rosny, S.J.

HEALERS IN THE NIGHT

Translated from the French by
Robert R. Barr

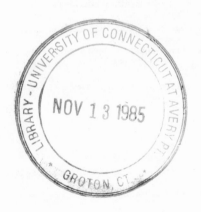

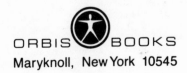

ORBIS BOOKS
Maryknoll, New York 10545

The Catholic Foreign Mission Society of America (Maryknoll) recruits and trains people for overseas missionary service. Through Orbis Books Maryknoll aims to foster the international dialogue that is essential to mission. The books published, however, reflect the opinions of their authors and are not meant to represent the official position of the society.

First published as *Les yeux de ma chévre: Sur les pas des maîtres de la nuit en pays douala (Cameroun)* by Eric de Rosny, copyright © 1981 by Librairie Plon

This translation copyright © 1985 by Orbis Books, Maryknoll, NY 10545

Manuscript Editor: William E. Jerman

Library of Congress Cataloging in Publication Data
Rosny, Eric de, 1930–
  Healers in the night.

  Translation of: Les yeux de ma chèvre.
  1. Duala (African people)—Folklore. 2. Folk
medicine—Cameroon. 3. Duala (African people)—
Religion. 4. Healing—Cameroon. 5. Duala (African
people)—Social life and customs. I. Title.
GR351.2.D82R6713 1985   398'.353   85-5659
ISBN 0-88344-199-3 (pbk.)

A ma mère

Contents

Preface   *ix*

Chapter 1
Douala by Day and by Night   *1*

Chapter 2
A Missionary Vocation Reconsidered   *15*

Chapter 3
The Battlefield of Ndimsi   *30*

Chapter 4
Loe and the Old One   *45*

Chapter 5
Ekong *Sorcery*   *58*

Chapter 6
Misfortune Is Malady   *68*

Chapter 7
The Trial   *84*

Chapter 8
Those Who Perform Cures in the Night   *108*

Chapter 9
The Healing of Dieudonné   *114*

Chapter 10
"Your Sister Is a Sorceress!"   *128*

Chapter 11
The Mountain Khamsi   *150*

Chapter 12
The Khamsi *Inspiration: Magic or Religion?*   *162*

Chapter 13
Order Lost and Restored   *174*

Chapter 14
Truth and Beliefs   *194*

Chapter 15
"Your Eyes Will Be Opened"   *203*

Chapter 16
Death of the Seer   *212*

Chapter 17
The Eyes of My Goat   *224*

Chapter 18
Afterthoughts   *246*

Appendix 1
*Glossary of the Most Important Douala Words Used in This
Book*   *261*

Appendix 2
Dreams   *266*

Appendix 3
The One Who Came Back from the Dead   *269*

Appendix 4
Two Ceremonies Compared   *271*

Appendix 5
Ekongolo Finds Her Jengu *Spouse*   *273*

Appendix 6
*The Various Manners of Preparing and Administering
Medicines*   *274*

Notes   *277*

Preface

This book has been written in the same way in which some of the Douala of the islands of the Wouri (in Cameroon, central Africa) build themselves a new house. They build it not alongside the old one, but right around it. When the old house, with its plank walls and thatched roof, is no longer large enough for the whole family, or threatens to collapse, they box it all around with stakes; then, without dismantling the old structure, they erect a framework and a roof on these stakes in such wise that the new structure covers the old one without touching it.

The owners continue to live in their former home while the walls of cinder block are being put up and the doors and windows fitted. They never really have to "move out." This molting period may take months, even years, if there is no reason for haste or money is in short supply. The procedure has the advantage that the family does not have to move, and that the new walls are impregnated with the old, familiar odors.

I have lived in this book, so to speak, for ten years—from 1970 to 1980— as in a house, giving it ever vaster proportions. From my first encounter with those I could call, for want of a better translation, "Africa's traditional medical practitioners," the *nganga*s of Douala land, I have written down my observations, in the conviction that I would have the opportunity to communicate them.

At first my notes consisted of accounts of night séances and transcriptions of tape recordings. The first pages of my first notebook describe a ceremony that took place in the city of Douala, near the quarter where I was living, without my being able to attend.[1] I reconstructed this material on the basis of interviews. But after that I recorded only events I myself had witnessed. When I thought I had observed a case of enchantment—a spell, for example—and that I had understood the behavior of the *nganga*, I wrote as complete an account of it as possible. Later I entrusted those closest to me—African and European friends, university students, priests—with these confidential notebooks, or sent them to members of my family. My concern for discretion is easy to explain: these passages involved persons I met on a regular basis. But I could not refrain from passing them on.

In 1974, persuaded that the work of these "masters of the night" ought to see the light of day, I took the risk of publishing the first accounts with Editions CLE, in Yaoundé, the Cameroon capital.[2] Had the persons concerned known they would appear in a book, under other names? If so, they had kept it to themselves. For their part, the traditional Douala chiefs welcomed the document, and I thank them here publicly, in this new book, for their rare spirit of openness. I had chosen a Cameroon publisher in order first of all to convince educated Cameroonians themselves of the greatness and competence of their compatriot *ngangas*. The book was to be objective, and I would express my own views but sparingly.

Two lines of argumentation impelled me to build a new book on my earlier one. The more I saw the *ngangas* at work—until indeed one of them caused me to "open my eyes"—the more I was taken by the desire to make them known to as wide an audience as possible. At the same time I was being called upon by those around me, especially by a Douala friend of mine, to air my own views more. "What do *you* think of all this?," he asked me one day.

In 1976 I sent my new manuscript to Jean Malaurie, director of the *Terre Humaine* series (Editions Plon, Paris). The purpose of the series is to throw light on the mysterious affinity between human beings living at one another's cultural antipodes. "The one who opened your eyes summons you from beyond the grave," Malaurie said to me.

The invitation to enter into myself, proffered by a person who had himself shared the life of a people at the ends of the earth, tipped the scales of my decision. It became clear that I must unmask myself in describing the *ngangas*, if I wished to make them as present to the reader as they were to my own eyes. Thanks to the pitiless light that accompanied my effort of writing, I understood that the experience I had had in contact with them had become one flesh with that of my religious life, and that I should have to let this oneness appear if I was to be faithful to the facts.

Like the buildings on the islands of the Wouri, I have sought to respect, beneath my new architecture, the basic documents containing the essentials of what I have to report. Here my tape recordings have a special place. Apart from a few brief expressions reported from memory, the words I here transcribe or translate, as faithfully as I possibly can, come from these recordings. This final draft, then, still rests on the original materials that fascinated and inspired me when I first discovered the world of the *ngangas*.[3]

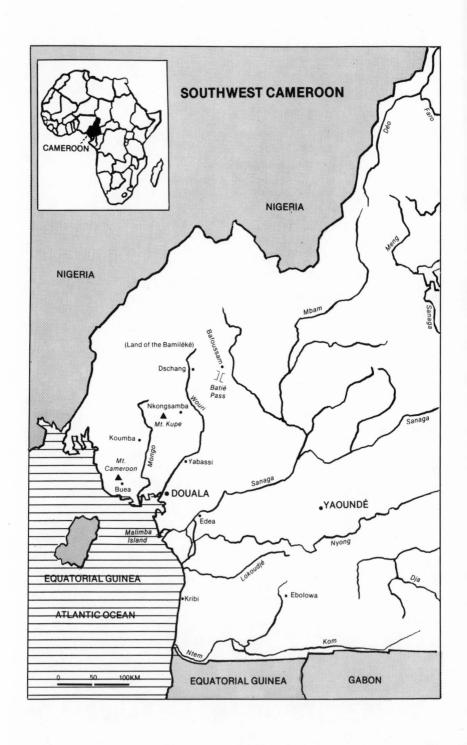

SOUTHWEST CAMEROON

NIGERIA

NIGERIA

Faro

Déo

Meng

Sanaga

Mbam

(Land of the Bamiléké)

Baloussam

Dschang

Batié
Pass

Wouri

Nkongsamba

Mt. Kupe

Sanaga

Koumba

Mongo

Yabassi

Mt.
Cameroon

Sanaga

Buea

DOUALA

Sanaga

YAOUNDÉ

Edea

Nyong

Malimba
Island

Lokoudjé

Dja

EQUATORIAL GUINEA

Kribi

Ebolowa

ATLANTIC OCEAN

Kom

Ntem

EQUATORIAL GUINEA

GABON

CAMEROON

0   50   100KM

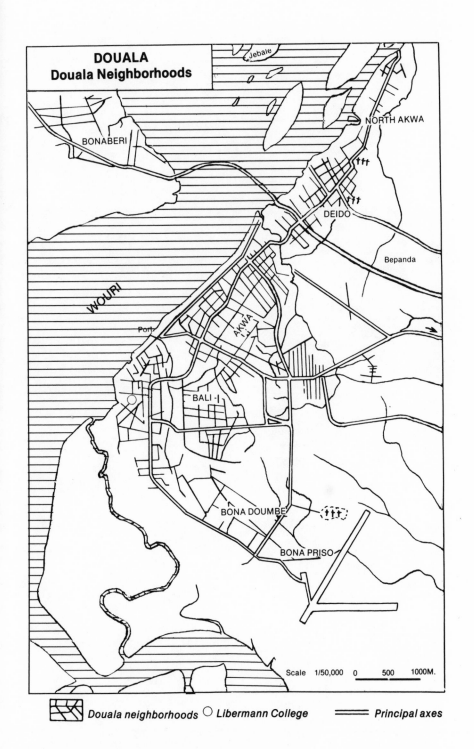

DOUALA
Douala Neighborhoods

Jebale

NORTH AKWA

BONABERI

DEIDO

WOURI

Bepanda

Port

AKWA

BALI

BONA DOUMBE

BONA PRISO

Scale   1/50,000   0   500   1000M.

Douala neighborhoods ○ Libermann College ═══ Principal axes

Chapter 1

Douala by Day and by Night

My First Séance

The magnificent old tree, called in French, curiously, *le Grand Fromager*, the Great Cheese Tree, was just a step or two away from the house I had come to visit. At night its mighty shape stood out so plainly from everything else that fishermen on the river sighted it to steer their course homeward. It was the dwelling place of the ancestors—living witness, in the heart of the city, of the persistence of the traditional beliefs. The symbol was all the mightier for the fact that its comrades on this side of the river were dead, long since.

Not far from the tree, a drum was beating somewhere, and I turned toward a neighboring house. It was nine o'clock at night. Nothing distinguished this house from the others. It, too, was unfinished. It had only the barest essentials: a plate-iron roof over a single-story structure, with walls, in unfinished cement, pierced by rectangular openings. I groped my way along the central corridor that divided the hut in two, and emerged in the rear court, where the drum—an empty hundred-liter barrel with an animal skin stretched across one end—was enthroned.

The young man beating the drum wore a red headband, his only special apparel. He had taken his position at the midpoint of a kind of path, or open space, along which some fifty persons had gathered—seated on little stools, lying on mats, standing, or leaning against the wall. The storm lamp shed precious little light, but I could tell that these men and women, who were chatting quietly, draped in their evening *pagne* (a sash wound around the upper legs, between the legs, and around the loins) were neighborhood residents. At one end of the path was a little enclosure—roofless, some two yards square—built of old iron plates propped vertically. At the other end I counted seventeen little bonfires, some thirty centimeters in height, waiting to be lighted.

I could discern no sign in those around me that they were in any way surprised to see me emerge in their midst in the course of this private night gathering of theirs. Did they already know I had received authorization to join them? In any case someone brought me a chair as if I had been expected and seated me in the front row, beside a man and a woman who were treated with a great deal of respect. They were dressed in the European style, and sat stiffly in their seats. The woman appeared infinitely weary, and did not return my greeting. The man was more willing to talk, and explained that he had come to learn the source of his wife's great exhaustion. Their presence would enable me to follow the events of the evening, for I was not yet fluent in Douala, the language spoken in this locality.

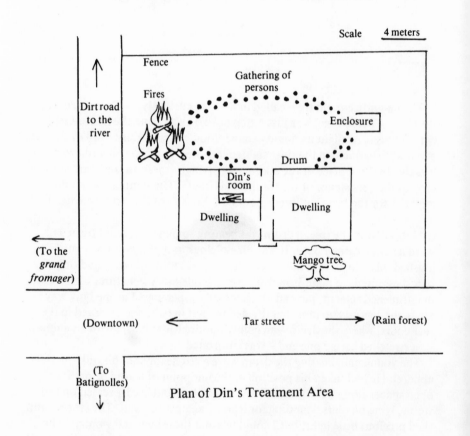

Plan of Din's Treatment Area

It was ten o'clock. Nothing was happening yet. The young man with the red headband beat the drum with one hand, in a dull, regular throbbing. From time to time a peculiar woman burst out into the path to do a couple of dance steps and a bit of clowning for everyone's entertainment.

I asked, "What are they waiting for? Why don't they begin?"

"But . . . they have begun," my neighbor answered.

A few minutes later I was given to understand by a sign that I should go into the house, and I was led up to the door of a room where something was supposed to be happening. A skinny man, rather tall, lay on a bed, his eyes closed. Like the young drummer he wore a red headband, with six little cowries sewn to it. (In earlier times, before money was known, these seashells served as a medium of exchange, and they still have a traditional value.) He was robed in a long red shirt, with a multi-colored sash knotted to his belt and wound about his legs like a shroud. I saw that he was Din, the master who had given me permission to come. For an instant I stood riveted to the spot. He had the ashen hue of a corpse, and his nostrils were pinched. I had to fix my gaze on his chest for a long moment to be sure he was breathing. At his head lay two little straw brooms resembling fly-fans—but they surely were destined for other use, to judge from the elegance with which their handles were set. From where I stood in the doorway, I cast a glance all around the room. The cement walls were bare, without even a trace of paint. A number of pans, or basins, stood on the floor, filled with heaps of various barks that looked all the same to my still ignorant eyes, with grasses and leaves in profusion, all marinating in a yellowish liquid. Bones, horns, claws, and other objects I could not identify in the semi-darkness lay all about. The room was filled with a strong odor of incense, oil fumes, and old leaves. I felt no distaste, fear, or surprise. Or more precisely, I made an effort not to. I was like a diver, holding my breath as if I were weighted to the waters below. And yet I felt in communication with this universe in some way other than by the sense of sight—in a way I could not as yet define.

Suddenly I became very tired, and I went back to my place in the rear court.

My neighbor now explained to me: "Yes, I have seen Din—or rather Din's envelope of flesh, for Din himself is in reality far away now, to the west, on Mount Kupe, to be exact, where the person to be saved tonight is being held prisoner. It seems that some sorcerers are making her work for them on their infamous plantations, where all their victims are gathered. Din is freeing her now. She is called Engome, the woman lying along the wall, just a few feet to our left over there. In appearance, she is there, but her essential person dwells on Kupe—unless indeed Din is bringing her back here at this very moment."

This explanation was given me in a neutral, courteous, subdued tone, just as I should have explained a Christian ceremony to a curious Buddhist.

My neighbor explained that the drum was beating not as a preliminary to the ceremony, but to call forth the water spirits that populate the depths of the river, a few hundred meters to our right. These spirits were a great aid and support in the struggle with the sorcerers. A minute or two went by. Then suddenly, in the rear of the courtyard, an old woman began to tremble on her bench. My neighbor exclaimed, "There are the spirits!" And indeed the old woman behaved like one possessed. Still seated, she would throw her arms forward and bring them back toward herself, rhythmically. It was as if an invisible force had grasped her by the neck, so that her head shook and bounced crazily from left to right, while her whole body was seized with steady, convulsive trembling. The others around her moved away, not interfering. The drum picked up its rhythm. At the same moment I noticed Din among us. He began to dance along the path. He approached the possessed woman, brandishing his two jeweled brooms and stroking her with them several times. He soon succeeded in calming her.

It was now past midnight. Several persons had taken their stations about the seventeen little bonfires, ready to light them all at once. Why seventeen fires? My neighbor did not know. He even hesitated to reply to me at all now that Din was on the scene. Din looked often in my direction, and made signs to me, but I did not understand them. Stepping across a number of reclining bodies, he approached Engome, at the wall. Now he led her to the center of the path. The assemblage applauded. She was a tall, very lean woman, half a head taller than Din. It seemed to me that one of her legs was swollen, and that she walked with discomfort. Here they were, then, the two travelers back from Mount Kupe. They were preparing to finish their circuit right where we sat. Engome, clinging tightly to her liberator's back, had her arms around his waist as if she were holding on for dear life.

With the woman holding onto him and dragging her leg, Din moved across the open space, in every direction and as quickly as he could, to show beyond a doubt that the escape had been successful. When they skirted the fires their faces and necks shone like metal, so heavy was their perspiration. Now the couple was upon us again, zigzagging along and ultimately vanishing into the little iron-plate enclosure.

Din soon reappeared, strutting gingerly, retracing all his steps—two little ones forward, and one to the side. Momentarily he would stop, look to the left, then to the right, as if he scented danger. From the moment he emerged, he was singing out little refrains, in a nasal voice, and the group would repeat them in chorus. I had the impression that the melodies were familiar to all, but that some of the words were being composed for the occasion. I recall: "*Wanea mo, wanea mo, Engome e nde o Kupe, wanea mo*" ("Bring her back, bring her back, Engome is on Kupe, bring her back").[4]

The heat—seventeen fires had been lighted—and Din's dance infected us all with a kind of glee. I was surprised to find myself laughing right out loud, then yawning. Even the woman next to me, my commentator's wife, appeared to smile and relax. Now little flat boards, like schoolroom rulers, were passed around, and we beat them together in rhythm, to accompany the chants. The night was pitch-dark, and I was still the only stranger. And yet, in this transfigured backyard, I felt completely safe.

From about two o'clock on, the joyous harmony began to soften. Demijohns filled with a milky juice, made from sweet, sugared sap drawn directly from palm trees, were brought in. Also served, alas, was some warm beer and bad rum, which could not be refused. There were long periods when nothing was happening. Many fell asleep where they were. I was unable to find a comfortable position: if I crossed my legs or feet, someone would immediately come up and uncross them. Did they find my attitude or posture offensive? I did not see how they could, but I submitted.

Suddenly it seemed to be "intermission time." Din kept disappearing and reappearing. Several persons, including the couple seated next to me, went to consult him in his room. I had a good number of questions to ask him myself, and I stopped him each time he passed. He allowed me to pose my questions, but his replies were always rudimentary. He looked as if he thought I had much to learn. Why all these fires? They discouraged the sorcerers, who were among us, from counteracting his efforts. What was over there in the enclosure? A powerful shrub, protecting Engome. I asked him whether the young woman would soon be well. He replied that she already was. I objected that she still limped, and I imitated her gait. He laughed, and invited me to inquire of those around us of Engome's condition when she had come to him a month before, all swollen and practically paralyzed. Din described, with his hands, a great, bulging body. And with a knowing glance, off he would be to drink and dance some more. How old was he, I wondered. I could not have said. Once youth is past, the African seems to be of an indefinite age, until sinking away into extreme old age.

About four o'clock in the morning I was roused from my dozing by drum rolls. From the far end of our ranks, Din's assistant was slamming his drum, with palms and elbows, for all he was worth. Everyone adjusted their clothing and stood up. A shiver ran through the assemblàge. Suddenly Din, barefoot, was trampling on the seventeen fires, extinguishing them, one by one, by dancing upon them. "Look, that's his miracle," my neighbor said to me. And indeed it was an impressive performance. I could see he was grimacing—but was that not the same face he had just been making when he and Engome had been "traveling"? We all followed him in procession, through the smoke of the smoldering bonfires, right up to the enclosure, where the young woman was standing to receive us. And now she was admitted to the assemblage that had swarmed into the path. Could I be mistaken? The "lame" woman seemed to dance normally! I went back and sat down. The couple next to me and I were the only three persons in the yard still seated. I was at once dumbfounded, overwhelmed, and . . . so tired.

The first gray light crept upon the roofs. Imperceptibly the balance of night was shifting. Near the equator, day breaks in one swoop. It was still dark, but I could feel the morning at hand. Still it would not have been possible to leave without displeasing Din. One could not leave before the final repast.

To enliven my legs a bit I went over to see where the meal was being prepared. Din's wife had been working for hours, behind the enclosure. "I've had a goat cooked, sacrificed last night," she told me off-handedly, "in place of Engome. This is what the sorcerers would have done to her." She had seasoned it with a kind of plantain called *miele ma sese*, as well as some edible herbs, which had cured Engome. She had mixed in condiments, and secret blossoms, that all *nganga* wives know. They give the dish its unique aroma. All was in readiness now. Din made off with several morsels and scattered them to the four corners of the court: the ancestors would be served first. Then he placed us around large pots: the meal would be a ceremonial one, and there were rules to follow. I had the honor of a place beside Engome.

All present squatted on their heels, plunging both hands into the common dish at once, fingertips together, and bringing the food to their mouths with a twist of the wrist that was easy to learn to do. I watched my neighbors carefully, then did as they, with clumsily folded fingers, but a heart full of joy. Only Din touched nothing. The meal was taken in silence and continued until there was nothing left over—a meal of great symbolic flavor, after all the hours I had spent with my companions, as they delivered one of their own from death.

It was daybreak, February 5, 1971, when I returned home from Din's séance. I felt an imperative need for sleep. The need I felt was not one of sheer physical fatigue. Ordinarily I do not try to fall asleep immediately after a long evening, especially when I have had some poor quality alcohol. But something was different this morning. I felt a special *desire* for deep sleep. I felt a kind of lassitude, and at the same time a great sensation of peace—a feeling of having emerged at last upon some beach, after a lonely journey through an endless forest, such as one finds along the Cameroon coast. The beach is access to the ocean. Of course it is not yet its crossing.

Before giving way to sleep, I attempted to analyze all that I felt. First, I noted a strong inner resistance in myself, surely owing at least in part to my fatigue. The slow pace, the slack periods, the lack of organization, and a certain feeling of having to "kill time"—all this had been trying to my nerves. A good part of the ceremony had been completely beyond my comprehension. I knew only a few words of Douala, and so the meaning of much of what was said had escaped me. Tomorrow I would go to see the patient and her family to ask them a few questions. Then I would play back what I had recorded tonight on my tape recorder. Then I would try to get Din to explain to me the ceremony as a whole and the meaning of each of the rites. I should have to perform each of these steps, in order, to try to understand. And I was aware of the extreme difficulty and degree of concentration of my powers that I should have to manage in order to attain this understanding.

I really felt split in two. I was beset with doubts as to the validity of the experience. Coming to the séance entirely of my own accord, I had stood surety for Din—been his endorsement—by my mere presence in the front row, from one end of the night to the other. Young Africans today have been drawn into a new world—the world of science, technology, and a global way of life. Why was I doing just the opposite? Why was I being dragged into a world of night, a world of symbols and rites of initiation? Why was I attracted by manifestations of a culture that was, so evidently, under condemnation henceforth and forevermore? It was an irritating question, and I thrust it aside as if it had been a temptation. The moment would come, however, when I should have to face up to it and answer it.

And yet I felt at peace. I had the feeling of having found something I had been searching for, however confusedly. Fourteen years after my arrival in Douala, I was discovering, for the first time, an electrifying expression of African culture; its benefits were beyond question and it owed nothing to Europe. On festival days, the population of Douala would be summoned to the traditional presentations in public places, where delegations from the various quarters of the city would perform dances and ceremonies of times gone by. Din's night séance was much different. It was not done to demonstrate the existence of an African culture. It was the very practice of this culture, in one of its principal functions: healing. No one there looked as if they were playacting. They were giving someone back her life—restoring the balance in a family. Even my presence had not modified the fixed order of the ceremony, still less its objectives. Din may have put a bit more into his dance, but he had not delayed Engome's liberation. Had I hampered him, he would have had a reason for getting rid of me. I was convinced of the authenticity of the ceremony. The door of knowledge stood ajar before me.

This healing ceremony was the first of a long series for me. I was to return to Din's house the following Saturday, and many other times, to the point where I would become a "regular" at his night séances. Then I was to come in contact with numerous colleagues of his, men and women, who practiced healing in Douala and other places. My gradual discovery of their universe is the subject of this book.

But this first night was also the end of a personal journey of mine, and I shall have to explain this before we go further. I had not come to Din's house casually. It was not a matter of momentary curiosity, as it was with tourists, or Europeans who lived in Africa, drawn by the sound of the drum and eager to see a private ceremonial celebration. They come and stand in a far corner of the court—despite invitations to be seated—take a couple of photographs, then discreetly withdraw, rather bewildered. I had come neither as an ethnologist nor as a critic. My case was quite different: I had been "called" to Din's house.

Vaulting the Gap

I had arrived in Douala fourteen years before—in September 1957—to join a team of five Jesuits who had preceded me by several weeks. We were to take over the charge of an institution of Catholic education, the Libermann School. We were new in the country. Indeed we had had no experience of black Africa. I had several years of the religious life behind me, which had been devoted to the study of literature and philosophy, but I was not yet a priest. Two years later, I would begin the study of theology. Meanwhile, it had been agreed that I should give courses in French and English to the pupils in this school. I had been sent because someone was needed, of course, but also because I had always manifested the desire to be a missionary.

I must also mention a certain experience that had left its mark on me, an experience still fresh in my memory as I arrived in Cameroon. It may clarify the state of mind in which I found myself. I came to Cameroon when the war in Algeria was raging its fiercest. I had been drafted in 1956, along with all the young men of my status, and attached to a unit of riflemen operating on the border between Algeria and Morocco. Shortly after my discharge I went to Cameroon. I still had dramatic, terrible sights before my eyes—all the more painful for my having also spent two years in Lebanon. The war had crushed me.

I shall recount only one thing that happened to me at that time, something I shall never forget, and something with a special meaning for my story. It was the experience of living in the Jebel region with a Berber prisoner for a number of weeks. We had managed to keep him with us instead of sending him to the interrogation center. We were helping the man to "play dead." After all, we could consider him dead—he had fallen into a night ambush along a wadi and had been fired upon by every man in our patrol, in a thunder of rifle reports by the light of the moon. He had been pressed into service by other fellahs to serve as their scout, and now scout and donkey together had collapsed under the rain of our fire. To our great astonishment, however, our target had suffered nothing worse than a bullet in the foot. Bad night ballistics? Deliberate misses? Miracle? In any case, there he was. We took pity on him, deciding he was "dead." He spoke no French, and we no Arabic. We looked on him, noble, impassive, with his shaved head and his foot in a plaster cast, and draped in his white jellaba. He returned our glance. Soon he would be gone. But all the while he was with us the distance was unbearable for me, and I strove to bridge the gap interiorly. From that moment forward, I was obsessed with the need for a genuine *encounter* with "the other."

I arrived in Douala a few days before the opening of the school year, bursting with a desire to come to know the world of the students who were to be confided to me. It seemed to me that it would have been unrealistic to wish to teach them anything, even English, without appropriate cultural preparation on my own part. My future would depend on these young persons, for they would be my first interlocutors in Cameroon. I had not come here for a visit. I had come to stay, for a great part of my life as a missionary. And so I would be concerned about the smallest variations in our relationship, or the slightest nuances in their confidence in me. A genuine time of trial was beginning for me. There would be strange oscillations on the barometer and I would not always know why. An unexpected barrier would spring up between my students and myself—not a hostile one, like the one I had known during the war, but one just as hopeless, at least on a certain level. I would have to learn to tolerate a permanent, subtle disproportion between the image they presented to me and their indecipherable personalities.

Incontestably, the very architecture of the school, as well as its organization, threw up a wall between us. There was nothing Cameroonian here. We had a carbon copy of a French school: two long white buildings, efficiently divided into dormitories, classrooms, a refectory, teacher's rooms, a chapel, and alongside them, a courtyard with a soccer field.

Libermann is a drab looking school for a part of the year, when great stretches of its walls are covered over with a black mildew. Some of the decor recalls colonial days—like the heavy, vertical shutters that you let down like a trap door, with a great clatter through the whole building, when sheets of rain pound down against the walls. But how else would you build a building to hold two hundred young persons working for their secondary school diplomas and their certificates of entry for the university? You simply had to build it that way!

The scholastic programs conformed to the standards of the University of Bordeaux, which determined the subjects for examination and the updating of transcripts. Besides, we were coming to the rescue of a teaching staff that was mainly French, teaching its courses in French, with students from all over southern Cameroon, whose common language, by virtue of modern history, happened to be French.

To be sure, I could have rested content with the expatriation afforded by nature itself—which reached right into the heart of the city, despite all the asphalt and concrete.

Fierce, speechless sign of a world different from mine, what would this nature reveal to me? We had 150 inches of rain a year—rain like an apocalypse, which, when no wind came to sweep away the clouds, fell heavily for hours, sometimes days, uninterruptedly. It was a warm, friendly-looking rain, and children would run outdoors to dance in its empire. But soon they would come in again, and spend the rest of the time crouching indoors. Eventually the rain would seem like a plague. Vegetation was rife, and a shoot of something appeared in every crack and cranny.

I recall my first class in the Libermann School. It was a small bridging of the gap between my senior students and myself. Thirty students standing at attention gazed questioningly up at me. I was so taken aback at their attitude that I could scarcely open my mouth. What I was about to tell them was that there would be no fooling me with this stilted first-day comportment! It was the same in schools everywhere!

They listened to me with extraordinary attention. I quickly guessed the reason. They were having some difficulty in following me. They had been accustomed to African teachers, and my accent startled them. That was all. Soon, however, their eyes would shine and sparkle, and we would have complete understanding. Not that the "military" approach would grow soft. True, the students would eventually relax a bit, but only a bit. And they would turn out to be the studious, patient learners that every teacher dreams of.

The weak point of our approach was that they would be interested only in the formal material of the course. They would care only about the textbook, and preparation for exams. My attempts to open their minds to the world of literature were doomed to failure. In their eyes, my only task was to dispense the knowledge that would lead to a diploma. The rest was beside the point. Each time I began to move away from the syllabus, they politely signalled their displeasure. I was being served my first notice of what I was to encounter again and again. I felt that they were like mobiles, that they obeyed inflexible laws, to which they expected me, too, to submit, without revealing to me their content.

It was easy to understand their tenseness, given the political climate of Cameroon. Before World War I, their country had been a German colony. After the war it had been an English and French mandate, and in 1957 it had still not gained full independence. But independence was imminent, and there was tension in the air. An armed rebellion was in progress in the rain forest, at the very gates of Douala. Commandos would appear in town out of nowhere. All this contributed to a climate of insecurity.

The students were electric. They loved to climb to the attic of the school, for instance, because the name "Libermann" was painted there in great capital letters, and they had chosen to understand the name in the sense of *homme libre*, the "free human being," even though it was really just the name of a famous missionary. To follow the course of events, the students were not content with listening to rumors in the various quarters of the city. They read every newspaper they could put their hands on, *Le Monde* in particular. The publishers would surely have been surprised to know they had such assiduous young readers in Cameroon!

Instead of distracting them, the political turmoil seemed to give the young students reasons to work. Even the youngest could appreciate that a free country would need new leaders, engineers, technicians, and especially politicians. They certainly believed in the value of the printed word. They were dreamers, but this did not interfere with their studies. At examination time the prefects had to prowl the corridors, looking for students working into the night with the aid of flashlights.

We newcomers were strangers to the spirit of colonialism, and we fraternized freely with our students. The fresh, brisk wind of liberty was blowing, and the strains of nationalism resounded in our ears like old choruses from our own history. These children would gladly discuss all these things endlessly—without revealing to us the least thing about themselves.

I had the feeling of missing out on whole broad areas of their lives. Between classes, our young pupils would remain in their classrooms, stand with their backs against the wall, motionless, intrepid—but with their eyes in constant, quick movement, which provided a very striking contrast. They were so observant, so perceptive, that they became automatic mimics. Some of them, when they greeted one of our colleagues who had spent a part of his life in China and had acquired certain affable Chinese mannerisms, made themselves look Chinese! This trait went beyond the common tendency of the adolescent to imitate adults. I do not think they had the particular sensitivity, the cast of spirit, that French youth have at their age, but I would be hard put to describe their own, so expert had they become at reflecting the world I had come from.

I was on the lookout for anomalies in their social conduct, and I did not have to search very far. For instance, I once punished one of them for regularly coming late to class. I expected an attitude of neutrality on the part of his comrades, perhaps, or even a certain sympathy. To my great discomfiture, the whole class faced off against the unfortunate lad, to the point where I had to take up his defense myself. The same class showed equal hostility toward the student who did best in the course.

One day we organized a table tennis tournament, to pass a rainy afternoon. The students' participation in the eliminations was lively—through the quarter-finals. But the semi-finalists displayed such indifference that no champion was ever declared. Why? Because any student who was either the best or the worst in anything was openly or secretly disapproved of by his comrades.

Thus I came by the surprising revelation that the lives of these young persons, above and beyond appearances, had an underside, a secret counterpart. Shortly after my arrival, a boy named Bona was suddenly seized in the dormitory by a convulsive trembling, as if he were suffering an attack of epilepsy. He shook with steady, violent spasms, and there seemed to be nothing we could do about it. He stretched out his arms and cried, "madiba, madiba!" One of the boys immediately translated this for us as a cry for water.

Sprinkled with water, Bona finally became calm. His comrades explained that this had not been an ordinary seizure. "It's the *jengu*, the water spirit. The *jengu* does not wish Bona to remain at the school." And indeed, in spite of all my efforts, Bona did not manage to pass his courses. He just sat in class, day after day, hour after hour, flaccid and absent. Finally, to get rid of "evil influences," his parents took him to the north and I never saw him again.

Following this incident, some of the students began to confide in me, and I heard stories of sorcery. They talked about spirits and their ancestors with a zest and detail, with such vivacity and conviction, that I felt my cultural rug being pulled out from under me. I listened to their accounts impassively, knowing that the slightest smile would have caused them to break off at once. But as a matter of fact I did not feel much like smiling. I was moved, more than I let show. It was as if these young Africans were already drawing me, blindfolded, into the deep caverns of their own beliefs.

Our situation had become truly uncomfortable. (I speak in the plural because several of my colleagues shared my feeling.) How, we wondered, was it possible to undertake the education of the young without knowing the underpinnings of their culture? Georges Balandier's *Sociologie actuelle de l'Afrique noire, Les Brazzavilles noires,* and *L'Afrique ambiguë* had been published, and Jean Rouch's film *Moi, un Noir* had just appeared.[5] We had read the historians of religion, too, and other classics of ethnology. All these had strengthened our faith in the substantiality of African civilizations. But they scarcely enabled us to create a pedagogy. Nor were our students themselves of any help. They resisted the idea of belonging to two cultures, theirs and ours. They were being penetrated by crosscurrents of modernity and of tradition so intertwined that they were unable to distinguish between them.

We were missing a trump: a knowledge of the world these teenagers came from. And we could not count on them alone to provide us with it. For lack of anything better, we made an effort to live as close to our students as possible, in order to progress by osmosis, as it were. We often shared meals and recreation with them, and our offices were always open. Our standard of living was as modest as theirs. We did not behave this way as a matter of strategy, but spontaneously, to close the gap between us. Their extreme kindness was an encouragement, but of course we could not learn anything from that alone.

Our situation was not exceptional. Most Europeans practicing a profession or carrying on a trade in Douala were in a less sensitive position still: they moved among the Africans and ignored them. Some of our French compatriots—there were some eight thousand in Douala—had come to the conclusion that the blacks had no culture of their own and defied us to prove the contrary. Unlike us, teachers, many of them had only superficial contacts with the people. Besides their "houseboys" with their conditioned reflexes, white women had only finicky post office, telephone, and telegraph employees and various art merchants to contend with. As for their husbands, they came home from work exasperated with what they called their workers' "inertia" and their African managers' "incompetence." A few aspersions cast on "African culture" were these persons' only reflections on the subject. Who was at fault? Surely the structures were more guilty than the persons on either side.

In conditions such as these, how would it be possible to come to a knowledge of another people's culture? I use the word "culture" with hesitation. I fear I may be misunderstood. I do not use it to denote a civilization's froth or luxury, but to denote the particular, ungraspable spirit of a people. How would it be possible to gain a notion of that except through objects of sense? This was a source of acute distress and irritation for me. I could feel the presence of this spirit—which would enable me to understand my students—but I perceived its traces only fleetingly.

I examined the oldest houses of the city, in the hope of finding some mark of an indigenous style. But I was surprised. These beautiful, sturdy huts, all in rust and mildew, only recalled the time of the German colonization.

The only writing that had been invented in this part of the world was that of the Sultan Njoya, who had lived in a region far to the north of Douala. He had created it at the turn of the century for the needs of his court. It was an object of curiosity, but of no practical value. Everything, or nearly everything, in this city and in this school took me back to my own history.

After a term of teaching, I was consumed by a furious desire to leave the place—to use my vacation for going all about this country and *learning* something about it.

Cameroon is divided into two parts, north and south. This seemingly rather self-evident observation is fraught with far-reaching implications. Except for their colonial characteristics, rooted in the past, northern and southern Cameroon differ in every way imaginable. Differing geographies, climates, languages, and religions make of the two parts of the country two mutually foreign worlds. To the north are the tropical grasslands, dry heat, Islam, ancient and tenacious African religions, languages of Sudanese origin, and tall, mahogany-skinned persons. To the south are the rain forest, humidity, Christianity, Bantu languages, medium-height persons of copper hue. Only recent history has compacted these peoples, more different from each other than Norwegians and Greeks, into a single nation.

First I decided to visit the north. I shall not relate in detail this earliest experience of mine, though I must say that I returned from it in utter astonishment and wonder. The north offered me everything I could wish for—a pleasant vacation, lush landscapes, adventure, but especially it gave me what I was searching for secretly: physical proof of the existence of Africa. And so I was most receptive to whatever might strike my senses—the melodious languages, the penetrating scents, the lights and shadows. I also arrived at the conviction that I could indeed find the original, unfamiliar Africa.

This experience, however, failed to move beyond the stage of first impressions. I should have followed in the footsteps of the Bororo and their flocks. I should have come to know the Banana by more than just their chants. I should have stayed in a village a few months. What were the concerns, the desires, the faith of these Cameroonians? The essentials eluded me. The splendor of the north was as deceptive as the European mask my students wore.

I spent all my other vacations, during those first two years in Cameroon, crisscrossing the south of the country, with the same eagerness. What did the south have to offer? Endless ocean shores, a 13,000-foot mountain at the gates of Douala—Mount Cameroon—and an impenetrable rain forest.

René Bureau, then a teacher in the Libermann School, was gathering research for a study he was doing, and I often accompanied him on his jour-neys.⁶ After so much traveling, in search of something too vague to say what it was, I finally came to this conclusion: vacation trips would not teach me much more than what I could learn in the Libermann School. I had to think of another approach.

There was a third type of encounter. I had experienced it many times, without ever guessing what promise it held. I had needed all these pleasant, but useless, explorations on the surface of the country to bring me back to the reality of Douala and open my eyes. As it happened, I often had visits of courtesy to pay to the families of my students who lived in the working-class quarters of the city. I would load up as many as a dozen students in my van, and we would stop for just a moment with each one's family. It could have made for a tiresome trip, given the number and the brevity of the visits and my own ignorance of local languages. But I returned home happy every single time. Hospitality had been total and spontaneous. I did not feel the same wish to tear away some intangible veil, as I did at the school. I began to perceive that my integration into this milieu was not impossible. I made a decision. I would endeavor to put down roots in a Douala quarter. I would live away from the school complex.

My project, alas, was not destined to be put into execution. The years passed, and I returned to France, as scheduled, to study theology and be ordained a priest. I finished the Jesuit course of studies with a second nov-itiate year devoted primarily to prayer. Then I went back to Cameroon for five more years, where my tasks, first at the Libermann School and then as a chaplain at the University of Yaoundé, left me very little free time.

Then something momentous happened. Briefly, students had staged a walkout at the university. When I decided to invite the university Christian community to meditate on the event, it caused displeasure in high places. In September 1969, I had to leave Cameroon.⁷

Chapter 2

A Missionary Vocation Reconsidered

In Paris, I tried to catch my breath and think things over. To be sure, I had obtained a return visa to Cameroon. The incident provoking my expulsion had not been serious enough to merit definitive exile. But *ought* I to go back? I had a question in the depths of me—a painful, obsessive question. It was not a matter of an incidental turn of affairs. It was a matter of my basic life orientation. Should I stay in France or should I go back? Would I persevere in my missionary vocation?

Leisurely and calmly, with the help of a Jesuit who had been a spiritual director of mine, I reviewed the motives that had once impelled me to leave my family and homeland for a land far away. It was not a question of an in-depth analysis of my childhood. I had no inclination for this, to begin with, and my spiritual director was not a psychoanalyst. I only sought to understand what this curious desire was still doing in me at the age of forty; *I wanted to go back to Cameroon.*

I reviewed my life, beginning with my birth, where my paternal and maternal families came together, to see to what extent my family and upbringing had influenced me to the life of a Jesuit missionary. When my parents, both of them of practicing Christian families of the nobility, had married, it was as if two rivers had found their confluence. I express it in this way principally to convey the harmonious understanding my mother and father exemplified all their lives. But they also had a common relative (for whom I barely missed being named—one Antoine-Nicolas, whose name I was excused from bearing because, at that particular time, Nicolas was thought of as a funny name to have). My parents had been reared in an identical gentle, disciplined atmosphere, though my father was from Boulonnais and my mother from Normandy.

On both sides of the family, for generations, the girls would grow up at the château and the boys went off to Jesuit schools—abroad, during the period of the Jesuit exile from France, while the antireligious legislation of Combes, dating from the turn of the century, was still in force, then to schools in France after the restoration. My father had first had his Jesuit primary and secondary education in this manner. He then graduated from the Ecole Polytechnique, after which he was commissioned an instructor in the artillery school at Fontainebleau, where I was born.

I was often told how the Jesuits of Normandy would visit my maternal grandmother's château, to work or rest. And my mother's youngest brother—to cite only my nearest relative in the religious life—had become a Jesuit (to no one's surprise) and spent a great part of his life in the west of France, tirelessly preaching in the "home missions." He was a fine, good man, and I regarded him with admiration on his rare visits to my parents.

As far back as I can remember, I can recall joining my hands in prayer, learning to read, and moving about in this large, traditional Christian family, where I drew deep breaths of freedom and peace. I recall matchless vacations with a tribe of cousins who seemed to have their special way of having fun.

But then it was 1940, I was ten years old, my father was a prisoner, and we had to leave Boulonnais—my mother, brothers, sisters, and I—to follow the columns of exile and take refuge in Sarthe. I suppose these events ought to have cut out part of the joy of my childhood somehow, and I should be hard put to explain how it was that nothing of the kind occurred, at least not in depth. This joy became invulnerable, so to speak, so that it is a part of me even today.

At the age of eleven I knew clearly—on a strange, calm, preadolescent threshold—that I was to be a missionary. On my confirmation day, I felt overwhelmed by an unutterable fulness that I simply had to communicate to the ends of the earth.

In 1949, after secondary school studies pursued in the catch-as-catch-can of the postwar years, in various boarding schools maintained by diocesan clergy or Jesuits, I entered the Jesuits, with the explicit request that I be sent one day to a mission country. This was the sole condition a candidate could attach to entry into this order, in which one's availability was supposed to be total. I had the unconditional approval of my family, and yet no one— not even my mother, who so hoped for a missionary vocation for me—had consciously influenced me, or so it seems to me. The family waters flowed in me as in an old riverbed.

Being sent to Cameroon rather than to some other country was purely circumstantial.

As I dug up the past, with the help of my spiritual director, I felt no discomfiture in searching for the roots of my missionary vocation in my upbringing and education. I was analyzing this religious experience from the point of view of my adolescent psychology, yes, but I was not seeking to reduce any irrational or mystical dimension. I was merely looking for the phenomenological reason why I had thrown myself, wholeheartedly and headlong, into a missionary mentality and life to the point of making it my whole reason for living.

It was thus that I discovered the power of equilibrium that this vocation

tion held. It had enabled me to effect a concrete reconciliation between my adherence to the Christian faith in which I had been reared, and my desire for independence. Both would be maintained if I left for another country. I could go and spread this joy and this truth, of which my family seemed to have given me such an intense, abundant store, to other human beings. I would perform the function of a missionary—in my eyes, the highest there was. And I would leave father, mother, brothers, and sisters, as the gospel counseled. Without a doubt, I had solved, in my own way and without calculation, in the particular context of a religious vocation, the problem of my emancipation. Was this what explained my perseverance?

Thus I submitted the call of my childhood to the crucible of close, rational reflection. And I found it still intact, like an ancient urn in an archeological excavation. I still considered my decision at age eleven as valid and viable, and the right thing for my future. My desire to "go far, far away" was no longer couched in the same terms, it is true, but it was just as imperative as ever. In Paris they said to me, "What are you going down there for? There's a shortage of priests in France. If you're looking for missionary work, you'll find it right here."

But that was not the question. I wanted to live in a world different from my own. To be sure, if my superiors had asked me, for strategic reasons, to stay, I would have obeyed. But one Jesuit in three works outside his native country, and I chose to follow the missionary tradition of my order. My vocation and my human desires coincided. Perhaps they were even confused with each other, as the future would show. Here I saw my highly integrated upbringing as the cause. And I had no regrets.

I often recalled the first scene in Paul Claudel's *The Tidings Brought to Mary*, when Anne Vercors explains why he is leaving. I saw an analogy between the situation Claudel was imagining and my own. The discovery of this spiritual relationship or bond between Claudel's character and me said far more to me than any analyses I might make on the subject. The reasons Anne gives for leaving his old wife after so many years of happiness struck a particularly responsive chord in me:

THE MOTHER: Lord! You are going away! You mean it? And where are you going?

ANNE VERCORS *(pointing vaguely toward the south)*: Down there....

THE MOTHER: But we are very comfortable here and nobody troubles Rheims.

ANNE VERCORS: That is it.

THE MOTHER: That is what?

ANNE VERCORS: The very thing; we are too happy. And the others not happy enough.

THE MOTHER: Anne, that is not our fault.

ANNE VERCORS: It is not theirs either.[8]

The decision to return did not depend on purely personal considerations. I was conducting my solitary debate at a moment when many were publicly questioning the opportuneness of sending new foreign missionaries to Africa. Between 1941, the year of the birth of my vocation, and 1970, the year I questioned it, the African church had matured. Pope Paul VI, on a visit to Kampala, had just made a most profound declaration, one with immediate repercussions for me. "Africans," he had declared, "from now on you are to be your own missionaries." And I was heading for southern Cameroon, one of the regions of Africa where the number of Christians and the proportion of native priests was highest. If I set out for Cameroon again, it could not be as a missionary.

My spiritual director assisted me in defining new conditions of presence for a foreign priest in an African country with a relatively high Christian population. My conclusions appeared in the review *Etudes*, in the form of an article entitled "Mission terminée?" ("mission accomplished?")—a title I had borrowed from a Cameroonian novelist, adding the question mark myself.[9] Anyone who knew me would not have found it difficult to distinguish between my own particular, personal considerations, and the pros and cons already being debated by other missionary priests of my generation. Indeed, I think I actually wrote this article mainly to make a definitive commitment in my own mind. The results of my several months of reflection, if put down in print, would represent a firmer commitment for the future than would a hand-written resolution. And this article was indeed to guide my conduct in the years to come.

The clearest of my conclusions were couched in two practical considerations addressed to non-African priests desirous of serving in Christian Africa today. First, they would have to be willing to accept a considerable "cultural reversal" in the regions where they were being called. That is, they would have to learn the language commonly spoken there, study the customs still pervading social life, become familiar with the ancestral beliefs that charged the culture from which new Christians were coming, and share the daily life of the people in all its truth.

Secondly, I counseled modesty and discretion. Church offices ought not be showy. Precisely at the moment when Africans were becoming Christian in their own way, it would have been absurd for Europeans to cling to their positions and prerogatives. And I concluded with myself very much in mind:

> I see a place in these countries for foreign priests who will no longer have the status they once enjoyed as officials, but whose network of personal relationships will make up for this by being more extensive. They will live without reliance on titles and institutions—as priests among their friends, as believers among other believers.

This conclusion would surely be criticized. It would be seen as retreat, abdication, *dé-mission*. And yet it actually demanded of the candidate a prime quality of the missionaries of times gone by: a compelling desire to communicate, to share, their faith. Courses of action would be different. But nothing would be lost of what constituted the essentials of missionary life.

The expatriate priest would preach less, baptize little, build no new churches in countries where that was in the hands of others—but would be a humble witness of the gospel in the very midst of life itself. He would not shine like a lamp on a mountain top; he would be lost like leaven in dough, and that was just as evangelical.

I sent a copy of this article to the superior of the Jesuits in Cameroon, himself a Cameroonian. I sent it without comment. I was sure he would read it against its dual background—the general one of the church today, and the particular one: mine. I had decided that his reaction would constitute the deciding vote. If he supported my thesis, I would return to Cameroon. If he basically criticized it, I would ask to remain in France.

This decision may seem rather abrupt, after all my soul-searching, and I suppose it was. But it lent my decision an objectivity I felt it lacked.

In the course of the following months, the Cameroon superior wrote me several letters, but he never alluded to the article. He must have received the manuscript, then the issue of *Etudes* in which it appeared, for he was a subscriber. This unexpected reticence puzzled me. I finally took his silence as an invitation to make the decision on my own. I decided to return to Cameroon. I asked his permission to spend a year in a Douala quarter to learn a local language. He most willingly gave his consent.

Life in Deïdo

In October 1970, then—a few months before discovering the intense activity of Douala by night—I found myself in the process of selecting a quarter of the city to settle in, and a language to learn. I chose the Douala language without hesitation, for two very simple reasons: I had begun its study during my other years here, and it happened to be the only genuinely local language—that of the old inhabitants of the Douala region.

This choice immediately eliminated most quarters of the city for purposes of residence. The city had experienced a great deal of growth since World War II, what with the expansion of the port, the beginning of industrialization, and the immigration explosion—strangers flooding in from all over the country in pursuit of a diploma, others coming in search of jobs. The population had increased from fifty thousand to six hundred thousand in the space of twenty-five years. The natives, in the true sense of the word— that is, the original owners of the land, the Douala themselves—had been lost in the deluge. They had not abandoned their traditional land along the Wouri—the river flowing down to the port—but they no longer represented, overall, more than a small minority: twenty-seven thousand persons scattered in three quarters of the city and some nearby villages. My problem, then, was simple: to choose one of those three quarters. I followed friends' advice and opted for the least central one, Deïdo. The Deïdo, where the Douala language was still dominant.

Most of the events narrated in the rest of this book happened in Deïdo. The name came from an English corvette, the Dido, which had lain at anchor a little way up the river sometime in the 1850's. The quarter was composed of several parallel subquarters, each opening out onto the river at one end, and what used to be Douala country at the other. In former times, the Douala nobility had lived along the river, where traffic and political power were concentrated; their serfs occupied the hinterland.This geographical division by social classes had totally disappeared, but the names of the subquarters had persisted, as well as their old boundaries, as originally determined by the language spoken there. One still heard references to the hierarchy of days gone by, whether at the traditional soirees, in discussions on property rights, in pleasantries, or the like. Even after the Republic was inaugurated, the Douala were still the aristocrats. I found something in them of the dignified simplicity of my own family.

I went to lodge in the inland part of one of the subquarters. I chose two little rooms I had found in a vast dwelling: one would be for sleeping and the other for receiving visitors. I moved in with a minimum of furniture. (I hoped I would be invited to meals by my neighbors, and had not even gathered any cooking utensils, other than a hot plate.) The house was not of a usual type. It had once provided lodging for the employees of the Batignolles Company, when the bridge was being built over the Wouri. Neighbors still called it "Batignolles"; they liked the sound of the name.

Batignolles scarcely marred the quarter's architectural integrity. All around were board huts, together with some large dwellings painted in a kind of theater decor. Stone cottages, which had never had roofs or been lived in, arose on all sides, black with mildew and overgrown. But there were no hovels, no slums. Only the main streets, which followed ancient pathways, betrayed that this out-of-place quarter was in the heart of a great city. Batignolles was right in the center, and cut an imposing figure. It was a fairly long building, built to accommodate a number of tenants. My rooms were in the middle. There was a bistro on one end, and a family of seven occupied the rest.

The first evening, as I shut the door and lowered the blinds, I discovered how much curiosity I had aroused. There was a kind of bustle in the neighborhood. I had moved in that afternoon amid polite smiles, but no one, apparently, had shared their impressions with others. With nightfall the chatter started up. I could hear it. Across the street, the gossips watched, for a long time—wondering, I guessed, who was going to keep me company that night. Then all was quiet. And the quarter and I fell asleep.

My neighbors would make their comments, and form their idea of me, soon enough. My connections with the Libermann School were good to have, even though I no longer taught there. Was a study of their language sufficient reason, in their eyes, to come and live in their quarter? This I would never know. I thought I had better be ready for them—I would be invaded by children and inopportune visitors. I was mistaken. The neighbors "figured me out" in no time. Somehow they had divined my tastes and habits.

The bistro in Batignolles, right next to me, was run by a young Bamiléké named Philippe. The quarter was predominantly a Douala one, but the little shops and businesses were run by the Bamiléké, an enterprising people down from the mountains in the west. Philippe had never set foot in the village of his forebears. He belonged to the new generation, born at Douala after the great demographic shift of the 1950's. He was sending off the installments that permitted his large family to maintain a traditional chief's residence in the mountains. Very much a homebody, Philippe was always at his place of business.

Technically speaking, he did not run a bistro, but a package store, a lower category, which had lower taxes to pay and was very popular. Theoretically he furnished no glasses, chairs, or tables, and no one was to drink on the premises. But all day long and a part of the night his customers drank, inside and out, sitting on the ground, leaning against the wall, under my window—a cheerful little group, sometimes a little tipsy, but never agressive. Philippe's even temper was extraordinary. In fact I got the impression that all here had a deep repugnance for violence.

The other tenants were less noisy: the family of six children and their grandmother. The mother had died at the birth of the youngest. The father was a hairdresser and would come from time to time to hug and kiss the little ones and give the old woman the money. He had another wife, and six more children, with him in a neighboring quarter. I wondered how he could feed and clothe all those youngsters and send them to school. But he belonged to a Douala family, so I supposed he had some income from some ancestral land. In a village, his second wife would have reared not only her own children but those of the deceased wife as well. In town, however, the burden of their upbringing fell on the grandmother, and the children were practically orphans. Every morning they would pass beneath my window, fresh as orchids, three of them on their way to the public school, three to the Catholic mission school. They had not far to go: the schools were side by side, down the block and across the street. Sending the children to different schools had nothing to do with religion—the family was Protestant—but was dictated by the number of available places in the schools.

Children were more calm and more patient here than French little ones at their age. Was it because they spent the first year of their lives in women's arms? Even orphans could find a back on which to perch and a bosom on which to fall asleep: their older sisters were their mothers. This prolonged familiarity with such hospitable bodies made these babies most jovial. They were little princes and princesses, waited on hand and foot. But at about eighteen months, they were put on the floor for good and deprived of this physical warmth that had been the prolongation of the maternal womb. Suddenly there they were, right down on the ground, equal to equal with children their own age, who would not be quite so gentle. This sudden discovery of rivalry is a terrible shock, and perhaps explains the latent anxiety that young Africans hide beneath such a jovial exterior.

I made the acquaintance of two very poor and very old persons, brother and sister, who had come from a village farther up the Wouri. When I was with them they made an effort to speak correct Douala. Our relationship was to become a warm one. Whenever I stepped across the threshold and through their low door—which was intended to be rectangular, but which now was in the form of a parallelogram that made you a little nervous, like all the doors of the broken-down old Batignolles house—I was received with evident pleasure. And yet I brought nothing with me, having decided to free myself of the burdensome role of benefactor. They did not know a word of French and had never had any dealings with whites outside of religious ceremonies. It was a fascinating new experience for them, just as it was for me. I had come face to face with a humanity I had been kept away from, by the formidable color barrier, by political circumstance, and especially by my ignorance of the language. They were as happy with my first stammerings in Douala as if they had been young parents. My condition of total inferiority afforded me the happiness of not frightening them. A surprising balance was struck in our relationship, rendering it an exceptionally pure one.

I was most concerned to let it be known that I was a priest, even though not one who was exercising a priestly ministry in the traditional pattern. In the south of Cameroon, the priest is part and parcel of social life. The population is half Catholic and half Protestant. This was something I must never forget, I told myself: even in the most aboriginal nocturnal ceremonies of healing, I would always be surrounded by Christians. (Here I should add, however, that some of the Bamiléké had held onto their traditional religion.)

I would regularly go over to the church, which was just down the street from the schools, to say Mass. Our church was one of the last places of worship that dated back to the German period. A rather more pointed steeple, a rather steeper roof, a Germanic credence table, and so on, recalled the nationality of its builders. On Sundays I helped the pastor, who was a native of the coast.

The parish consisted of two natural communities that were not easy to gather into one assembly: one made up of Douala faithful, like my two aged friends, and the other of the Bamiléké, to which Philippe belonged. These two groups had strong reasons to stay apart. The Douala, and their allies, the riverbank dwellers of the Wouri and the inhabitants of the coast, feared the peaceful invasion of the Bamiléké, who already occupied half the town. And the Bamiléké reproached the Douala with leasing their land at exorbitant prices. The pastor was kept on his toes keeping the two communities together in the same church. He alternated the hymns—first one in Douala, then one in Bamiléké, and so on.

That was the extent of my public life, unless I count the visits I paid to the traditional chief under his tree, *le Grand Fromager*. (Which was more important in this quarter, the chief or the tree? Doubtless the tree.) The chief, a man of my own age, had lost, like many of his peers, many of his privileges—first, repeatedly, in colonial times, then under the Mandate and the Protectorate, and now under the new government, which had been running the country since independence in 1960. He continued only to collect taxes, arbitrate internal clan quarrels, and enjoy a certain popular prestige.

I could always depend on finding *ludo* fanatics in the chief's home no matter what time of day I arrived. The game of *ludo* looks easy, but I was beaten every time I played it. The players are very skillful in turning the probabilities of the dice to their advantage. Unemployed or retired, once the game was over, they sat under the tree and looked. What were they looking at? They seemed to stay on the alert, like soldiers resting on guard duty. What interior struggles were theirs?

I took my meals with various families, learned the language, and soaked up all manner of ordinary customs that make a culture. I was lost in a sea of guests whose main concern was eating. I regularly visited a dozen homes. I would arrive, without forewarning, at mealtime, and partake of the food that was placed on the table. The extreme simplicity never ceased to amaze me. For a year, I would be fed, now by these families and now by those, and it was unthinkable that I should offer a single franc in return. Poor families often had to be content with only one meal a day, and so I preferred to dine with Douala who were better off. These were persons who had succeeded in modern life, had finished their studies abroad, and had adopted new lifestyles. It was they who best understood what was at stake in my work. Up to a certain point their journey in life resembled my own. They too were in search of the past. Some of them would become real friends of mine.

The ritual of the evening meal in simple households was unalterable. Only the men sat at table; the women dined right where they did the cooking. Douala men are in the habit of raising their voices in debate, or in giving orders, but they know that it is their soft-spoken wives who really wield the power. All the dishes are served at the same time, by the women, in little multicolored enamel pots, "Made in Hong Kong," or "Made in France," now being part of "traditional" tableware. You serve yourself, a morsel at a time, from this pot or that one. The children stay with the mother—except for an occasional frontal assault on the men at table, with everyone, big and little, reaching into the pots at once.

Cultural initiation begins with cuisine. I was fortunate enough to find myself among persons who loved to eat, and who did so in excellent and varied style. The vegetables, spices, and condiments that lent flavor to the meats and fish had no equal in Europe. I counted seven kinds of spinach, five ways of preparing manioc—in little cubes, in slices, in soup, raw, and cooked—and so on. And of course there was the holiday meal, with the famous *ngonda mukong*, which required three days to prepare, and which I would have to compare with pistachio cookies except that they are so much more wonderful.

A Douala house retains the fragrance of its cooking—the odors have filled it for so long—to the point that its walls are fairly impregnated with it. Whenever I approached the house of any of the inhabitants of the quarter, whether it was the home of someone well off or a little hut where poor persons lived, I recognized the familiar odor of raw manioc and smoked fish. Powdered manioc, sold in stores as tapioca, may not have much taste, but the root itself, when marinated in water and fermented for several days, permeates the air, the walls, and everyone's clothing with a heavy, musty odor. It reminded me of the cellar at home during the war, at the time of the "soldiering," when we were keeping potatoes as long as possible, until new supplies arrived. The aroma of fermented manioc is disagreeable only to those who do not eat this kind of food. It blended with the smoky smell of dried stockfish, and dominated the subtle perfumes of the peppers, spices, and condiments. It was an organic odor, maintained by heat and humidity, as if of moist vegetation, and one's sense of smell quickly became accustomed to it.

I soon fell in with the rhythm of life in the quarter. The days were always strewn with new happenings, sometimes dramatic, often picturesque. One day, for example, as I was showering, and just about to rinse, soapy from head to toe, someone turned off the water at the supply valve outside. Later it happened again. The third time it happened, I took the neighborhood children to task. But they simply replied, "It was the crazy man." And indeed there was a happy-go-lucky "crazy man" in the locale. No one made fun of him, for his strange behavior was evidence of his communion with the spirits. So I mentioned it to him. He laughed, and did it again. The elderly brother and sister I visited every day proposed a solution to my problem, and initiated me into the language of signs. I was to cut a long blade of grass they showed me and tie it around the valve. This would show my displeasure better than would a long speech. Never again did the "crazy man" disturb my shower.

Another time, a herd of zebus filled the quarter. The animals had been driven down from the north and were on their way to the stockyards, accompanied by their herders, and surrounded by swarms of children having the time of their lives.

Another time we had a hurricane. Without waiting for the winds to subside, the schoolchildren were out under the trees gathering the fallen mangos.

Another day, when we were celebrating the birth of a baby, a child died next door. Beside herself, the mother of the dead child hurried out into the street, unmindful of the rain or the traffic, moving in little dance steps and trilling a plaintive, pathetic incantation.

Then there was a great drama. Cholera had killed seventeen persons in a single night on a little island of the Wouri. Cameroon had known numerous epidemics in its history, especially smallpox—but never cholera, until now. Rumor had it that pharmacies had been raided for their vaccine, and that secondary school students had gone on strike to protest official apathy. But I saw no signs of panic in my quarter. I had the opportunity to form an idea of the people's power of resistance. Some call it passivity or indifference, but to me it looked like self-control honed to razor sharpness.

The radio broadcast hygiene instructions, telling everyone that the germs multiplied in unsanitary water—whereupon the mothers, several times a day and with the greatest of care, washed their children, then washed them again. Endless lines formed at the town pumps, and yet there was no disorder. Still the disease persisted. A short distance from Batignolles it carried off a man in his prime. His relatives were prevented from attending the corpse, and it was laid out at once in a zinc coffin, to prevent infection. At nightfall we beheld an agonizing spectacle. The coffin passed in front of us, carried in a small cart. A dozen persons followed at a good fifty yards' distance. There was no traditional funeral cortege. Later, the ceremony of mourning would begin.

At last the residents of Douala were invited by radio to come and get their vaccinations; at seven points in the city—seven places for six hundred thousand persons. The residents of our quarter were to gather at *le Grand Fromager* for their vaccinations, to be presided over by medical technicians, the new priests of health. Beginning at six o'clock in the morning, I watched silent groups passing beneath my window, walking to the appointed place.

Each group formed a tight cluster of grandparents, parents, and children. The family unit presented a homogenous appearance, as if it were a single human body—a striking image of the African social structure. About eight o'clock, I saw the same families, in the same order, but on their way back— silent still, but disappointed. The crowds had been so huge that the medics had called off the vaccination and sent everyone home until further notice. In all, the pestilence took a hundred victims in the city of Douala, all adults. The number could have been ten times greater, had it not been for the discipline and sense of responsibility maintained by the families. The battle against cholera was to occupy the quarter for another month. Then appropriate hygienic measures would be added to the list of precautions taken against better known diseases, such as measles and swamp fever. Cholera had become a medical concern in Douala.

I was part of the quarter now. The neighbors no longer paid the attention to me thay had in the beginning. They absorbed me as they absorbed everything else—a rumor, a novelty, an eccentricity, the child of an unknown father. I led a quiet life and disturbed no one. Each morning, under the guidance of a retired church functionary, I studied Douala. There are a good number of books in Douala, first published by the Germans, then continued by the French, and now perfected by the Douala themselves—dictionaries, grammars, anthologies, and so on. There are over eight thousand listed words in the language. It has no orthography of its own, but the Roman alphabet has been adapted to it, and this is the system I have used for the Douala I have reproduced in this book. There is a phonetic orthography as well but, outside intellectual circles, no one uses it.

At eleven o'clock in the morning, I would leave my house and move from theory to practice. Even apart from those wonderful moments of my meals and my conversation with the brother and sister, I never let slip an opportunity to practice my Douala. I would catch a phrase on the fly, try out an expression on some children at play, speak to someone in the street, or mingle with groups of persons who were chatting. My efforts often ended amid bursts of laughter. Douala is a language with multiple intonations: use the wrong tone on a syllable and the meaning of the sentence changes completely.

Despite the many advantages of my situation, weak points were appearing. Living in this quarter, I found myself completely cut off from academic and professional life. Students and workers would head off every morning for parts unknown. In the evening, when they returned and I could speak with them, they made hardly any allusion at all to what they had done during the day. It was as if they had spent their time in another world. Their silence was disappointing to me, but not surprising. I knew about the inevitable rupture between the domestic life of a quarter and that of the workaday world. But the modern world, the world of work, was of no interest to me at that time. Was it not precisely to get away from it that I had withdrawn to Deïdo?

And now a new question arose: What was my real place here? I was spending my day with women, children, the elderly, and the unemployed. The only person I saw at his work was Philippe, my neighbor who ran the bistro. Even the pastor left his rectory every morning, to teach in a downtown school. I was a child in this quarter—no more, no less; it narrowed my field of information.

I was very surprised that I had not yet observed, after four months in Deïdo, any flashing irruptions of the African world-in-the-background whose presence I had felt at the Libermann School. True, I did not know the language well enough yet to grasp any allusions that might have been made to sorcery, or to revelations of ancestors or the water spirits. My status as a child forbade my access to the secrets—if there were any secrets. Be that as it might, I came to a provisional conclusion: manifestations of the spirits and the scandals of sorcery held a smaller place in daily life than I had imagined. Perhaps my recognition of this fact would be the most useful lesson of the first months of my peaceful stay in hospitable Deïdo. So I thought, for the moment. Once I had discovered the other face of reality

that is the subject of this book, I should not forget this time of observation—keeping my ears open, and, well, "taking my ease," in this simple,
straightforward quarter so similar in many respects to a small village of the
French countryside.

The Antisorcerer

On certain Saturday evenings, I could hear a drum beating not far away.
It would stop, then it would start up again. If I awoke in the middle of the
night, I could distinguish every beat in the deep silence. Sometimes its
rhythm was very slow—then suddenly it would pick up.

It is difficult to describe the sensation I had on hearing that drum. It was
like the agitation I felt when I remembered certain, you might say, "sacred"
moments in childhood, when I used to tiptoe up to the smooth, brown surface of our pond in the evening, to pull in my fishing line. I felt agitated and
excited back then, just as I did now. Beneath the calm and murky surface,
which in my mind's eye covered an enormous, dark abyss, I imagined the
whole intense life of a strange aquatic world. I would force myself to a total
interior solitude, and the most profound silence within me—then I would
approach the banks of the pond, where the line sank into the waters. If the
line were jerking about, I would be paralyzed with fear and joy. Other kinds
of fishing—with fly or plug—did not overwhelm me in this fashion. Only
the line that went all the way to the bottom. Only this drum in the night.
Calls—signals—from what depths?

I knew that funerals could last until very late in the evening, and that it
was the task of drummers and singers to console those present. But this
drum was not accompanying a wake. I could tell by the beat. It was accompanying some other activity. Something was going on. And yet no one had
told me about anything that went on at night. I had been familiar with
Douala for twelve years and had no inkling of what that nocturnal activity
might be. I was deeply disappointed that my neighbors, otherwise so hospitable and understanding, should have hidden it from me so well. The
wooden walls were thin here, and the cement ones echoed loudly, and evidently there were things they did not talk about.

I asked Philippe about the drum. He told me right out that the drum
master was a *sorcier*, a sorcerer, who officiated in the vicinity of the great
tree of tradition. Waiting no longer, I paid him a visit.

His name was Din. And Din granted my request to be allowed to assist at
the coming Saturday evening séance, the one I have described at the beginning of this chapter.

Philippe had called Din a *sorcier*. And indeed this is what this sort of
person is most frequently called in French. But Philippe was not using the
word in a pejorative sense, and I would soon understand why. He simply
meant that Din was someone who healed the sick—although, admittedly,

the preternatural character of his powers was a source of fear to Philippe.

Whenever I heard the activities of Din and his colleagues discussed in French, I would hear this word *sorcier*, but it would always be accompanied by smiles, or an uncomfortable look—or, on the contrary, pronounced with affectation, as if it needed to be corrected somehow, in order to be properly understood. The expression is not flattering. Strictly speaking, it designates a category of unsavory individuals—and then everyone who practices esoteric, nocturnal rites is simply lumped together with them. It is a particularly unfortunate expression in Din's case, because he incarnated, in his person, the very opposite of a sorcerer. He was really an *antisorcerer*, one of many, and it is high time we did them justice.[10]

In the Douala language, Din is classified among the *bato ba mianga*. *Bato* means human beings, men or women. *Mianga* refers to the secret remedies they know, remedies charged with a power that goes beyond that of pharmaceutical medicine. These persons are at the pinnacle of the traditional medical hierarchy, above the many lesser healers who possess the secret of a particular herb for curing a particular malady. Every family knows some recipe or other, handed down from generation to generation, to alleviate stomach pains, for example, or to promote fertility. But rare are the families with a *mota bwanga* (the singular of *bato ba mianga)*. He or she is an exceptional person indeed.

In this book I have decided to use the term *nganga*—Douala synonym for *mota bwanga*. It has the advantage of being shorter, though it is less commonly employed than the lengthier expression. *Nganga* is the generic name, and is common to numerous Bantu languages from Douala to Cap.[11] And so we shall be speaking of *nganga*s and sorcerers—and they will be opposites, adversaries.

But would I be able to "get away with" going to visit *nganga*s? After all, they were surrounded by a special aura, and that aura was charged with a great deal of popular emotion. I was sure I could rely on my closest associates for their help: my neighbors would know how to tell the others what I was doing, and why. I counted on my Douala friends, the ones I took my meals with, to let their neighbors, as well as the traditional chiefs, know the innocent purpose of my nocturnal activities.

The only remaining problem was the approval of ecclesiastical superiors. A priest who comes home at daybreak, after a night in another quarter, awakens suspicions, especially when the adventure is repeated. But the bishop accepted the honorable (and honest) explanation given in advance: research into traditional medicine. Father Essombe, Deïdo's pastor, who had come from the same village as Din, and Father Endene, the Douala priest who had introduced me to other secular priests, would take care of the rest. They had an ethereal network of friends and acquaintances, a network that could be locked quickly into other networks. It gave them a power understood by all, and allowed them, I had no doubt, to follow my activities at a distance. As for the Jesuits, I had no misgivings. My Came-

roonian superior himself did similar research in the region he was from—
the Bassa forest—and a long tradition in our order made my work look
practically routine. And so a consensus gradually took place regarding my
work: I was doing research.

Having taken these precautions, I now had the illusion that I could return
to Din's house in all tranquility and confidence.

Chapter 3

The Battlefield of *Ndimsi*

The religious dimensions of existence have long seemed to me to be identical with the quest for basic truth. To be sure, methodological materialism or atheism seem to me to be a prerequisite for all modern science, which reduces everything to the quantifiable, to space, and which must play to the hilt the game of demystification. I employ this methodology unstintingly. But, essential as it may be, for me it is simply one area of human intellection. A religious inquisitiveness has also animated my thinking. When all is said and done, I believe it has served a purpose. For I fail to see how one who has had no experience of worlds-in-the-background, continuously present and sometimes sensible, nor any practical idea of transcendent powers and absolute imperatives, could be on an equal footing with human beings who bathe in such certitudes, and whose lives are permeated with them.

—Philippe Laburthe-Tolra

Family and *Nganga*

All through that first night at Din's house, I had had eyes only for him and his patient Engome. Otherwise, among the persons assembled there, I noticed only the drummer, the couple seated beside me, and the cook. The others seemed to me to form a homogenous, docile group, eager to encourage the *nganga* in whatever he might seek to do.

It was during the visits I paid to Din in the course of the next few days, and the later night séances in which I participated, that I came to grasp the crucial role of the patient's family in the success or failure of an attempt to heal someone. When all went well, as in Engome's final treatment, the family stayed back, lost in the crowd. But in crisis or conflict, the importance of the family became clear.

I came to appreciate the great power of the family group in the course of two treatments that failed, occurring several days apart. Din was the un-

30

happy organizer of the first, and another *nganga*, whose acquaintance I would make, was the victim of the second.

Fortunately, between the first night and the lost battle I am about to recount, several weeks intervened, during which I was able to come to know Din and the world around him better.

My visits to Din were almost daily. I found him most often on his doorstep, when he was not busy with clients. He would push a little stool toward me and I would sit on it, just a couple of inches above the floor. Everything in Africa happens a little closer to the ground than in Europe.

Usually we sat in silence. A whole hour could go by without our exchanging a word. Those long periods of tranquility reminded me of leisure time at sea, in the navy. But Din's apparent inertia masked an acute attention—to passers-by in the street, words spoken somewhere behind us, insects creeping out of the earth, or strange configurations among the tufts of grass at our feet. At times he would prick up his ears at something that I could not hear at all.

I observed the movements of the persons that this house, by some miracle of compression, contained. It was a medium-sized house, all on one floor, with six rooms. Din lived with his youngest wife and Barthélémy, or "Bata," his 17-year-old son, whose mother, Din's first wife, had remained behind in the ancestral village. Din was not the owner of the house; he was the tenant of Ekwala, a minor Douala notable, who also lived there with his seven children. When everyone was home, with the mother, grandmother, and elderly aunt, there were a good dozen persons. Then, besides the two families, there were three patients who stayed there, confined to bed or shuffling slowly about in the backyard—each with a relative. Engome, the lame woman of that first night séance, was there, completing her cure, and Ndolo, a little 6-year-old girl, was waiting there with her mother, not to be discharged until her father could pay the bill for her treatment. Finally, in this already overpopulated dwelling, there was Din's young assistant. Only the use of suspended partitions made such cohabitation possible. Thanks to them, no space went to waste. They would be let down at night, and rolled up in the morning.

I watched Din. Unique among the rest, he moved about as if he were alone. He would sing:

Na boli ebolo, ba yana nde
duala Mbedi, na bole nde ne?

"I work, but they scorn me, those Douala *Mbedi*—what am I to do?"

Din's isolation was explainable first of all by his origins. His native village was a remote island of the Sanaga, some 150 kilometers from Douala. Not to be able to practice in the land of his ancestors was certainly a handicap.

Even *le Grand Fromager*, that venerable genealogical tree, towering over his house only a few steps away and extending its protection over the whole quarter, held no interest for him. At any rate, I never heard Din, in any of his refrains or incantations, allude to the headless giant of tradition, with the wonderful protuberant roots that formed its buttress and kept it erect. Nor had I ever seen him solemnly pour out a bottle of wine at its foot, or perform any of the other little attentions that went with cultic reverence.

Din made sure, however, that he was surrounded by numerous means of self-defense, and these counterbalanced his isolation. He was like a stranger on guard. He had so many talismans I could not count them all—pieces of bark, seeds, clasps, the teeth of wild beasts, old coins, and the like, hidden in his house, buried, or carried on his person. Once I surprised him in the act of slipping a small object of some kind, the size of a die, into a glass I had served him in my lodgings. He recovered it at once, surreptitiously.

Of all these "pieces of armor"—the best way I can think of to translate Din's Douala expression—the mightiest was the shrubby tree that grew within the plate-iron enclosure in his rear courtyard. It was called *njum bwele*, and everyone agreed that it was the most excellent of trees in its power against the onslaughts of sorcerers. In the wild, this plant prevents everything around it from growing, and so it always stands in the center of the clearing. Actually, Din's *njum bwele* had grass growing all around it, and so I was inclined to doubt its authenticity, although perhaps I was mistaken.

Next to his isolation, Din's worst enemy was the doubt in others' minds. Times had changed. *Nganga*s could no longer count on their systems of signs and beliefs as in times gone by, however much they might themselves continue to cling to them. Not all their clients still held these beliefs as earnestly as they. Nothing was taken for granted anymore.

The ones who were the most difficult to manage—and to heal—were students. "I don't believe in all those things," a student at Collège Saint-Michel said to me one day. His mother was currently under Din's care. "The treatment is going to cost 24,000 francs—not counting the wine.[12] How is my father going to pay my tuition next year? But what can you do? They're convinced that Din is going to cure her!" Only one family member's consent is required for treatment to begin. When one is sick, one must try everything.

The erosion of belief had annoying practical consequences for Din. Persons with money were not always the ones with faith and gratitude. Some would quarrel with Din: Had a *nganga* asked for money in the old days? "In town nowadays," Din would reply to them, "everything costs money—even certain medicinal barks that I could have gone out and searched for in the forest, but the forest is far away, and getting farther away every year!"

Sometimes patients would try to leave without paying Din his fee. What was he to do? He could not sue. He had no juridical status. A lawsuit would boomerang. So he simply refused to discharge patients who failed to pay—under threat of a relapse—until the amount originally agreed upon by both parties had been tendered.

Behind these doubts and protests loomed the shadow of what grounded and maintained them: the hospital, pharmacy, and infirmary. Din could not compete with them. I had seen him face to face with the reality of it all the day when thousands of Douala citizens trooped past his door to receive their cholera vaccinations in the shadow of *le Grand Fromager*. No one, of course, stopped in on him instead. It took all our efforts to get him to go and be vaccinated like everyone else, for he claimed to possess the means to stop the epidemic himself. I once heard him sing, during a treatment, "I have closed East and West to this malady called cholera." (He pronounced it "kol-ra," instead of *choléra*, which made everyone laugh—but he would retort, "If you want a drink in my house, you'll pronounce it the way I do.")

But this was obviously mere resentment. Din did use "the whites' medicine" for himself and for his family. He was a realist. Only there were taints and blemishes that did not show up on an x-ray: *maya ma bobe* ("bad blood"), and *mbeu'a nyolo* ("bad luck"), provoked by the *ngada mudumbu* ("mouth pistol") or by the dangerous snake called *nyungu*—which will haunt the tale I am telling in these pages. When these types of sorcery appeared, Din knew that the family did not take the victim to the hospital. They came to him, the antisorcerer.

"I am like a soldier fighting against the underground," he told me once, alluding to political events in Cameroon in the 1960s. He was on his guard day and night. I had come upon him too often, alone, in an attitude of extreme attention, to imagine that he was just gameplaying. Even when he was telling stories, and laughing with all his might—which did not happen often—he never slackened his vigilance. Anyone at all, you see, might be a sorcerer—a passer-by, someone in his own family, or myself. Din kept a very close eye on me. He knew that the sorcerers wished his death: "*Na mea nde onyolam*," he would sing while treating someone—"It's me I weep for." Or: "*Mulopo mwa machine mu bambe bebambam na byei pe*" ("I am the head of the machine [locomotive]; I pull the cars and all the scrap iron").

For all these reasons, Din lived in Douala in a climate of insecurity. And yet, rarely have I met anyone so seemingly sure of having power. Din had the conceit of a boxer. In fact, at times his attitude annoyed me a bit, even though I understood it. To keep his own faith in his charisms he had constantly to reaffirm his own certitude of it, for his efficacity depended on it. One had the impression that all of Din's power resided in the art of convincing his patients that he had more power than did the sorcerers.

I once witnessed how contagious his conviction could be. A lodger of his had been knocked off his motorbike by a taxi. He came home with deep gashes in his shoulder and arm. Everyone who lived in the house rushed out to meet the victim with cries and lamentations. Din alone remained imperturbable, seated on his little bench. The man recounted his misadventure, with one good arm for gesturing. Then he saw Din—without a trace of fear in his face. And he too became calm. Later he confided to me: "If it hadn't been for Din, I'd have fallen on my head and broken my skull. I have a cousin who wishes me ill, and he knows it." The man was but one of many who firmly believed in the efficacity of Din's interventions even from a distance.

Except for times of treatment, such power of fascination seemed most unlikely. By day the little faith clinic looked quite shabby. Grass, rags, and a great hodgepodge of props lay everywhere. But when night fell, Din would have the fires lighted, would put on his red tunic, brandish his little brooms, the symbol of his power, and set a whole universe in motion, just by dancing and looking. Unlike other *ngangas*, Din used few instruments—and none of the sleight-of-hand with which some of them momentarily snatched preternatural glory. He never lost his good humor for a moment. This was the supreme mark of his self-assurance. His secret was to concentrate the attention of all on his own lanky silhouette.

If you asked him where this confidence of his came from, Din would unhesitatingly reply that he owed it to the water spirits, the *miengu*. "No one sees them but me," he declared, and this gave him a singular power. Their chieftain was called *Ndoka Bewudo*, the Stubborn One of the Herbs, presiding at the end of the bridge over the Wouri. *Dambo Dam*, My Thing, is the chieftain of the Kribi riverhead. "These are the 'great doctors'—the others are less important, and too numerous to be summoned all at the same time."

Din ascribed to the "great doctors" the same titles that he claimed for himself, so that it became difficult to distinguish, in his chants and other formulas, whether it was to them or himself that he was giving all the laudatory titles—Caterpillar, Revealer of Secrets, Leader of the March, Lord of the Medicines, or even "Prostitute" (meaning "one who gives oneself to all").[13] Spectators could not tell the difference. One night I asked the man next to me, "Why did that woman fall into a trance like that all of a sudden?"

"Din asked her to," replied the disciple. Then after a moment's reflection: "No, I misunderstood the question. The spirits pushed her into the trance. . . . Din sees, and the disciples do the work."

Then I asked Din, and he responded, "Yes, the spirits do the work, but so do I!" Actually, neither of them liked my questions very much. Was it because they had never occurred to them?

Din's self-assurance never left him. I saw him drunk, I saw him without money, and without patients. Still he proclaimed the same confidence in his own power. Indeed, this certitude was indispensable. It was itself proof of his knowledge of invisible realities, and of his gift of "double sight," which allowed him to divine the machinations of the sorcerers. It was his own patients who obliged him to believe in himself, to believe in his own abilities as a battler. They had no other recourse to sustain them in their quest for a cure. If Din gave way to a doubt, he would lose his credibility and thus his power. *"Balemba na munja ba bele mba Esomawuta,"* he would sing ("The river sorcerers call me The One Who Reveals What Is Hidden").

Ndimsi

Ndimsi is the name given to what is beyond the vision and knowledge of the ordinary run of mortals. It is the hidden face of things—the world of secret intent and veiled design. Those who have received the gift of penetrating these invisible realities possess an awesome power, permitting them to effect health and sickness, for simple mortals' weal or woe.

The initiated have a special vocabulary to describe their gifts of perception in terms of spatial and temporal dimensions. In this invisible world, too, one travels thousands of kilometers, on foot, on horseback, or by plane. Dantesque battles are waged in people's houses without the inhabitants' knowing anything about it. The water spirits, *miengu*, and a whole series of beasts—including the serpent, *nyungu*, of whom I shall speak later—are there, but only privileged eyes can see them.

It would be erroneous to postulate that the *ndimsi* vocabulary is "made up as you go along." It obeys precise laws, and if you do not abide by them you will not be understood or be taken seriously. It is not a figurative language. Still less is it a mythical one. It is the expression of a profound reality, but with only surface manifestations.

How might one translate the word *ndimsi*? "The practice of the occult" conjures up a strange, closed world. "Mystery" seems better to me, in the sense of the hidden heart of reality.

When Din spoke to me of *ndimsi* he always made an effort to convince me that he was not describing what Christians would call an "evil" world. He was fighting the good fight there. His explanation is a redoubtable apologia for *ndimsi*.[14]

"I want to tell you something worthwhile. You know, we have the means to open our eyes at night, in *ndimsi*. What *ndimsi* is, then, is as if we were in the light. That's *ndimsi*. *Ndimsi* is something good. You can see over to Europe, you can see that far, and other places too, without even leaving home. That's the way *ndimsi* is: you see evil and good. It's as if it were broad daylight.

"*Ndimsi* . . . you have to know there's nothing evil about it. I was reared in the Catholic religion. I give to the church. It's not because I use *mianga* [objects charged with power; medicaments] that I don't go to communion any more. It's because I have two wives. As far as I'm concerned, *ndimsi* is a good thing.

"If a sick man comes to see me, I just pray to God to help me to cure him, because God has given me herbs and barks for this. If it's a sickness I can cure, I say, 'You're going to get well!' But if I see, in *ndimsi*, that I can't do anything for him, I tell him right out, 'Go to the hospital!' And I know that man is a dead man.

"But nowadays some Douala are going around saying that *ndimsi* is bad. But *ndimsi* is bad only if you want sorcery *[ekong]*, if all you want to do is kill someone. In this world God lets everybody act the way each one thinks."

There was no doubt whatever in my mind that Din believed in *ndimsi*. I found him one day in his sanctuary room, his *dibandi*—the same room where I had contemplated him, stretched out, when he had gone, invisibly, to Mount Kupe to find Engome. This time I approached him from behind, and I could see only his back, as he leaned over a table. He could not have noticed that I was there. He was wearing his red shirt and was totally preoccupied in tapping on a plate with the tooth of a wild boar. The rhythm was irregular. It was like Morse code! I recognized its crisp, syncopated click. His long magician hands, silky and dark brown on top, rough and yellowed on the insides, with their coarse, jagged nails, were imitating the rhythms of an old-time telegrapher sending a message. Had he watched the German postal telegraphers in his childhood? Or had his own master transmitted to him the secret of long-distance communication? Bewildered, I asked him what he was doing.

"This is to see and communicate long-distance."

"Do you do this often?"

"No, only when the disease is serious."

"With whom are you communicating?"

"With the ones I have at work. I have spirits *[miengu]*—I talk to them. I have ancestors *[bedimo]*—I talk to them."

"Do they answer you?"

"They answer me. We can do this work, or we can stop doing it."

I peppered him with questions, delighted to have happened upon him when he was alone and applying himself to a healing. There was certainly no question about his sincerity.

The wild boar's tooth was a precious instrument to him, as I already knew. It was a symbol of strength and power. He had brought it back with him from his apprenticeship among the Pygmies. In the plate he was tapping upon, he had gathered a number of meaningful objects. There were tokens of sickness: a hook, on which the victim hangs; a chain, for fettering the victim. There were tokens of treatment: various pieces of bark; an old halfpenny; two small, polished, oval stones, one white and the other pink— perhaps meteorites—called by Din "God's thunder." There were tokens of vision: a piece of a broken mirror; a piece of broken glass. Each of these different sorts of objects had the value of a "sign" for Din—understanding "sign" in the sense of something not only signifying, but having genuine operational value, a meaning of which it is generally devoid in our modern Western languages.

Such was my picture of Din, the *nganga*, after several weeks in his company, at the moment he sallied forth to hunt the *nyungu*, on the battlefield of *ndimsi*. I had participated in several of his night séances, and spent a goodly number of hours, with him or without him, on my little stool at his front door.

Nyungu, Serpent of Mishap

You see the *nyungu* only if you have double sight. He enjoys the privilege of invisibility in *ndimsi.* It is he who executes the high designs of the sorcerers. He creeps right into persons' houses, to steal for his masters' profit or to commit a murder by eating the heart of a designated victim. You do not see him, but you feel his presence in disturbing signs—a commotion in the hen house, strange noises, lines in the sand. On the little island of Jebale, in the Wouri, one end of which lay opposite our quarter, they dug no wells, for fear of the *nyungu.* Several persons had told me this, including Jacques Mudiki, himself a practitioner there, and Simon Musinga, a fisherman. The Douala attribute to the *nyungu* the properties of a boa, which was still actually seen sometimes in town, but of an invisible boa. On Jebale belief in him was so strong that the inhabitants simply refused to dig latrines.The *nyungu* would be sent there by the enemy to drink women's blood and thus prevent the child in their womb from coming into the world. How powerfully the notion of the serpent can strike the imagination!

All *nganga*s have their own way of driving away the *nyungu.* A Jehovah's Witness claimed to use only those remedies authorized by the Bible—herbs and barks—without having recourse to demonic magic. Still he gave me a recipe. Bring water to a boil in a 50-liter barrel. Add a great quantity of salt, and pour the mixture on the floor of the house. "The snake will not come," he explained, "for he thinks he is faced with an invisible ocean. The salt keeps producing more water, and the beast does not like the deep water of the sea." This treatment, against the *nyungu*, is expensive, because it is performed against a formidable type of sorcery.

Din had a patient living in his house who claimed that a *nyungu* was living within her. What frightened the poor woman out of her wits was that the snake could be as small as an intestinal worm or as big as a dragon. "He actually has the power to live inside you without your knowing it," Din declared. Here was the mythical serpent of all civilizations—symbol of evil, tempter of the gardens of earthly paradise, sea monster, seven-headed hydra.

More recently, the *nyungu* had acquired a brand-new advantage: confusion about him in the popular mind. Belief was less common now, and less strong, and the *nyungu* profited from it. In times gone by, if we are to believe the elders, or the few writers on the subject,[15] this snake had a more precise form and shape: *nyungu*, in the Douala language, also means "rainbow." In the old cosmology, heaven was full of treasures. A rich person had the privilege of climbing to the skies, and the *nyungu* would be his or her guide. To obtain this assistance, one had to belong to a certain society called *Ekong*, and to belong it was necessary to sell a member of one's fam-

ily. With the *nyungu* in your possession, you had a chance to see your fortune grow, or even eat the heart of your enemy.

The family that had invited Din to put an end to the machinations of the
nyungu that was haunting them had not taken this extreme decision from
the outset. The step of going to Din was a last resort in an unfortunate series
of events.Two years before, there had been an accident on the riverbank. A
little girl in the family had fallen out of a pirogue and disappeared in the
waters. When she came to the surface she was dead. But a curious detail
gripped everyone: she was not wet. All evidence pointed to a death by mysterious causes. Suspicion gnawed away at the family. Some accused the
grandfather. He defended himself, accusing his eldest son—who in turn
accused the youngest. The family arranged for various ceremonies to reconcile its members, but in vain. One course of action remained open: to have a
specialist come in to neutralize the maleficent activity of the *nyungu*, sup-
posedly responsible for all these misfortunes, and to deliver the family from
its devil. And they called on Din.[16]

The house the *nyungu* haunted was in our own quarter, along the main
street that ran past Din's house. Judging by its exterior—painted pink, with
an unsophisticated little balcony—it would have been impossible to imagine
that such terrifying things went on inside. We arrived at eight o'clock in the
evening—Din, his wife, a few lodgers of his, cured or convalescent, including Engome, who still limped a little, a friend we had met along the way,
and I. Din's main helper, the indefatigable drummer, was not with us, and
his presence would be sorely missed.

The men of the family were already gathered in the sitting room, waiting
for us. The room was spacious—it must have taken up two-thirds of the
house. It had windows and doors facing out on three sides; its fourth wall
separated it from the bedrooms. The kitchen and toilets were two little separate huts, outdoors, as was customary. A large table took up the whole end
of the room where the courtyard began. Armchairs and straight chairs were
lined up, theater-style, starting at the door to the street. Seated waiting for
us were the owner of the house, the elder son—under suspicion—and his
youngest brother—also under suspicion—who had insisted on this meeting,
and who evidently was the more worldly-wise of the two. One would not
have thought that this fat man slouched in his easy chair had plodded
through not only every part of his own country, but Europe as well, and
that he had held a number of government posts.

The two brothers were the principal protagonists, and it was they who
had invited the *nganga*. They were surrounded by some old men—feeble,
deaf, or blind, but consulted on everything—a young schoolteacher, who
was not involved in the affair, and, at the end of the room, around the
table, a band of secondary-school students, sons of the family, who were
paying more attention than they wished to show. The grandfather, the main
defendant, was not present. (His absence would determine the outcome.)
The women—in doorways, in adjoining rooms behind closed doors—

followed the action without taking part. Custom forbade their participation. It was a matter for the fifteen men present—representing at least three generations—and the *nganga*.

In accordance with a prearranged scenario, the evening began with a good omen: before entering the sitting room, Din discreetly received the 25,000 CFA francs he had demanded. He immediately sent his women to the rear of the building to light the protective fires and to prepare the *dindo*, the shared repast, with five chickens and appropriate herbs and barks. The *dindo*, closing any ceremony or treatment, was taken in order to counterbalance the one being eaten by the sorcerers. I was already familiar with the ritual from having shared in this meal after Engome's treatment.

The women set to work, and almost at once four fires were protecting the rear of the house. We saw the glow of their flames at the windows and heard their crackling. There was a whole strategy in Din's method. The number of fires varied with the degree of danger or the severity of a disease. "You can have twenty, or you can get along with one," Din explained. "They're to block what the sorcerers are doing."

Soon I noticed Din speaking to the younger brother in reference to me. Was he justifying my presence in his entourage? I had no idea, but no one paid any special attention to me afterward.

As Din turned to be seated, one of the men, of the grandfather's generation, rose and said, "This is not the way to drive out the *nyungu*. He is driven out by day, not by night!" And the old man stamped noisily out of the room.

Din waxed wroth. His oval face lengthened even more, and his color changed, in a few seconds, from dark brown to slate gray. His eyes turned red. Unmistakably, he was in a rare frenzy. At the same time his expression hardened, reminding me of a wooden mask that hung on the wall of my room. What would happen now? I could feel his very credentials under attack. From this moment, Din could be neutral no longer. He began to enter progressively into conflict with the family. His habitual strategy was compromised now. He did put on his red shirt, and grasped his *janjo*—the little broom he used in his evening séances—but he let it hang at his side like any ordinary utensil.

He went into the bedroom that had been prepared for him, remained prostrate for a good long moment on a chair, and went through the motions of a dance, but without conviction or inspiration. He repeatedly blew his nose noisily, as if to gain time: he would place his right index finger on his right nostril, then his left index finger on his left nostril, until he finally expelled, with a great blast and a goodly measure of insolence, a particularly stubborn chunk of mucus. And he stuck out a yellowish tongue besides. He no longer looked himself at all.

Finally he asked me to plug in my tape recorder, to let the group hear certain samples of his repertory that I had recorded in his house. This gesture of honor to me gave me a chance to set the tape recorder, so that I was able to record what followed.

"When you came to my house the other day," Din began, addressing himself to the younger brother, "you said to me, 'You listen to what comes out of my mouth to go sell it' [a term used in sorcery, stronger than 'to betray']. Well, I'm going to tell you the truth. The *nyungu* you see [the younger brother, then, had double sight] relies on many things. . . . The truth is, they're afraid of you because you are full of power. They say you have eaten certain powerful things you don't even remember."

"I've got mange all over me," said the younger brother, ironically, meaning that any ills of his were superficial ones. "If that's bad, remove it."

"What I just said is true, too!" Din expostulated, turning to the group of old men.

"No, it's nonsense," they replied.

"Let him be," said the younger brother. Then turning to Din, he added, "Get to work. It's nine o'clock."

"That's what I'm going to do," Din answered. "Let's get this over with. Let's begin!"

"If we're all going to have to sleep here, say so," someone said. . . .

A little later Din called out: "Now I'll tell you something. There are three *nyungu*. Two are females, the third is a male, in an egg. If he hatches, someone in the family will die. Now I have to drive them out. I'm going to chant. . . ."

"Your brother has taken some *mianga*," Din told the elder brother later on. *Mianga* are *ndimsi* medicines. "He has eaten a lot of things he no longer remembers. He has a *janga* [an onion with evil powers] but he doesn't remember. He doesn't need your money. He hates you only because you are good to him. He is 'against you without reason,' " he added—the very definition of sorcery. "What he wanted to do was kill you, but he couldn't do it. You ate things that kept him from seeing you. If he'd seen you, he'd have killed you. There they are, the *nyungu*! Your brother can tell you if I'm lying. They're there, and there." And Din pointed to two places on the floor. "You told me to show you the *nyungu*. Is it true or isn't it?"

"You do a lot of babbling. We want you to get to work," interjected the younger brother.

"God have mercy on us," Din replied. . . .

Around midnight, the five students seated around the table at the end of the room grew restless and began chatting about something having to do with *nyungu*—*nyungu* this and *nyungu* that. They had been fairly calm until then—attentive to the joust without wishing to seem to be, concerned as they were to keep their distance from a tradition they were ill-acquainted with, but which still impressed them enough to make fun of. After an hour they had started to doze off, seated at the table with their heads on their arms, but with one eye on Din. Now they were seeing how far they could go.

One old man took them to task: "You think you can talk about *nyungu*?

I'm eighty years old and I haven't seen a *nyungu* yet!"

Din was beside himself. "What are you laughing at?" he barked at the eldest of the boys. "I have a son who's worth more than you. Don't you know I can punish you this instant if I want to?" They boys laughed nervously. "You and your friends there—who told you to show your teeth? Who has allowed you to laugh in front of me? Your father may have killed someone, but he's still your father. Now let me do my work. Isn't this work?"

"Yes!" chorused the old men.

"Look there!" Din went on. "There's the *nyungu* hunting members of your own family. Are you crazy? Members of your own family were just about to cut each other up with knives—for a truth it's about time to discover. Here it is—it's going to happen now, this truth is! Now you'll find out what it is! And then what will you do, when you know exactly whether your father is the killer or not? . . . Go ahead and snicker! I'm doing my work! Your grandfather's *nyungu*, that's what we're after now!" And Din repeated this last sentence three times.

"Tomorrow," Din continued, still addressing the boy, "what *nyungu* might kill *you*? Tomorrow, what *nyungu* can make you not even know where to live anymore? You're too dumb. Your studies—you can see you can't go on with your studies because your grandfather's *nyungu* has disturbed your intelligence! Look, you don't even understand that all this is serious. . . . So stop laughing like a fool. I declare that that man has seen the *nyungu* [pointing to the younger brother] and knows him, and sees him!"[17]

I felt more and more ill at ease. How could this family let me stay on? They must not know that I knew sorcery terminology. I was particularly uncomfortable for Din. So proud, so sure of himself— and here he was with his back to the wall, failing pitifully before the eyes of the person he had invited to come along. Toward one o'clock in the morning I made a little sign to the schoolteacher and slipped into the darkness, leaving this hunting party to wind down however it might.

The next day I made out the heavy silhouette of the younger brother far down the street. I had seen his zest and sensitivity, his truculence, and his self-control under the *nganga*'s repeated assaults, whereas his elder brother, whom the *nganga* respected, had remained so mute and impenetrable. I hesitated to approach him, lest I be going beyond the limits of discretion. But my desire to hear how the night had ended overcame me and I went down to talk with him.

After some preliminary hesitation, he began to talk, as we stood together in the street. "Din didn't do any work. He only drank, he didn't work. He complained about everybody. He hadn't brought anything [any weapon] along. After the *dindo* we thought he was going to start, but he chanted a bit, and drank, and—that was all! He had to give the money back, and now he has to find somebody who'll get rid of our *nyungu*. Once there was a white man, a fire fighter [he gave me his name], who was very good at it. He used to come and say, 'There . . .' And he would catch the snake behind the head and carry it off and burn it. Or else he would dig here, dig there, and keep looking, and find the *nyungu*—then he would take out his pistol and shoot it. Din may be good at other things, but not for *nyungu*."

I tracked down the white man. He had resigned from the fire company since independence and was back in technical services. He was a chubby little man, his face all swollen from alcohol abuse. He was quite affable, and delighted to be able to talk about his thirty years in Douala. He was a typical example of what Cameroonians called *les anciens du Cameroun*, the old colonials. He lived with an African woman, whom he had had to marry in church. ("They'd have killed me with their machetes!") I could tell that his racial slurs were not to be taken too literally, and that he was actually capable of being very considerate. I told him I was doing research and took notes as he was speaking.

"I have the gift of magnetism," he said. "I'm the seventh boy in a family. It started in 1951 when I became a fireman. If there was something scary and they couldn't find it, they came to me. This magic serpent belief comes from planting their outhouse seats in sand. The sand shifts. Or some of them pour calcium carbide in there and that gives off acetylene and burns their behinds. Magic snake? All you have to do is roll a tire through the sand and tell the guy, 'Pay me, and the snake is gone forever.' Actually there wasn't any. Blacks are so naive!

"I never went after a magic serpent, but I've hunted some real ones. When there was a real snake, a python, I would catch it. I've seen them nearly twenty feet long in Deïdo. But the magic snake is just a trick—a money maker. There isn't any such thing. If a man's intelligent and knows what's going on, he doesn't get tricked by things like that. I never saw anything out of the ordinary. I don't take money for it myself, otherwise I'd lose my gift. . . . But I've found bodies—a well locked up with a chain, and a baby's body inside."

His Cameroonian wife served us a drink, with a smile.

I found Din seated on his doorstep, imperturbable, watchful, and with his stern self-assurance back in the corners of his mouth. He did not hesitate to give me his viewpoint on the matter. It was very different from that of the others. I started up my tape recorder.

I asked him, "What did you do after I left?"

"I tried to get rid of the *nyungu*, but they had me surrounded. I decided to wait and do my work some other time."

"But then why did they call you over?"

"They called me over to drive out the *nyungu*. They're killers. They're sorcerers *(bewusu)*. I tried to find a way for the *nyungu* to get out, but more and more of them came to battle me in *ndimsi*. So I decided to quit. If I'd kept at it, somebody could have died—somebody who'd come along with me, or even me."

"Did you find the sorcerers?"

"Yes. They live in that house, but they weren't there last night. They had a plan to surround me."

"So are you going back?"

"I told them I'd come back and chase out the *nyungu* when there was nobody home. But the owner [the elder brother] told me not to come back."

Din had lost 25,000 francs. He could have lost my confidence as well, had I not seen him in action on other occasions and been so sure of his sincerity and his powers in other circumstances.

Of these three interpretations of Din's failure, his own seemed best to me. His language might confuse the European that I am, but it shed the most light on the affair. I agreed with the fire fighter on one point: there was no such thing as a *nyungu*. But I could not agree with him that it was a matter of trickery and deceit. All these persons shared the same belief in the existence of the *nyungu*. I agreed with the younger brother that Din had failed to set the stage—a tape recorder is no substitute for a drum—and had lost control of the séance, but not before he had seen that his efforts would be in vain. I especially agreed with Din that all conditions necessary for exorcising this family's devil were not integrally present. It had not taken long for a misunderstanding to arise between Din and the family members that ruined any chance for success.

Now I considered the viewpoint of the younger brother, the leader of the opposition. In his opinion, Din should have done as the fire fighter would have, and shoot at it point-blank, or catch it and burn it—with an appropriate magical technique, to be sure, because the *nyungu* was not an ordinary snake. From where he sat ensconced in his easy chair, caught in the middle of a dramatic family conflict, the solution would have to be in a deft stroke from the hand of a specialist.

For Din, the case was the exact contrary. Scenting a family difficulty, he had sought to resolve that before moving on to the exorcism. Many treatments began in that way, I had often been told—by an invitation to confess one's wrongs. The action can simply mark time, for hours, waiting for a confession to be made. As it turned out, the younger brother refused to make a confession. The *nyungu* do well in the weeds, and Din could not kill this one until he had caused signs of reconciliation to appear. The family thought it was to be an audience at an exorcism, and Din was watching in vain for a change of attitude!

But to my own way of thinking, Din was missing a key factor for success: the grandfather. It was well known that he and his two sons did not accept responsibility for the drowning and for the family disorder. In the absence of one of the adversaries, how could anyone expect confession and reconciliation on the spot? The brother's behavior was all too clear: in the absence of their father, they decided to adopt a negative attitude, the elder seeking refuge in absolute silence, the younger playing the ironic antagonist. But why had Din agreed to work in such conditions? Had it been the money? The alcohol? The hope of seeing the grandfather arrive? Thirst for a battle? A mistaken judgment? Or simply an unshakable confidence in himself and his water spirits?

There seemed to be a moral in this story. The *nganga*'s cannon hangs fire if the family withholds the powder.

Chapter 4

Loe and the Old One

A short time later, I found myself the witness of yet another case of formidable resistance, and once more the power of the family was confirmed. The *nganga* who had to pay the price was called Loe (pronounced "low-ay"). Persons with whom I had taken meals had described "low-ay" to me as a very competent practitioner. I noticed a certain hesitation about encouraging me to go to see him, however, which I ascribed to a habitual caution or suspicion surrounding this type of person. I found someone to accompany me.

Loe was a native of Deïdo. He belonged to the family of the high chief there, but he had long since decided to live on his own, in order to be able to perform the function of a *nganga* more independently—out in the country where the herbs and medicinal barks were right there to be gathered. Loe had not reckoned with the rapid expansion of the city. To see him now, in the quarter called Bependa, lost amid the houses, it was difficult to imagine that he had been living in the wild ten years before.

But he had taken ill luck in good part and continued to consider himself lord of his surroundings. He was an enterprising person. He had built a chapel for the faithful of the Cameroonian Baptist Church, of which he was a member. He had constructed his buildings with his own hands—rather strange buildings, put up without any concern for their relationship to one another, all of different sizes and lying hither and thither like dice, in a vast courtyard, with their roofs of aluminum sheeting, their frames in brown wood, and their walls of gray cinder block.

Loe was a thin, serious little man, lively, and fragile-looking. His features were fine, with very slightly flaring nostrils—and a little mustache along his upper lip, which was unusual for an African. He was not especially dark, and I wondered whether there could have been some Portuguese, French, or German in his ancestry, with so many sailors having passed through this port over the past two hundred years. To be sure, I refrained from asking this at our first meeting.

When I entered Loe's house, with my friends, the *nganga* "sized me up,"

45

as if I had come as a prospective client. He understood French. He spoke in a determined, somewhat aggressive way, unlike his compatriots. This would keep our relationship simple and direct, but would thereby also allow us to be less defensive with one another—something Din and I never seemed to be able to manage. I introduced myself rather abruptly, said I was a priest, had taught at the Libermann School, and was interested in traditional medicine. Loe called for some of the "strong," meaning whiskey, and a local distillation called *ha*! (because you always choked on your first swallow.)

We were chatting along when Loe suddenly asked me whether I could get a car. He had to go to the outskirts of Douala the next evening, he told me, for a little ceremony with a colleague at an hour when it would not be easy to hire a taxi. I asked for more information, and Loe told me he wished to respond to a personal request from a *nganga* he called the Old One— someone who had been working as a *nganga* before Loe was born. The Old One was importuning Loe to come to see him, on the occasion of the new year, to breathe new strength into him—for his powers were waning, and when he attempted to treat his patients his efforts no longer met with success. Loe would have to demonstrate his own strength and restore his colleague's failing vigor. The proposal seemed so simple and logical that I had difficulty believing that this was the only thing involved, what with all the complications I had just witnessed in the attempt to drive out the *nyungu*.

The following evening, then, at the appointed time, I arrived at Loe's house with a car. I found the master seated on the floor on a mat, and his whole family squatting or lying around him. A storm lamp, set on the floor, lengthened the shadows and gave the bodies strange forms. The atmosphere was humid and hot, but there was no threat of rain. I could see by the fixed, matter-of-fact expressions on the faces that we would not be going to the Old One's rescue that evening.

I was disappointed, of course, but this was also an opportunity for me to get acquainted with the whole family, because the women were present. Unless you live in a quarter day and night, it sometimes takes several weeks to find out who is who—who is this one's sister, that one's father, and so on. It was a delicate investigation, especially because it would be "uncouth" to ask too precise questions. Introductions were not customary, so I sat down beside Nkongo, a disciple of Loe, and he very quietly identified each member of the family for me.

Loe, I learned, had married four times. His first wife was dead, and the third had left him. The second and fourth were still with him. Each of the four had given him one child. The list was easy to remember: four wives, four children, two boys and two girls. The eldest daughter, who was not present that evening, had had two babies, fairly close together, of different fathers. "She is not well regarded by the family," Nkongo commented. There they were, the two babies, naked little chits, climbing on backs, finding a knee here and a lap there, bawling at the slightest annoyance, and taking unfair advantage of an extraordinary climate of tolerance shown toward them.

The group's attention was focused elsewhere—on a couple, the *nganga*'s elder brother and his wife, quarreling violently right in front of us. Loe had to restrain his brother, drunk out of his mind, from physically assaulting his wife. A lazy, irascible man, a drinker, as Nkongo told me, the brother lived in this same cluster of houses with his wife and five children. "I could not have left the neighborhood that evening," Loe would explain to me later. "My brother would have killed his wife. He claimed she was hiding their savings." Relationships between the two brothers, I could see, were intimate and explosive. And yet, as a *nganga*, Loe had to allow the center of gravity of the family to find its natural place in his own home.

The last to arrive was Nkongo. About twenty-five years old—he did not know exactly—Nkongo had the slight ruddy cast of persons with a touch of the albino. (Real albinos, a common sight in Douala, have a milky white skin that makes them look from a distance like Europeans.) He worked as a manual laborer in the Mikès warehouses where he spent eight hours a day carrying sacks. He was sturdy and muscular. After work he would come to Loe's for supper and to spend the night, even though he was not a member of the family. He had once been cured, right here, and had become so attached to Loe that he had become his disciple. Unlike Din's drummer, Nkongo was privy to the secrets of the herbs and barks. The only thing he was missing to be a full-fledged *nganga* was double sight. Something blocked him from moving on to this step—some deep hesitation, doubtless, arising both out of his Christian convictions and the three years of accounting courses that had initiated him into the modern world, although unfortunately he had failed to graduate.

When tempers had calmed, I asked Nkongo a question that had been burning in me ever since the evening before. With my little tape recorder on my lap I recorded his answer, as I would be doing systematically from now on.

I asked him "How can a *nganga* lose his power?"

"There is a time for everything, you see. Nothing is eternal. The grass, the herbs. . . . The power of the medical practitioners of ancient days is gone now. Trees and herbs don't have the force they used to. Just as belief in God's word isn't as strong any more. Before, God would do miracles out in the open, in broad daylight. The world received proofs. Now, because God doesn't reveal himself any more, and there is only the Bible"—Nkongo was a Protestant—"and fewer miracles, fewer proofs, the world doesn't believe much any more. It's the same with the work of the *nganga*. They had very great power, and the power has shrunk. There are fewer proofs."

Loe's brother had collapsed in exhaustion and fallen asleep on the spot. I steered Loe back to the matter of the old *nganga*. According to Loe, he was neglecting his family and his wives had nothing to eat. This, perhaps, was the reason for his failure, and Loe said he would declare his wrongs to him at the proper moment during treatment. But I could tell there was something else. Loe said neglect of family duties. Nkongo said general unbelief. I was soon to learn the real reasons why the old man was obliged to ask his young colleague for reinforcements.

The next evening I found Loe ready to leave. He was taking his elder brother along—he did not want to leave him at home—as well as his youngest wife and his disciple Nkongo.

Before the expedition, we all had to go to the *dibandi* to "put our armor on." Din's *dibandi*, for want of anything better, was his own bedroom, but Loe's was like a little sanctuary, a separate building. There was nothing on the outside to indicate that it was a sacred place. It was a shed, with windowless walls of cinder block and a single door. Inside, however, I beheld an altogether amazing spectacle. In the back was a nondescript heap of things some six feet square and perhaps six feet in height, consisting of several mushroom-shaped termite hills that had been carried in and set up on the cement floor, bark strips up to three feet long, some empty bottles, vials of inexpensive perfume as you might find at a market, half-burned candles all covered with wax drippings, eggshells, all sorts of skins and horns, and some rusty old daggers. The whole collection was cordoned off by strings with little bells and faded pieces of dyed cloth hanging from them. There was also a kind of platform, black with the blood of countless animal sacrifices, broken eggs, and wine libations over the years. I had had the impression of a single, homogeneous mass the moment I entered. Although there was some ventilation, there was an intense odor of oil lamps and ointments, as if you were in a crypt where candles were always burning.

After the first shock, I tried to imagine the effect of this fantastic concentration of objects on the minds of my companions. With solemn gestures, and perfectly at ease, Loe now addressed himself to what he had to do there. The others stood behind him, well behaved, but without the least sign of fear or even reverence. Was this impassibility or incredulity? I did not yet know.

Loe pulled on the string that separated the group from the heap of things, and the little bells rang, calling the water spirits to the rescue and asking them to follow us. Then he did homage to the ancestors by pouring a bottle of red wine on the termite hills that marked their presence among us. Then he rubbed his body with an oil he called *ndima*, "the invisible," a word with the same root as *ndimsi*. Then he invited all except me (and his brother, who had slunk away into a corner) to do the same. Then he swallowed a powder concocted of various grated barks (*ngando*), which had the power of protecting one on a journey. I got ready to take whatever he would give me, but—was it out of respect for my sensitivity, or did he think I was "armored" by nature?—all I got was a spoonful of honey.

Later I asked how honey could provide "armor." Loe responded: "How can you ask such a thing? You know what honey is, don't you? It's because a bee gathers her honey everywhere. There is a lot of strength in that stuff.

She even gathers it on corrupting sores, the slime of a corpse, the froth of a poison, rotting meat, and even on *mianga* [*ndimsi* remedies]. . . . Honey is the result of that whole mixture."

Now Loe called for his red battle robe, a leaf as large as a platter (called a *dibokuboku*, used in reconciliation rites), and some small objects that I did not recognize. "I don't have double sight, so I don't always know what they're for," Nkongo remarked. But he did seem to know what a simple candle was for, and he took one with him. Indeed it was going to have much to "say," he assured me. All these things were for what the Cameroonians call, in French, *contre*, "armor."

"We are going to a foreign land," Nkongo explained further (an outlying village). "We don't know whether we'll be attacked during the treatment or not. We have to be ready. This is not the first time we have gotten ready like this and gone and treated a sick person in his house. You have to have a lot of strength. We'll have the whole village against us down there, all the sorcerers. We'll need to be well armed."

The journey began. We drove through the Bepanda and Deido quarters, leaving them already wrapped in sleep. We crossed the 1,800-meter bridge over the Wouri, passing through a fairyland of boats with burning lights along the piers to our left and the somber shapes of the riverbanks and islands on our right. My companions neither glanced in either direction, nor uttered a single word. Once across the bridge, we turned to the right, passed through the Bonabéri quarter, and were in the wild. We came to the village almost immediately. Loe directed me along the sandy paths to the old man's hut. It was a moonless night, and we could scarcely distinguish the clusters of huts and larger mango trees along our route. We were seven kilometers from our homes, but we were in a "foreign land," following a Douala *nganga* on a visit to another Douala *nganga*.

Family Confrontation

The old man was asleep. He rose, declaring himself flattered that we should come to see him. It was unfortunate, he said, that he had been unable to gather the funds he could have wished, so as to be able to receive us in a worthy manner. The reason lay in a vague adventure having to do with lines and fish. Thus without money Loe's treatment would perhaps be ineffective. Loe, with the air of a great lord, replied that he had come to work, not to drink. After all, he added significantly, his work consisted in the rescue of one who suffered.

Even as Loe was speaking, the village chief made his appearance on the scene. The contrast was striking: the puny old *nganga*, reduced to a frail bundle of bones, but with his two malicious brown eyes in perpetual motion in a skull like a death's-head, and the tall, imposing chief, of harmonious mien and with something earnest and just in his glance. I was altogether taken with him at once. To my surprise he simply withdrew a few paces and sat down. He even declined to take the whiskey Loe brought over to him ("You'd better know what you're drinking," Loe himself had told me once.)

Suddenly, the door flew open and in burst the chief's son. He was opposed to this meeting, he said, this ceremony of healing of which he had not been informed. And then besides, he and his father were of the old man's family. "What ails you?" he demanded of the aged *nganga*.

"My parts were failing," replied the old man ironically, "so I called the doctor."

"Who is this white you've brought along?" continued the chief's son, turning to Loe.

Before I had a chance to reply myself, Loe explained that I was a friend of his, visited him often, was interested in what he did, and followed him everywhere. Then he repeated his reasons for being there himself. He intended to wash the body of this person who complained of having lost his power. He would "wash him of misfortune" (*mbeu'a nyolo*).[18]

Now a neighbor came in to ask what all the shouting was about. He was astonished that a *nganga* had been called in: generally it was the sufferer who sought out the *nganga*. Loe explained patiently that he was there to bring peace to the family. He was "president of the *nganga*s of the region," he said—what a sonorous title—and could not leave his colleague to suffer, even if the Old One was his senior and surpassed him in experience and in the knowledge of the laws of *ndimsi*. Loe's young wife began to show uneasiness, and sought to persuade her spouse by signs that he ought to adjourn the gathering. An old woman attempted to say something, but she was silenced: it was not the moment for a woman to speak.

Then the chief's lieutenant spoke up. Finally we heard right out what everyone knew all along—the real reasons for family opposition to the old man. He had recently taken a sick woman into his house. Then, no later than a week ago, this woman's child had died at Douala. The old man was accused of having made a pact with the husband, demanding the child in exchange for healing the mother.

Nkongo was whispering all this to me. "The child that was sold did not really die. He simply had his breath withdrawn from him and they buried him. But he is not among the ancestors (*bedimo*). He is alive, in *ndimsi*. He helps his new master [the old *nganga*] by working for him."

The family was in the following position. A *nganga* who kills someone automatically loses his or her power. That was well known. That was the crime of crimes, because it was what distinguished a *nganga* from the opposite, a sorcerer. In turning to sorcery, then, he had lost his powers of healing. And in permitting the old man's treatment, the family was, in effect, admitting the truth of the rumor. Now it was clear that the old *nganga* had sent for a colleague to give him back the powers he had so shamefully forfeited.

The old man protested his innocence. The chief's son—decidedly a most aggressive person—violently attacked him, reminding him that this was not the first time that he had fallen under suspicion of killing someone. The old man now thought they might kill *him*. (*"O ma pula bwa mba"*—"You want to kill me!" I understood him to say.) Things had taken such a bad turn that Loe's brother, silent until this moment, rose, and solemnly declared that the family alone would be the judge. No healing would be attempted without their consent. Loe turned to the chief and left the decision entirely in his hands.

At once the chief made a sign that we should all leave. Even were Loe to undertake to heal the old man, he said, it would do no good. There was no point in wasting his talent. He was willing to recognize that we had not come there with evil intent. Otherwise we should not have been able to leave. "God grant you safe return!"

Here I broke in, introduced myself more precisely, and explained the reasons for my ignorance. I did so as calmly as possible, in my still very stammering Douala, more to hide disappointment than fear, as I considered myself "armored," being a priest and white. I proposed to come again another time to pay them all a visit. Here the chief pronounced the only amicable words spoken that evening: "You shall be received as a son." Everything he said was spoken almost ritually, after the fashion of an official pronouncement. The chief had chosen to adopt a reserved attitude in the beginning, to let each one have the floor. His final decision, decreeing our departure, fell as a logical, inevitable conclusion, without his seeming to have taken sides.

Over the course of the next several days I repeatedly discussed the event with Loe. The accusation lodged against the old *nganga* seemed incredible to me. But the important thing was to know what Loe thought about all this, and what meaning he gave all this in his universe.

"Whether it is true or false nobody knows for sure," Loe told me. "At least none of us foreigners [foreign to that village]. By doing my work I could have found out if it was really sorcery. We weren't allowed to do what we should have had to do. They are convinced. I'm not so sure. If the old man dies I will know it was his family that killed him. No need to conduct an investigation. Before, to have absolute proof, you gave someone a dish of *mianga* [a mixture of medicinal herbs having a special relationship with *ndimsi*]. The accused person had to drink that and throw up. But now, the way things have changed, it's forbidden. It was called *kwa*."[19]

"Accusing someone that way" I asked Loe, would you say that is a good or bad custom?"

"With us it's a good custom. It's for correction. It holds sorcery down a bit. It's not for the pleasure of accusing someone."

Loe had no doubt about the responsibility of a third party (even the victim) in a case of illness. I tried to discover a flaw in the system—not to prove to myself that I was right in considering it naive, but in order to get an idea of its resistance and consistency, in order to understand it better.

I said to him, "Surely there are diseases where it's obvious that nobody in the village is responsible! For instance, take the cholera epidemic that broke out at Jebale. You have to admit they falsely accused an old man of having caused the death of the first seven victims!"

Loe knew, just as I did, that cholera was a new disease. It had come from the Middle East with travelers—more precisely, with Nigerian fishermen and their families coming in from the Wouri estuary, that is, from the south.

Loe was unperturbed. "And why was it so bad precisely at Jebale? The Jebalese live in the north. The Douala are more to the south. Why did the attack begin at Jebale? Our sorcerers are always on the lookout for a chance to practice their trade. Then the chiefs put a stop to that cholera. First the island chief at Jebale protested against the sorcerers. Then it was Deïdo's turn. Same thing at Bonabéri. They had the *esa* [a collective rite for the expulsion of evil]. They said they didn't want this disease, and they stopped it. It's our custom. Even if the Europeans hadn't given us the vaccine, it couldn't have continued: the populace was against it. Besides, the people wondered why the vaccine was brought out only the day the cholera started and not before. You don't call that sorcery?"

Shaken, I stopped questioning Loe. I still could not believe in the death pact that was supposed to have made a sorcerer of the old *nganga*. I was stupefied that the interested parties could have found it plausible, and have had recourse to logic to defend it. (Little did I suspect that I should soon have the opportunity to pass from astonishment to experience!)

"When Loe receives a patient, he always seeks to have the family present," Nkongo told me, "and he gathers them together before starting the healing, so as to know if the family is against the patient or not, if they don't want treatment, or if they are doing something that would keep the patient from being cured. Then he makes an effort to persuade the whole family to accept the treatment. If they don't agree with his arguments, he doesn't start the treatment. It has happened.

"But if it's very serious, and he sees that the patient is on the point of death, and it's the family that's the cause of the disease, and they don't want him freed, then in that case he forces his will on them. Whether they like it or not, he cures the patient. He couldn't do that over there because he was in a foreign land. At home he has more power."

Din and Loe had left their fortress to expel the *nyungu* or to restore an old man to health. They had failed. They had collided head-on with families who awaited them in familiar precincts. The complementarity of these two stories is no illusion. The words the tape recorder faithfully preserved do not give the whole picture. There was also a tacit, untranslatable exchange established between the speakers, one that was inaccessible to a foreigner. I was unable to perceive the communication that was taking place between the lines. But at least I could see that it was there. Would I achieve this level of perception one day?

In any case it had gradually become clear to me that the families had refused to cooperate with the treatment. This little, at least, I had accomplished. Two forces were necessary to conjure this type of sickness, conventionally called a "spell": the family and the *nganga*. If a conflict arose between them, to the point where the *nganga* failed to attract enough allies in enemy territory, treatment was impossible. How can someone be nursed back to health against the will of their family?

Rumor Has It . . .

"Ba na. . . ."

"They say. . . ."

I had been warned. A Cameroonian sociologist, Cosme Dikoumé, had said to me, "You'll be watched, you'll be observed. Then one day you'll be part of the system; they'll have formed their idea of you."

Slowly his prediction materialized. I was watched, I was observed and sympathetically. I could not have hoped to pass unobserved at those meetings where persons healed one another, and where so few Europeans, let alone priests, are ever seen. I had been genuinely touched by the warmth and tact shown me by my hosts, on every visit, even in conflictual situations such as I have just described. When it came to being "integrated one fine day into the system," I had not seen that this had been taking place, unless it had been by the slow osmosis to which I had been submitting, a labor of patience for them as for me. I felt immunized, unassimilable, over the short term. And yet, suddenly, unexpectedly, this integration was to take place, in the village where Loe had sought to restore the old man. Surely it could have happened elsewhere just as well, and just as abruptly.

Loe had warned me: "It was I who took you there for the first time. Now I have to tell you not to go back. I shall not go there again myself. We are outsiders, and I have told them so, several times. They have told me that of course they believe me. But this being said, it really is not possible to go and do more research."

In spite of Loe's cautions, I returned to the village as I had said I would, to pay a visit to the chief. His residence had nothing particularly traditional about it. It was a broad, solid, one-story dwelling, such as notables had had built for themselves after the war—a sheet-iron roof, slanting so that the rain would not get through, a raised floor, against the floods and the snakes, little stoops, and windows with wooden shutters. The date the residence was finished—1951—appeared in large figures in the pink cement.

The interior, consisting of not much more than a vast meeting room, was more characteristic. Here were armchairs, straight chairs, and tables, grouped in circles for receiving visitors and taking account of their rank. Along the walls were ranged numerous photographic portraits: three generations of persons looking into the camera and stiff regardless of their age, exactly the contrary of what they were in real life—jovial, relaxed, and impulsive. In each picture, the present chief appeared. After all, he was the central figure of the village. Over one of the doors, in Gothic characters, was a proverb recalling the law of genealogy and hierarchy: *Muna a si ma ya pon sango tom* ("a child will never engender its father").

In broad daylight and plain reality the chief was even more imposing than I had seen him to be. He was a fine-looking old man, tall, with an air of the warrior about him, like the image of the "black king" I had had ever since I was a child, when I had collected cards with explorers' pictures on them. He wore a white, sleeveless singlet over his torso, from which his two marvelous arms projected with sinews like plaited cords. His sash was tied about him— a rich one, with stripes in black and gold. Three-quarters of the material formed a great bunch about his belt; the remaining quarter barely covered him to the knees, like a short skirt or Scottish kilt. The instant seduction exuding from this man was doubtless owing to the harmony of his fine features—something of a surprise with such a physique. Every part of his face—his ears, his nose, his mouth—was perfectly proportioned. The wrinkles, the furrows, even the little blisters were like the grain in fine wood. In the magnificent, melancholy eyes of this man, sixty years old, I read now intransigence, now sorrow, and sometimes gentleness.

He received me generously, offering me an alcohol of his own distillation, tempered with the sweet flavor of barks. His name? Caïn Dibjunje Tukuru. We spoke about the Libermann School, where he wished to enroll his grandson. He had nothing to say on the subject of the failure of Loe's healing expedition. He only expressed his surprise that it was a "foreigner"— Loe—who had brought whiskey and poured it for the company. The drinking rites had great meaning, I saw.[20] I left the chief at nightfall, promising to return to record the *ngoso*, the traditional Douala musical repertoire. He was among its best interpreters.

Driving back, I suddenly came upon a roadblock, a barrier of lumber, logs, and stakes across the broad, main road that ran through the village. It had been thrown up hastily, during my visit to the chief. There was no way through! On guard were perhaps fifty young persons and children in scout uniforms, or rather pieces of uniforms—one would have a hat on his head, another a kerchief about his neck, and insignia of rank on everybody's shoulder straps. These were the famous scouts you saw in holiday parades, responsible for a capricious style of order along the route. I asked them to clear the way. They replied that, in the absence of the police, the task of guarding the road was theirs, and that I would not be allowed through without first meeting with them in a nearby hut. A taxi came along, then a truck, and they were allowed to pass without difficulty. I began to wonder what this strange scene meant. I supplied identification and references, but to no avail. It seemed to be the wiser course to make an about-face and go back to see the chief. Surely he would know how to open the road. And so I did.

First the chief was surprised. Then he was angry. He and his eldest son and heir, with a couple of guards, all managed to stuff themselves into my little car. I realized the gravity of the situation abruptly when I saw one of the chief's wives hurl herself at him, all in a frenzy, trying to stop him from getting into the car.

Soon we reached the roadblock again. A dense crowd had gathered. Some women had joined in with the scouts. In a few minutes, the atmosphere had become different. A thick dust had arisen with the arrival of newcomers and the commotion of the scouts. A buzzing began to be heard, as in a marketplace, but more disquieting, and punctuated by shouts and shrill cries. Two women had undone their hair, opened the tops of their dresses, and begun crisscrossing the road, with wild gestures of lamentation.

The chief ordered me to keep the motor running and the headlights on and to stay in the car, there in the midst of the crowd. Calmly he addressed the scouts, ordering them to open the barrier. But it was of no use. His son feigned a terrible rage, but without result. Now the chief gave vent to his anger in earnest, thrusting back the foremost logs of the roadblock with mighty blows of his bare foot. The scouts repositioned them immediately. In other circumstances I should have relished this epic scene of a furious old giant, naked to the waist, his *pagne* solidly bound to his belt, confronting, alone and at nightfall, a troop of youths who were doing all they could to avoid direct conflict. But the road was still closed; the gesture of authority on the part of Caïn Dibunje Tukuru had had no effect.

It was then that I learned from one of the chief's bodyguards, who had remained at my side, that I was accused of connivance with the old *nganga*, now considered a sorcerer, and that I was thought to have come to buy men and women from him, whom he would sell me at a very high price. He would then undertake to have them die by the mysterious ways of sorcery. Thus I would acquire human beings at my service in the world of invisible realities. The rumor was going about that I had already been thrashed for sorcery the previous week. I was said to be Mukala Ndedi, a Greek merchant accused of carrying on a traffic in human beings in the region.

The chief returned to the car, leaving his son to debate with the recalcitrant youth, and I turned the vehicle around once more and headed back. Once in the meeting room of the chief's residence, I simply awaited the result of the negotiations. Several persons in the chief's entourage encouraged me to call the police, but I had no inclination to do so. I distractedly turned the dials on the radio in the meeting room, as if to maintain contact with the outside world.

I considered the effect my calling the police would have. It would ruin my plans. First of all, I would be denied my nocturnal comings and goings, and consequently any study of traditional medicine. Above all, I would be completely undone in the eyes of the people. So I decided to follow the advice of Caïn Dibunje Tukuru, who wisely counseled me to wait for the emotional excitement to die down.

An hour passed. Time seemed to stand still. Then the son returned, greatly agitated and bathed in perspiration. He had persuaded the youth of their error and obtained the reopening of the road. But woe betide me if I ever returned to the village. He was willing to listen to me, and weary as I was, I recounted for him the origins of the affair. We returned to the car, the son and I, and drove between the two silent columns of scouts where the barricade had been. As I drove through the crowd I gave a great wave of my left hand out of the window. A few of the scouts timidly responded. I deposited the chief's son at the edge of the village, with some money to celebrate his diplomatic success.

Thus the adventure had seemed to come to a harmless enough conclusion. But I could not hide its importance for me on the emotional level. Here I was all of a sudden, as the result of a misunderstanding, on the side of sorcery, on the side of the shameless white exploiters, on the side of persons deserving of society's excommunication. I felt the hurt in my innards. I was in no physical fear—I had been in more dangerous situations during the war in Algeria—but I felt a cold shiver, as if I had been a child whose playmates have driven him away. No explanation I could give, no words from my lips, could possibly change a single thing. A terrible collective reprobation weighed on my shoulders.

I knew very well—after all, I had seen and heard about it often enough—how a society, after a long cultural development, manages to work out a manner of behavior in the face of the anguishing reality of evil. It ascribes to certain individuals, whom it flushes out of hiding, the responsibility for disease and death. And now I was actually experiencing the power of this mechanism. How very much a group can feel relieved and consoled when it thinks it has found the one responsible for the evil it suffers! For the group, it is a veritable collective liberation. But what mortal anguish for the marked person! I thought of the old *nganga*, who had become a sorcerer, to be shunned by his own village for the rest of his life.

Still, we should not forget that today sorcerers enjoy a more enviable position than in days gone by. They have no juridical status, and so cannot be brought to justice simply for being sorcerers. They would have to be caught in the act of poisoning someone, for example. The old methods of truth by trial (*kwa*) have long since been outlawed. The sorcerer is off the leash. Even Christianity is an indirect help: at least in this village, where everyone is Protestant, there was hope for the Old One, if he earns it, and little by little the people could learn to tolerate him.

Another stroke of luck for sorcerers is doubtless their relative, and paradoxical, usefulness to society. Sorcerers enable society to localize its ills in their person. Evil, which otherwise would remain an anonymous force, and hence a far more disturbing one, is concentrated visibly in the person of the sorcerer. Do away with all sorcerers and you run the risk of being confronted with evil on a daily basis.

My own troubles rapidly reached alarming proportions. A few days later I learned that the rumor had actually reached a distant village. I had gone to a village more than thirty kilometers from Douala, to meet with a renowned *nganga*. I went with a friend of mine from the Dedo quarter who had once been a schoolteacher in this village. The episode of the roadblock was not a week old, and I should never have thought that a rumor could spread so rapidly. We had arrived in the little village, set back from the high road, in the evening, and the old *nganga*, having been informed he would be paid a visit, had received us agreeably. It was evident that his preparations suffered from improvisation, and I shall not stop to describe them here.

But suddenly, just as in the other village, the chief appeared. He professed himself mightily astounded that a white should dare to come to his village without informing him. I acknowledged my error and begged his pardon. He sat down to have a drink with us. "You teach in the Libermann School and you are a priest," he told me. "So I am reassured. You see, there are whites who do good and whites who do evil. Just the other day, down around Douala, a white was caught in the act of playing the go-between for an old sorcerer and the chief, to buy certain persons. They say he was called Mukala Ndedi."

He named the village. There could be no doubt. He was talking about me! Once the formalities were over, I hastened to take my leave, citing the lateness of the hour, and fled without further ado, along with my schoolteacher friend.

The next day my friend brought me up to date as to the status of the rumor. "The moment we left that village, persons started dying. I'm certainly not going back there!"

Once I could get control of myself I inquired into the causes of such dramatic consequences. It was then that I learned of *ekong* sorcery.

Chapter 5

Ekong Sorcery

"They say I was going into the villages to buy persons."

"That's called *ekong*," I was told.

The same thing would be said to me, just as spontaneously, all over the southern coast of Cameroon, as well as in the backcountry all the way to the edge of the rain forest. *Ekong* is the most widespread sorcery in this part of Africa today. I could cite numerous testimonials to the reality of the *ekong* procedure, which consists in going to a sorcerer and offering money in return for human beings, whom the sorcerer will then undertake to deliver to you to make slaves of. This is *ekong*. Engome, the first person I saw treated by Din, had been a victim of this kind of traffic. Din had made himself invisible, betaken himself to Mount Kupe where Engome was already toiling for her new master, and delivered her, in the very moment of her death agony.

Ordinary mortals see victims fall ill, waste away, and die, whereas certain other individuals grow wealthy and prosperous at their side without apparent reason. It is supposed that there must be a causal relationship between these two abnormal situations. No other proof need be adduced. There is, in addition, the testimony of certain ones who have returned from death. [21]

By contrast, the initiated, those endowed by birth or by ceremony with "double sight," are deemed to contemplate this traffic in human beings as if it were transpiring in broad daylight, and to intervene to further or hinder the transaction. I recorded the testimony of the oldest and most revered of the Douala people, Etame Dika, on the subject. Etame explained to me why, although believing in *ekong*, he has nevertheless always refused to have his eyes opened.

"Selling persons? Yes, that still goes on today. They're sold for prices that are different from ours. They're sold for *ndimsi* money. Someone can be sold for anywhere from two to twenty-five francs. [22] You can go out behind the village and find persons who've been sold. When somebody knows how to go about it, he puts drops in your eyes, and you can see them talking away the ones who are going to be sold. It's their invisible power. I can show you somebody who can go to sleep and then tell you everything that's going on, even in Europe. But if you learn to see, it's dangerous. There are too many forbidden things; if you transgress them, you can die. It can happen that somebody comes to you and asks for a person. . . . They wanted to open my eyes, but I refused. There are too many forbidden things about it."

Etame's language was based on an anthropology a Western will find passing strange. For Etame Dika, every human being had a double. This was a fact as self-evident and irrefutable as the soul-body distinction for a European. The soul-body distinction is not missing from the Douala anthropology, but it is of secondary importance in comparison with the doubling of a human being into a visible and an invisible person. While one is asleep, for instance, one's double can be kidnaped by sorcerers—body and soul—while one apparently remains lying on one's bed, in sight of everyone. I had to keep this datum well in mind in order to understand what I was told. It constantly presupposed the doubling of an individual. By way of illustration, I shall give Loe's own words, as he sought to explain, in French, and with powerful word-images, the technique of the *ekong* sorcerers.

"They pick your name; you are going to die. The ones who kill you purchase something that resembles you perfectly. They copy your shape, they build a sort of big doll. It's a perfect picture of you. It's there on the bed, and everybody's crying. But you, you're over there, and you see everything. They've put something over your mouth and you can't talk. You're like a dog that's obedient to its master who's killed it. And the family is going to bury the perfect copy and think it buried you. After the burial the *ekong* practitioners come with their amulets. [They exhume you] and carry off your form, with all the winding cloths. The coffin will be empty. They take you to the one who bought you. [They reconstitute you] and from that moment on you work for him as a slave hand."

Ekong and *Ndimsi*

The sale of human beings through the *ekong* network is but one operation among several in the vast domain of *ndimsi*—a world that laughs at distance, time, and darkness. I managed to get Loe to situate *ekong* for me in this universe, and to compose and contrast it with the other form of sorcery, cannibalism, with which I had not yet come in contact. Once more I preferred to interview him in French, in order to oblige him to create some of those spicy, pregnant expressions of his.

"There are four slots [categories] of *ndimsi*. The first is the Lord's *ndimsi*—the *ndimsi* of God the Creator. You've died but you're going to live with God. That's one *ndimsi*, as we call it. The second is a criminal *ndimsi*—*ekong*, where they kill and sell. The third, as far as I know, is where they also kill you, but they eat you up. They eat you in their mouth like meat. One meat eats another meat. Then there's a sorcery that's stronger than anything, sorcery in the water, the crocodilian [caiman] sorcery.[23] It's the first sorcery of Cameroon. They don't sell you. You keep living, walking. But you feel a little pain, you start singing softly to yourself or something like that, then they take you to the hospital, you just can't understand it. You don't know it's *ndimsi*.

"My work—that's in the fourth *ndimsi* slot. The medical practitioners, the *ngangas*. I sleep—I sleep and I have a kind of dream, and I see the nonsensical things people do. I stay still. I don't move a muscle. I have dreams. And sometimes I get this thing from God, like a light. And if the light comes back, then I'm really happy. I see how I have to work the cure. I see how I'm going to have to scuffle in *ndimsi*. I see they've tied a fellow up over there. But if I start shedding a person's blood, if I sell a person's hair or fingernails, if they come to ask me to kill somebody, and if I shed blood, it's my own death. This is the fourth *ndimsi*; there's no other, in my experience.

Ekong is essentially bound to wealth and money. Prosperous persons are suspected of maintaining slaves, to work for them on invisible plantations. As far back as the oldest members of the community can remember, belief has undergone no evolution on this point. In former times, *ekong* was the name of an association of businessmen, outstanding members of the community, and chiefs—in a word, the wealthy class. In those times—again, as the elders recall—*ekong* did not have the odious connotation it has acquired today. There was a clean-cut difference between the sorcerers properly so called (*bato ba lemba*), who were considered cannibals and genuine incarnations of evil, and the members of the association (*bato b'ekong*). The former had the reputation of doing evil for evil's sake; the latter at least had an excuse for their behavior in their love of money. They had the invisible snake, the famous *nyungu*, at their beck and call, to carry out commando operations on their behalf and increase their wealth.

But nowadays *ekong* has evolved. It is no longer the prequisite of people of great wealth, but is available to all. It has become democratized. And as it has become more general, it has become more alarming. It has taken its place in the hierarchy of horrors, and is as firmly censured now as are the other practices of sorcery.

Wages and paper money may be one of the causes of its reappearance in force, and of its generalization. The power of buying and selling is no longer a monopoly of heads of families or wealthy business persons. In principle it is shared by all now. As a consequence, the need for money, growing with the cost of living, creates, surprises, jealousies, and dangerous temptations. The incomprehensible laws presiding over the distribution of money, the secret world of the coining and printing of money, and those fortresses called banks—all this contributes to maintain, in the popular mind, the idea that an invisible, disturbing reality exists somewhere here, and fosters belief in *ekong*.

If belief in *ekong* had not managed to assimilate the mystery of economics, doubtless it would have practically disappeared by now. It would have been unable to account for the facts of experience. Its persistence among the masses is evidence that it continues to furnish an explanation of wealth. It keeps "the lowly" from feeling totally confused in the monetary rat race and will thus continue to enjoy a certain usefulness, until such time as the schools begin to give a better explanation of the laws and taboos of the new kingdom of money.

Ekong and the Slave Traffic

After my visit to the *nganga* I went to see the chief, convinced that such a visit would preclude the imaginative interpretations the other visit had occasioned. This was an unfortunate mistake. In both cases, the three persons present were suspected of having entered into a conspiracy— the *nganga*, myself (taken for a Greek merchant given the Douala name Mukala Ndedi), and the chief. The scouts had been surprisingly disobedient to the chief at the roadblock. I was to learn that, in the other village, its chief, too, had been suspected of complicity, for he had drunk the whiskey I had offered him. The rumor fed on any of a thousand little signs. One who drinks an alcoholic beverage of especially fine quality, in such circumstances, is a comrade. There are no alliances without libations.

But why such readiness to suspect the chiefs? In the anguished times of the slave traffic, certain chiefs had served as intermediaries, entering into negotiations to supply whites with compatriots and reap a profit. Commerce in slaves was not so extensive along the coast of Cameroon as it was along the shores of neighboring countries, but its memory has not been effaced. A white who shuttled back and forth between a *nganga* and a chief awoke the collective memory of an infamous tragedy.

Thus the slave traffic, a historical fact, and *ekong*, a popular belief, are interrelated. The whites came to buy slaves. Blacks were taken away to work in a distant country and were never seen again. Cameroonians still believe that whites can acquire persons to work for them and they disappear forever. Sorcerers cause them to pass to another world, far from the gaze of those close to them. What must have been the impact of the slave trade on belief in *ekong* sorcery? I do not claim that it was at the origin of *ekong*, but I do maintain that it invests it with singular force and power today.[24]

Finally, there was another factor that helped lend substance to the rumor circulating about me. The white person in question was readily confused with someone already familiar, one about whom disturbing rumors had long since made their rounds—Mukala Ndedi. Inasmuch as I was being taken for this person, I decided to go and look for him.

Mukala Ndedi was a Greek merchant in Douala. His fame had gone to his head a little. It was not that he did not know the reasons for his renown, for it occasionally happened that someone would come to him and offer to sell him a family member. At a loss as to what to do, he had finally decided his strategy: he would refuse all private conversation with everyone, no matter whom—and if someone insisted, he would threaten to inform the police. Of course, Mukala Ndedi was not a disadvantageous nickname to have. It meant "the white who has pity," the good white. He had the same name in the Bassa language—*Nkana Ngo*—for he had the reputation far and wide of selling his fabrics at lower prices than those of his competitors.

I found Mukala Ndedi, and he and I discussed the possible origin of his redoubtable reputation. First of all, his rise had been rapid in the world of business. He had arrived in 1963 with 250,000 African francs—about $1000. Less than ten years later he could have anything at all on credit, and was one of Douala's most prosperous merchants. His fortune, he said, was not as great as those of other Greeks of the city. But the riot of fabrics he displayed was very impressive. It was clear evidence of his wealth. This person, who had seventy employees (visible ones) in 1972, and sold his wares at such low prices, must have an army of workers in the other world! There was no other explanation.

"But why me? Why not some other European? I'm not the only merchant doing this well around here!"

Clearly, Mukala Ndedi was paying dearly for the stroke of genius that had made him so successful. His business was located in the very center of the African quarter, in one of the busiest parts of Douala. "I looked for the locale where the most shoppers came, and set up a little business." With an enormous capacity for work, and good business sense, and then specializing in something that happened to be popular at the time, Mukala Ndedi had not had long to wait for fortune's smile.

The spectacle presented by his shop was fascinating and superb. His fabrics fairly spilled out onto the sidewalk. What waves of muslin for the passer-by to swim through! Breakers of blue, purple, yellow, and bright red splashed everywhere, blending in the gracious light. Behind these billows of color the sashes were piled, methodically folded into squares, and stacked in pillars that reached to the ceiling. Hanging among them like murals were one of each pattern, unfolded. You made your way among these columns as if you had entered a temple, and you instinctively lowered your voice to address the high priest of cloth, Mukala Ndedi. He spent all day rubbing elbows with his customers, who were dumbfounded at such brilliance, such success. And so he was "absorbed," you might say—his deeds, his exploits, became the subject of interpretation. Rumor contributed its accustomed share and Mukala Ndedi was rechristened "Ekong Man."

His shop, which looked like something out of Ali Baba, was frequented by one of those lovable street persons, in continuous dialogue with themselves, whom one sees going about bedecked with medals and amulets, at once respected and feared. Between Mukala Ndedi and this street eccentric a genuine friendship had formed. Mukala supported him with modest alms and paid his rent. In return, the eccentric obliged him in various ways—for instance, by imperiously halting the stream of passers-by whenever his master wished to sally forth. But to my view the presence of this person, known as his "sorcerer," contributed to the false rumors circulating about the merchant. Mukala Ndedi, the man of pity, passed as well for a slave dealer.

Ekong and Rumor

What was to be done now? To continue my research outside Douala by conferring with *nganga* would have been to expose myself to popular disturbances even more violent than the ones I had already provoked.

I consulted various persons in my perplexity, but received quite conflicting advice. One told me he simply did not know how to proceed in cases like these, because the Cameroonians in question were Protestants. If the villagers had been Catholics, he told me, a solemn high Mass could have been arranged, and the whole community could have been assured of my identity as a priest. And yet there was the old story of the German Catholic missionary who had been mistreated in this village when the allied soldiers had arrived in 1915, and there was still a children's song, "And who burned the priest's beard?"[25] Another person I consulted thought I should simply wait. Tempers would cool with time.

I recounted my misadventure to Din. He advised me against returning to the village alone. With a logic of his own, he declared that there was not a single person in that village capable of standing up to the sorcerers. The whole village was a kingdom of sorcery, for the *nganga* corps had lost the battle. Furthermore, "You travel too much," he told me. "You must be provided with talismans." And he offered me a number of objects for my protection.

Then, quite to the contrary, another chief spoke more encouragingly. This was a minor matter, he said, one easy to rectify. All that would have to be done would be to go to the village and convene a meeting of the leaders of the people, with the support of the highest popular authority. I should leave administrative officials out of it, he said, and settle the matter with the support of the traditional popular and religious leaders alone.

I opted for this latter solution. Let the machinery of tradition run, I thought. One of the high chiefs of Douala, the one within whose general jurisdiction that particular village came, agreed to take the matter in hand, and we formed a delegation: the high chief, a neighboring chief who was a popular figure, Father Endene, who was a Douala priest, Endene's cousin, who was a chemical engineer, and I. Undeniably, here was an imposing group. It would pay Caïn Dibunje Tukuru, the chief who had been incriminated, an official visit, and summon into his presence all the principal dramatis personae.

Then we sat, chatting with Tukuru, depository of tradition and master in the art of digging out pirogues, as the sounds of the frolicking of the scouts played in our ears, coming from somewhere nearby—whistling, the signal to muster, patrol cries, even old tunes from the grand games of my own childhood—in a word, the whole acoustical tradition of scouting.

Here they were—after their lengthy preparation somewhere, a little way back in the brush—the village youth en masse, marching past in full parade—with three banners at their head: the flag of the Unionist Scouts, the flag of the Cameroonian Scouts (with "Boy Scouts of France," *Eclaireurs de France*, ill concealed), and the flag of the Republic of Cameroon—banners enough for a regiment. The flag bearers were followed by a motley group—which kept ranks pretty well, however—of little boys of cub scout age, several girls (scouts, no doubt), and a dozen older boys and young men, all in the most improbable get-ups.

Here, then, were the scouts of the locale, demonstrating their might and discipline for us—an outlandish little army of irregulars, in the very precincts of the chief's official residence. Now they encircled us, and performed an undecipherable pantomine, which consisted in squatting and rising and emitting little cries, all executed with a macabre kind of playfulness. Father Endene and I looked at each other in consternation at this childish, grotesque display. First, dignified tradition, then, shoddy Europeanism. These youngsters were proud of their relationship with a great international movement and had decided to stand up to the chief as the guardians of a new order. They were the same ones, I could see, who had believed the rumor and thrown up the roadblock.

The village chief, who spoke French with difficulty, now held forth in Douala. "What a happy coincidence! We were on the point of convoking them, and they have come of their own accord!"

And that was his whole speech. In fact, he ordered the reconciliation flask to be carried indoors. Clearly, the village youth and Caïn Dibunje Tukuru were in confrontation.

But now the scoutmaster (who also bore the title of chief!) began a discourse of his own: "Let no one take it into their head that our youth wished to do the white man any harm!" Then he gave us to understand, by way of an old story, that a village chief is always held responsible for the evil committed in his territory. King Bell, he recalled, supreme chief of all the Douala, on a visit to this village when the colony had gained its independence, had had to listen to the challenge addressed to him by one of the local elders: "You have abandoned the presidency of the republic to another. But know that it is you who are responsible for the country. Whether it dies or survives is up to you." Our conflict today clearly was a conflict of generations, a conflict of cultures, and it was the old culture that had the upper hand, at least on the emotional level.

Now speech followed speech. The high chief of Douala played the scouts' own game. He declared himself their protector, and enjoined upon them obedience to Caïn Dibunje Tukuru. Then he explained the reasons for my visit to the *nganga*—my interest in the study of healings. I had a visible orientation to the modern world, a world to which the local chief had no access. Then Father Endene took his turn and explained the meaning of our work, which he described as "scientific, religious, and peaceful."

It all ended in an atmosphere of reconciliation. The high chief's whiskey sealed all the protestations of friendship. There were greetings, promises to see one another again, and congratulations all around. Everything seemed in good order now—except, it seemed to me, the relationship between the village chief and the scouts.

At that moment I saw the Old One—sorcerer? *nganga*?—discreetly mingling with the curious crowd. I went to shake his hand. Another man approached me to ask, "Did he sell persons to you?"

"Absolutely not!" was my prompt reply.

Then I turned back to the old man with the question, "Did anyone hurt you?"

"No," he said. "But they made me pay a goat and a pig."

Here our conversation was interrupted by one of the leading men of the village, who wanted to drive the old man away, telling me, "I don't like you to speak to him. He's an evil man. He wants to kill my son."

The old man and I looked at each other long and earnestly. Did he understand how much it hurt not to be able to intervene on his behalf? I thought I read a lesson in resignation in his tranquil eyes. Never again could we meet or speak together.

On the road back, the high chief of Douala gave me a piece of advice. "You can come back to this village. But do not come alone at first. And if it happens anywhere else . . . you had better run the roadblock."

Power over Rumor

I returned to the house of the grand elder of the Douala, Etame Dika, who had informed me earlier about *ekong*. He was one of my surest sources of information, and the most spiritual, as well. He described the bombardment of Douala by the English in 1915, when he was himself a functionary in the German administration. His oral sound effects made his great-grandchildren break into peals of laughter.

He made a very realistic statement to me. "Chiefs no longer have the power (*nginya*) they had before, because the government has taken this power. In our ancestors' time, when someone was named chief, he had the right to make any decision at all with regard to a malefactor. Today even the chief must use government channels. His only purpose is to see to the observance of custom. Chiefs today are but symbols (*eyembilan*) of tradition."

But the most surprising thing of all was this: deprived of any juridical role except that of gathering taxes, the chiefs still had a popular prestige and position that all still had to reckon with, even the youth.

I wanted to know the viewpoint of the other camp, so I arranged to meet one of the young scoutmasters, the one who had prevented me from leaving the village. He had me walk across the sandy streets, among the guardian mangos, as proof of my innocence and our reconciliation, and he explained what we were doing as we did so. I can recall some of his self-assured statements:

"The secret of this quarter—win the youth. . . .

"There are many young persons here. Some of them are at Douala, but they come back on Sundays. . . .

"The chief doesn't do anything for development. . . .

"What we want to do is have a revolution. . . .

"We're going to make parents listen to reason. . . .

"The chief hadn't informed us that a white was going to see the old *nganga*. That's why we threw up the barricade. . . .

"The chief wanted to break down the barricade, when he should have discussed it. . . .

"His son, the heir, is young; he understands us; he debated with us. . . ."

Was dialogue possible between a vigorous chief, confident of his traditional values but not very well able to express himself in French, and these young persons who had not succeeded in integrating themselves into modern society, but who nonetheless refused to return to pirogues and fishing? This little village was more town than country. But it still lived as if it were country. Cultural conflicts were more acute here. The provisional solution to the standoff between the two authorities was that the scout officials at Douala suspended the scoutmaster for six months for insolence to the village chief.

There was no question of anyone's discussing in my presence the rumor that circulated about me. Indeed there were two radically different languages here. The same event was reported, by turns, in two lights, lunar and solar. Circumstances—or the person who happened to be reporting—determined the passage from one to the other. The youth themselves, whose social raison d'être was their rejection of the old order, nevertheless held fast to the reality of *ekong*. The scout commissioner, with a scandalized air, expressed to me his shock "that scouts could believe such things!" It was evident that they did believe such things. But their language at a roadblock, at night, would not be the same as at 4 P.M. during an amicable get-together.

Now everything was reduced to a struggle for influence between the village chief and the youth. The latter had eagerly seized the opportunity to rebel, knowing that the people would be on their side when it was a matter of denouncing an affair of sorcery. Today they were whitewashing me of all suspicion—but only because we had done them the honor of an official visit. They had incurred a sanction—but they had offered a demonstration of their power. Score: one to one.

Rumor varied, then, at the good pleasure of different interests. But once it had broken loose, mighty indeed was the one who could throttle it, for it was founded on the emotional power of beliefs.[26]

As I was relating the resolution of the affair to Loe, who had been present at its inception, he replied, "The scouts didn't believe you were a priest—

even though I'd told them you were—and that's the reason they didn't let you through." And indeed, as experience had shown, when my identity was known—in town, for example, where, after all, I would go to see *ngangas*— the attitude toward me was very different. The churchman (*mot'ebasi*), the person of God (*mot'a Loba*), enjoyed a certain respect. But this prestige depended in large part on the powers attributed to the priest.

I wanted to know if Loe considered the priest a *ndimsi* personage in any way. Opinions differed on this point. Some had told me that a priest would not be part of *ndimsi* because a priest was a "white of God" (*mukala Loba*). Others said the opposite: yes, on condition he had "armor."

Loe was the founder and builder, and a parishioner, of the chapel of the Cameroonian Baptist church in his quarter. He was emphatic: "There are priests in *ndimsi* because there are priests who kill. They wear a string around their waist."

"Their belt?" I asked. Certain missioners wear a knotted cincture, or rope, and a knot in popular symbolism is a sign of murderous intent.

"Yes, the belt. It's for killing. Or for instance, if you take your Bible, and read it, you might go crazy."

"What? I've never heard of such a thing!" I said indignantly.

"That's what I am telling you. There are good priests and there are bad priests. Priests that kill. Besides, Jesus himself killed."

"You don't say! Give me an example."

"One day Jesus saw a tree. He was hungry and thirsty, so he went up to this mango tree.[27] But he didn't find any fruit. You can't have a tree growing on the earth and not bearing any fruit. So he made it dry up."

"But Jesus didn't kill a person!" I responded with relief.

"A tree is the same as a person. The grasses and herbs, the trees, the birds, the beasts are born of the earth exactly as a person. God created everything."

"That's one way of looking at it. But tell me—the good priests, what do they do with their power?"

"They have a power like mine—forgiving, consoling, giving advice."

The dialogue was like a friendly joust—which I obviously was losing. What idea could they really have of me?

Chapter 6

Misfortune Is Malady

> Misfortune comes from (the
> relationship) between you and
> me.
>
> —Din

After my adventure, of such dubious outcome, I decided to stop running
about the countryside for a time and let the rumor die down. Even if villagers who felt sure of my identity were to accept my presence at a treatment
séance, I would risk causing such excitement that the treatment would
doubtless not follow standard norms. So the backwoods were out of
bounds. But in town I would be able to find peace and security, especially in
the Deïdo and Bepanda quarters, where my patrons, Din and Loe, practiced. And so I resolved to continue my research right where I was. My visit
had begun to bear fruit. Here I would be recognized and safe.

I wanted to solve, finally, a little vocabulary mystery. Conversations I
held were frequently frustrated by misunderstandings about the meaning of
the word for sickness.

I was forever hearing the word *maladie*, "sickness." Engome had been
"sick" in Din's home. Then she "got well." Loe had sought to come to the
assistance of an old *nganga* who, it was said, suffered from a strange "sickness," which had pared away his powers. I began to wonder about this
word, "sickness." It seemed a kind of master key to so many things. A
child would have measles. Loe knew how to treat this *maladie*, this "sickness." And of course it was a sickness. And I was certainly willing to consider a lengthy physical indisposition, with a fever, but psychosomatic in
origin, as a "sickness." But if a man dislocated his shoulder, and misfortune was cited as the culprit, it too was called a "sickness!"

Was it that they were merely simplifying—translating several different
Douala words by the one French word, *maladie*? But after a little inquiry I
realized that when they said "*maladie*" they always meant *diboa* (plural,

68

maboa), so that the Douala word had exactly the same extension as its French equivalent. It seemed to me that the reasons for the amalgamation were not purely semantic, that they sprang from a certain way of looking at life (and death) that still escaped me.

Then Loe unintentionally gave me enlightenment on this question, and the opportunity to advance one step further into the logic of his universe at the same time. Elimbi, his only grown son, who was twenty years old, and whom I rarely saw at home, was out of work. Actually he had never had a real job. "Look at this fellow," Loe said to me in desperation, "he quit school and doesn't work!" And so he decided to treat the young man for misfortune, in his *nganga* fashion, as he would have treated a disease, so that Elimbi could find a trade.

When I expressed my surprise, Loe told me, in French: "Misfortune is a sickness like any other. Only it is more terrible. If you have no money, you're in a fix, aren't you?"

"You mean misfortune can be treated like an ordinary illness?"

"Ordinary illness! It's a—it's a provoked illness! What do you mean, 'ordinary' illness?"

"You think misfortune is always provoked?"

Loe gave me a whistle of assent. In his logic, three situations were practically equivalent: sickness, misfortune, and unemployment. That is, they all translated the same word in Douala. It would not be easy to find a word in our languages that would carry all three denotations.

A question came to mind. "If Elimbi has no work," I asked, why don't you have him become a *nganga* like yourself?"

"A son does not automatically follow in his father's footsteps. To be a *nganga*, you have to have a heart that doesn't grow angry quickly as other hearts—a patient heart, that can take anything. One must not kill. That's why it's the *bedimo*, the family ancestors, who choose a successor. Your character is measured, to see if you are respected, if you have heart, if you are obedient. I don't want an apprentice. There's no such thing as an 'automatic' science of tradition. If I die, my *bedimo*—my vanished ancestors—will give the secret to someone else."

For that matter, Elimbi was of the same mind. "I don't want to do what my father does. You have to have heart. I don't have his heart. It's dangerous; you can die. And my father nearly died; he fell down once when he was doing a treatment. Sometimes visitors come to him who wish him evil. Someone like papa, you will know—he sees things I can't see. It takes courage to see all those things. He says there are things that don't exist in our world that exist over there—monsters, and plenty else. It's easy to see how somebody could get killed. You can understand how it's not a pleasant thing to do! Because there are laws, too, but you musn't talk about them to anybody. If you did, you could be the cause of your own death. That takes courage!"[28]

Elimbi had attended elementary school, but without finishing. Then he enrolled in a trade school, but very quickly ceased to attend classes. Next, his maternal uncle found him a little job in a business called SEPIC. But after five months he was let go. The secret passion of this big, somewhat effeminate, unfortunate boy was electricity. In desperation, he wanted to take some correspondence courses to get an electrical engineering license. I sought to dissuade him, knowing how useless and costly such an undertaking would be.

Elimbi was one of those unemployed secondary school dropouts who know too much and too little: too much to be willing to be manual laborers, and too little to have any professional aptitude. "We have a difficulty here in Cameroon," Loe sighed. "A child like that is a 'secondhand book,' somebody without work." Here was a real case of misfortune!

Elimbi's position at home was not very solid either. He could have considered himself the eldest son, a position that commanded respect. But his mother, Loe's third wife, had left them when Elimbi was a baby and had gone to another quarter of the city to live with another man. In reprisal, Loe had always refused to recognize his son legally. He had married his mother validly in the eyes of custom, but without a civil marriage license. "It's something that touches me very deeply," Elimbi told me. And for his part, Loe confided to me, "My wife is another man's blood. Elimbi is my blood."

Pilgrimage to the Tree

Theoretically, a treatment for ill fortune begins in the forest, at nightfall. But is this the forest? The city had showed no more respect for the forest than it had for the *nganga*'s house. The tree at whose foot we gathered grew in a ravine, already surrounded by new houses. In fact, it owed its continued existence to the fact that it grew on a slope unsuitable for construction.

This tree fell far short of the majesty of my own quarter's *Grand Fromager*. Its trunk was all twisted, and at first sight there was nothing special about its reddish bark. To the eyes of the simple layman, such as I was, it could be distinguished from its neighbors only by a series of gashes near the foot. "Other *nganga* [plural] come here," Elimbi explained to me. "This tree is rare and famous. It's the family's tree, and it can kill you or grant you your request. Nobody goes up to it. Everybody knows there are . . . there are things about it. Nobody ever says the tree's name— that's a family secret. Even some members of the family don't know its name."

Loe and I had come in a little Vespa. I drove, seated on Loe's suitcase, with one arm carefully extended so as not to break the pair of raw eggs he had asked me to keep in my hand and take good care of, for some purpose of which I was ignorant. And so, as we drove through these quarters, where everyone had gone to sleep, along streets that were nothing but paths of broken earth, with holes and bumps like an old battle-field, I felt as if I could have been mistaken for someone doing a balancing act. We were following a car driven by Elimbi, who accompanied his father when Nkongo, the disciple, was absent, and the prim little man who was to receive treatment this night. We left our cars near the edge of the ravine, and the little man had a long, animated conversation with Loe. He was refusing to go down the slope, and was not hiding his fear. He asked me in French what they were going to do to him—a question that I was hard put to answer. Irked, Loe left him where he stood, and invited Elimbi and me to follow him to the tree.

On the way down, Loe confided to me, "He's more afraid of you than of the tree." In view of recent events, that was plausible. Once we got to the foot of the tree, Loe decided to begin treating his son—something that he had had in mind to do for some time.

Later, Elimbi told me, "I wasn't going to be the one treated. It was going to be the other man. But he didn't have any confidence. He refused to be treated. Papa was ready to go, right? He couldn't just let his power sit idle. He had to work. It had to come out. The reason he treated me was to release the power he had. It was to let out the power he already had that he had gained from the tree."

At his tree at last, Loe did not hide his happiness. He was not in a "foreign country," as he had been on our previous expedition, but quite at home now in this ravine, which led down to Mbanya Creek, a tributary of the Wouri, and sacred to Douala tradition. Loe was in the habit of speaking to his tree, to ask it for things as if it had been a person—the person of his ancestors. Then he began to chew up a certain sugary condiment called *nsote*, which then he spat against the bark. This was a gesture of good intentions. It was also a form of blessing practiced toward members of one's family. Now Loe inserted a lighted cigarette in a crack in the bark. Then he dashed one of the eggs against the trunk. By these very simple actions, Loe involved the basic materials and elements of nature in his rites: water, fire, breath, and vegetable and animal matter.

After having blessed the tree in this fashion, and made some new notches in the wood itself, Loe stripped completely, as did Elimbi. They anointed their bodies with perfume from head to foot, then began to embrace the tree with their whole bodies, pressing their flesh against the bark, in order to be impregnated with its sap and life.

Elimbi later told me, "When you rub against the tree, you're supposed to be thinking inside yourself. If you think you're going to die that night, you die that night. I always think of having good luck and a long life."

I asked, "To whom do you speak?"

Elimbi said, "To the tree."

During this ceremony, the *nganga* would murmur an incantation to the tree in quick staccato phrases. I stood a few paces back, and off to the side, on the slope, and tape recorded his words, though they were scarcely audible. Then the forest began to speak, and my tape recorder was filled with the sounds of thousands of insects, the rustling of leaves, and the creaking of trees. Here was Loe's prayer, which Elimbi later helped me transcribe.

> We learn no divination (*bedinge*) without recourse to thee. . . .
> Give me the gift of strength (*nginya*) that God (*Loba*) has given to thee. . . .
> Absolutely all strength. . . .
> Gird me well with my sash.
> Truly art thou in the hand of Jehovah, the God of heaven (*a Loba la moyn*)!
> If anyone thinks of evil . . . this is a matter for God (*a Loba njom*). . . .
> For that one knows not God's love (*ndol'a Loba*).
> I beg the luck (*musima*, "grace") and blessing of God (*bonam ba Loba*).
> The one I touch, whoever it may be, must really get well (*angamen nde bole*)!
> Whatever the disease (*diboa*)—leprosy, madness, epilepsy, paralysis— no matter what it is. . . .[29]

Once father and son had honored those at the source of all "good fortune" ("grace")—that is, God and the ancestors—they walked back toward the house in silence. Climbing back up the slope, we were neither to look around nor utter a word. At the top the little man was waiting for us. But the power of the tree would not come to him that night.

Our procession found its way back to Loe's courtyard where we came upon some twenty persons, all either singing, beating a drum or gong, or clicking a kind of castanets. They had accompanied us at a distance during our visit to the tree. These few neighbors, patients, and close relatives of Loe were seated along three sides of the square closed off by the *dibandi*. When it came my turn to be seated, I took my place beside my fellow pilgrims on the men's bench, the other benches being reserved for the more numerous women.

These benches were merely unsteady planks, resting on cinder blocks, practically at ground level. I always preferred this type of seat to a chair during the long treatment sessions.

A chant was begun. I picked up a pair of castanets, the only instrument within reach. They were cut of bamboo, and were flat, like a schoolroom ruler, only rather wider. The idea was to smack them together in rhythm, using both hands. The gong was a kind of triangular bell, struck from the outside with a little stick. The drum, with its leather head, and the gong were much too difficult for me, with their offbeat rhythm.

During the chant, Loe and Elimbi went into the *dibandi*. I was never to know what actions they performed, or what words they uttered, in this center of energy—of which I have seen the inside but once in my life. Loe, who has been known to coin a phrase, called it his "central commissariat."

The affable man seated on my left was a retired public official. He was ending his days in this quarter, and never missed a night séance. While we struck our sticks together to the rhythm of the drum, he gave me, in elegant phraseology, his opinion of Loe.

"I assure you, he cures persons. I always come here. I wouldn't come if he played tricks on the imagination. He always gives the name of God first priority. He knows that herbs have their power from God. He often cures someone. Like this woman here, for instance," and he pointed to a young woman dressed in a white sash. "She was crazy. She went to the hospital again and again, but she kept having relapses. I'm not saying the hospital didn't help. But she kept having relapses. And she was convinced a sorcerer had cast a spell on her. So she came here. And there you see her, cured."

"There are *nganga*s who mix a bit of the European into their dances." My neighbor was alluding to the new astrological practices. "But Loe's cures are unadulterated. He uses herbs, as did the ancients among us in bygone times, when whites were not here. There have always been *nganga*s. Of course, real ones are rare, but you can still find them. It's too bad they can't get together—some cure the insane, some cure epilepsy, some cure other sicknesses. If they could all get together they could have a kind of team, you know, and the government could use them. There should be rules and procedures for treatments. But these *nganga*s are all individualists.

"Getting cured—it's a matter of conviction. When you're sure you want to be cured, you're cured. And so, too, when persons are convinced they're going to die—even with the best medical help in the world. . . . It's a matter of conviction. That's the way it is with the things of God, too—faith, belief. . . . When you believe, you're saved."

These reflections reminded me of Loe's disciple Nkongo—not present this evening—who admitted (with a certain spirit of criticism) the efficacity of all conviction as such—apart from the reality of the objects of belief. Despite their difference in generation, both these persons believed in the intervention of the ancestors and the water spirits, even though they had the intellectual formation that could have permitted them to doubt it. These beliefs, I could see, had formidable staying power.

Now Loe, accompanied by Elimbi, came out of the *dibandi* and took advantage of the respite that ensued to open a bottle of rum, from which he poured a drink for each of the men present. When he came to me, he remarked cynically that the bottle had been brought by the little man for his treatment, which had not taken place. "They'll buy him another one," he added. Whereupon I said—in a loud voice, in the hope that the little man would hear me—that I was sorry I had been the unintentional cause of this failure. "It's a matter of blood," Loe replied. "He doesn't have

enough blood"—with no reference to what I had said! A few minutes later
the little man discreetly slipped away and disappeared in the quarter, and I
would never see him again.

A lengthy family ceremony then got under way, in the space marked out
by the square along which the visitors were seated. It would keep us in the
courtyard until dawn. Loe bade all his relatives stand in a line: his brother
and his sister-in-law—the reader will recall their disputes—his own two
wives, and an aunt on his father's side. He himself stood facing them, with
Elimbi, who was a head taller than he, on his right.

The ceremony was divided into two parts. First, there was an animated
conversation, in which all the protagonists spoke at once.[30] Then there was a
stately, solemn rite in which each spoke calmly and distinctly. My neighbor
made the following commentary.

"Loe is asking the family members if they agree that Elimbi should be
treated. The uncle [Loe's elder brother] is asking, 'Will it be my fault?' His
wife has just said, 'Yes, because he's your nephew.' See, it's like a confession! The uncle says he gives his consent to treat the young man. You might
say he had thrown in a kind of wedge [a brake, an obstacle], because Elimbi
wasn't up to snuff."

I learned much in a few words. Any disease, no matter what it was, even
bad fortune, always had a cause. Loe's elder brother must have been responsible. In the first place, he was obviously an aggressive person. After all
those quarrels, his wife was now going to let slip the opportunity to indict
him publicly. Secondly, the Douala know very well that the relationship
between a paternal uncle and his nephew is structurally conflictual. When a
man dies, his brother and son have to compete for his estate. In case of
illness, then, the sufferer's paternal uncle is spontaneously, almost ritually,
accused, because he could profit from the disappearance of his rival.

My neighbor, the retired official, went on: "Right now Loe is trying to
convince the whole family that the young man ought to be treated. His
youngest wife just said, 'Anyway, he's a child of the family'—so their husband ought to try to bring him back to life. If it had been somebody from
the outside, there wouldn't have been any need to get all the family together."

Up to this point, what was at stake in the treatment seemed to me to be
the well-being of an individual. A young man had been unable to find work.
His family was now seeking to get it for him by the means their tradition
offered, means I was trying to analyze and understand. But thanks to my
neighbor's commentary, I began to appreciate the collective dimension of
the problem. Would not the fate of Elimbi as an individual be a by-product
of the solution of a family difficulty? And at the moment, the finger of
suspicion was pointing at Loe's elder brother.

"Now Loe is rebuking his elder brother for not having spoken frankly,
and for having 'thrown a monkey wrench into the machinery,' " my

neighbor went on. (That is, he was accusing him of having interfered with the normal course of things, of having "blocked" Elimbi by sorcery.) "This proves that he doesn't have a serene heart. Loe's asking him what he wants exactly. Loe's saying that this is a child the family should bless, but that the uncle is putting up resistance and not wanting the family to give the boy their joint blessing."

But the elder brother solemnly protested that he wished his nephew well. And now the second part of the ceremony could begin.

"Forehead, Open up to Luck!"

Muto a si manea,
mumi nde a manee.

A woman ought not to command;
a man ought to command.

Now Loe intoned a majestic, tranquil, melodious chant in Douala. It contrasted sharply with the incantation rhythms that we had been hearing over and over for an hour now. I should say the melody was probably inspired by a Protestant hymn. As for the words, they began: "I have received the strength of God. I am the person who suffers."

Elimbi stood in the center of us looking like a coconut palm, straight and supple. He obeyed his father's orders. "Woe to you if you tap your feet!" Loe cried to him. "Look me in the eyes!" And Loe began by making little pricks on the boy's forehead, considered the seat of good fortune and happiness.

"Forehead, open up to good fortune and happiness! Forehead, open!" Loe cried. And he did the same on Elimbi's ears, mouth, chest, arms, and legs. When he had finished, he brought up a great pot, filled with water, in which "special family herbs" were marinating—in particular the *diboku-boku la wonja*, a large, thick leaf, round as a plate, which is always used in these ceremonies to signify and effect reconciliation. Now each family member present took the leaf and, one by one, without spilling any of the liquid it held, brushed it back and forth all over Elimbi's face, improvising a little sermon made up of reproaches and good wishes.

The ceremony as a whole, including the family council part, is called *esa*, and is without doubt the rite most familiar to the Douala people. It is practiced on all occasions, little and great: when danger threatens, when there is cause for joyous celebration, when greater group unity is desired, and so on—in public life as well as at the home. The words spoken, then, contain nothing canonized or particularly solemn. I report them here because they give the key to this "medical" treatment of an unhappy, unemployed young man.

Except for a few flowery phrases pronounced in French, the whole rite took place in Douala, mixed with expressions from other Cameroonian languages and Pygmy. Loe sometimes used as many as eight languages in the course of a single treatment. This recalled that the water spirits had given him the gift of tongues, which in turn was a demonstration of his universal calling. He once told me he had even, during an herbs and bark treatment, spoken several European languages that the spirits inspired in him. A *nganga* knows no linguistic or racial barriers. I should like to have heard those "voices," for the Cameroon languages as used by Loe were not always intelligible even to those who spoke them fluently.

Next, then, in his florid language, Loe invited each of the four women present to take her turn to speak during the ablutions.

"O coconut, beautiful lady," said he, in French, "my beautiful love, my beautiful darling." The he went on in Douala: "Dear to my thoughts, dear to me as the fruit of the sloe, O thou who love not riches, who art beyond beauty . . . but do my wives not recognize their names?"

Loe enjoined his brother to speak first. As Elimbi's uncle, he passed the leaf across the young man's face, saying: "You are the heir here. Your family wants you to find work. You're standing here because of bad luck. Your bad luck comes from me and no one else. I say this because my heart is very, very pure within me. May God (*Loba*) help you to go forward. That's the way our ancestors did it: if you're angry at your child, you ought to tell him so. If you keep it a secret, you kill him. As I told you today, I believe that I love you. God have mercy on you."

Then there was the chant: "Tis not by pride that I am here; I wait for war."

Now the first wife took her turn with the leaf. "In the name of God, I wipe you too. You are a child, born of Lord Loe. It is not the woman who commands. It is the man who commands. I wipe you with great care—may all misfortune go away, go away. I am urging your heart not to come back to your father's house, and then if you have this thought yourself, may your heart turn around. Son, recognize your father. May your hands serve you well. May God have mercy on everything you touch in order to work."

This speech, then, took a sharp turn, which the others would accentuate still more. It showed me the key to Elimbi's treatment. The first wife had made no allusion to Loe's brother—the uncle who had been the object of suspicion until now—but to Elimbi's own family situation. One after the other now, in perfect unanimity, everyone stressed the abnormal side of Elimbi's behavior. How could this boy live apart from his father? Everyone knew Elimbi's mother had long since left her husband's household. Now I learned something of capital importance. She had taken their son with her. And so, contrary to custom, he had spent most of his time far from any paternal influence. Was this not the main cause of his misfortune?

The other three women now took their turn at giving a speech like the one the first had given—on the need for a boy to be with his father.

Then Loe took his own turn with the ritual leaf, and touched his son's face, saying: "Our ancestors say that a child is not bought with money. One does not steal a child. A child is a generous gift of God. My son, glory to God the Father, to the Son, and to the Spirit that I was able to engender you. I am not content with you, my son, for you were not at my side. I walked down the road alone. If I went out, who would stay home? Death does not take away a piece of wood, but a human being, with arms and legs. If it had taken me, would you have even known? If you say you will not recognize the family—to each his own, O man! But if you say you recognize the family, may the words coming out of your mouth be sweet as honey, and your heart within tranquil as the heart of a true man.

"For there is competition in Douala [for employment], if you don't see it yourself. In the name of the little wisdom God gave you, know that it is your own hands that must feed your mouth. You know very well that your father has money. I want you, too, to earn your own money. The French say, 'Everyone for themselves, and God for everyone.' May your feet do your searching, may they carry you, may they carry you off where fortune (*musima*) is! May they not take you where bad luck (*mbeu'a nyolo*) is!

"Misfortune, get away, get away, I drive thee away! Amen, Alleluia!"

Each of the officiants had punctuated his or her statement by spitting upon Elimbi the little seeds of the condiment called *nsote*, the same seeds that Loe had spat upon the tree of the ancestors. They have the capacity to reforge unity.

During the final rites, Loe used the same materials or elements that he had used at the tree. First there was fire. For his son, Loe did not spare the blasts of fire. He lighted a fistful of straw, took a mouthful of gasoline, shot it across the flame, and thus caused a brilliant flash, or explosion, in the air above the head of the young man. After each bomb, Elimbi responded: *"E!"*—that is, "Yes, it's me!" The fiery puff prevents evil from rising up, it removes trouble, Loe explained to me later. Elimbi has to answer to show whether he is dead or alive. After this ritual trial, Elimbi still had to leap over the pot where the "special family herbs" were marinating—that is, Loe told me afterward, he had to "leap over the bad luck all around him"—and receive, full in the forehead, the second egg, which I had carefully brought back from the ravine. As he did so, Loe pronounced the following words in a loud voice, and I did not have to ask him what they meant: "This chicken [in potency, that is] loses its life for you. May the anger of this chicken rise up against you if you do not hear! May the anger of this bird [now with our ancestors] halt anyone who shall seek to oppose your journey! There. Lift your head up. You've got a dirty face, like your uncle."

The chanting and dancing continued until morning. Meanwhile Elimbi waited silently in a corner. The only thing he had said all night was *"E!"* after each fiery blast. "He's not supposed to speak," Loe told me. "It's forbidden. He's just been blessed. He has to stay quiet. Even in my presence he keeps silent. No one may ask him anything."

The following day I invited Elimbi to my lodgings. It was not difficult to persuade him to come, perhaps because he had had to be silent for so long the night before. I sat him down in the only easy chair I had, and Philippe, the bistro-keeper, brought us a couple of beers. I could feel that Elimbi was relaxed, confident, and eager to talk. I tried to interrupt him as little as possible. I wanted to be most careful not to distort his testimony, especially because it was being given in French.

"So," I began, "you think what they did last night can bring you better luck?"

"I think so," Elimbi replied. "I don't believe so, but I think so."

Surely this distinction between "thinking" and "believing" indicates a difficulty Elimbi had in reconciling a great number of experiences. But it also recalls that "believing" implies commitment, a gift of self. This is the sense in which Elimbi was drawing a distinction between the two words, thus felicitously clarifying his position with regard to the treatment he had undergone. Nkongo, Loe's usual assistant, and the retired gentleman I had spoken with during the séance, had already expressed their own positions.

"I didn't say it doesn't bring luck," Elimbi went on. "There are times when it brings luck directly and times when it brings luck indirectly. For instance, you're looking for a job. That can come directly. It can be Papa or anybody else. There are other *nganga*'s. You want a job, you go to a *nganga*. He works on you—he sends a letter to the employment agency himself, and you're called right away. That proves there's a certain power in all this.

"Sometimes the science [of healing] doesn't work directly, let's say it doesn't work directly enough to attract customers to your shop. It works, but not that fast. It starts a little bit at a time. It can take a month. But in the meantime you can feel you've been worked on.

"My father has a certain manner of treating. You know, in this city life is full of enemies. I don't know how it is for the Europeans—I'm talking about the blacks. There are families that don't get along. One member or another can go to a fetishist [a dishonest *nganga*] and say, 'Try to block that particular person for me!' Well, everything you have, your things, start disappearing, right into thin air. You think you're not sick?[31] Well, just watch your luck disappear. Sure, in a case like that, you can be treated. But I don't think they can *add* more luck to the luck God has given to each one.

"For instance, in the same family you can have one father, but different mothers. Then I'll say, 'I'm the one to manage my father's things.' Another will say, 'No, you're not.' It happens that way all the time. So then I might go to a marabout [a Muslim healer] and tell him I haven't got the courage to kill the one who doesn't agree with me, but I'd like him to drive him crazy. This kind of thing is done! But I don't think a marabout or a fetishist can *improve* the luck God gave us—I really don't think so."

"How can you tell the difference between a real *nganga* and a false *nganga*?" I asked Elimbi.

"A false *nganga* has to be smart, very smart. Some of them, when you visit them, ask you how you feel. 'Don't you hurt anywhere?' they'll ask. Well, then, you'll say, 'Sure, sometimes, my back. . . .' 'Aha!' the *nganga* will say. 'That's it! Your brother who lives with you, he's the one who causes you all this pain!' "

"But to go back to the last séance," I said, "—do you really think luck is going to smile on you?"

"I know one thing. All those things they did to me will do *something*. It was something important. It was something. . . . Everything they wished for there is all going to happen. Because, really, my father has a power. But myself, I'm saying I don't base everything on that, I don't entirely commit myself, I don't entirely give myself. I mean, I don't put my whole will power on that. Because, even me, when I do anything, I can't say, 'O spirits, help me!' I have to say, 'God, help me!' Because . . . because God said, 'Thou shalt have no other God before thee.' Because when someone gives their whole self, that's 'adoring.' So if you give yourself completely to something, you're adoring it."

Nkongo told me something once that was a real surprise coming from an apprentice *nganga*. "When you believe in something," he told me, " when you believe down deep inside in what a *nganga* does, it has too much of an effect . . . . When you believe in them completely, you don't believe in God any more."

Elimbi was full of things to say, so I prodded him on. "If you sit quietly at home and not move a muscle, can good luck come?" I asked.

"Ah! Ah! That's just the problem! That's just why I always say: when it's magic, I don't believe in it. I know it has power, that's for sure. But me, I've always thought, all you have to do is have self-control. If you can get self-control, you can go to an office yourself to look for work. You've got self-control? Great! Then give your will. What you're going to ask for, maybe God will give you the good luck to have."

"Where did you learn that?"

"You know the Great Ones [highly placed persons] are always discussing things. That's where you hear the best stuff. You have to be curious, kind of. If I see you discussing an intellectual subject, I just can't pass by without listening.

"God can give good luck. There's proof of it. I had it happen one time, when mama had a baby, one night, in the middle of the night. . . . She was four months late, so this was very serious. So I went off into a corner and prayed and cried. I saw God had mercy on me. I don't know what you call it in French. . . . It started to form and it came out. The son was breathing. I saw that it was really God helping me, because there are others who collect death like it was nothing! I knew that if you give yourself completely, if you really pray, you get satisfaction."

"Why were you willing to be treated?"

"I was living with mama, and she had three children after she left Loe.

She lives with a fisherman who doesn't make much money. I have to find work. But there are things only a father can take care of. And if I stay with my mother, my father won't bother finding me work.

"Here they're jealous of me, I think, because I'm the oldest. All the others are still children. If my father dies now, there's only me to take charge of things. So then I'm responsible for three women. My uncle would be there only to guide me; he can't be the one responsible."

"You think the treatment is going to get you a job?"

"I'm not sure yet. I've just been treated. I still haven't seen if . . . . Even if I found work now, I couldn't state that it was because of this power. It'd be God that helped me."

Elimbi's misfortune was that his parents were separated. If this big, soft young man continued to live with his mother, he would not be considered a man, as far as custom was concerned, but a vagabond. Vagabonds did not find work. But if he resumed his place as eldest son at his father's side, in line to succeed him, he would gain social status. In the street he would be considered an upstanding man. And there you had the conditions of employment!

Elimbi appreciated this. It was not love for his father or his father's wives that brought him back to his father's house, but wisdom and prudence. He submitted to treatment, placed God at the source of all good luck, prayed to the tree, and willingly offered ablutions and sacrifice. But he did not "give" himself completely. He performed his role in the *esa* ceremony with docility and was reconciled with his relatives. He hearkened to the lavish advice. He even allowed his family to warn him against his mother. This was the price of reintegration. Until now he had not been lucky enough to find work, because he was being kept in a family situation that was in imbalance.

The uncle had been challenged by his wife to accuse himself. "Accuse yourself!" she had said. "You're his uncle!" And the uncle responded, prudently, "I repent, for I have a very pure heart within!"

Even Loe did not believe the uncle was culpable. "The evil comes from the mother's side," he told me when I asked him about it. The evil came from the fact that this son had been kept in the maternal family, away from the father's influence. "It is not for a woman to command, but for a man!"

And so, this ceremony would not give Elimbi a job. He still must look for one, but this time the chances were on his side. I asked Loe about the way things were going. "What if your son doesn't find a job?" I asked.

In reply, Loe first asked me to find him one. Then he added: "I'll see. If he doesn't have any luck, I'll ply my trade. But now I have nothing in my brain." (That is, he had taken no decision as yet.) If Elimbi were not to find a job, his father would go back to the *dibandi*, don his red battle robe once more, call the ancestors and the water spirits to the rescue, and undertake to discover, during another night of dancing, what sorcerer, man or woman, wished his son evil.

Elimbi's story had been for me like a photograph being developed. At first it had been fluid, nebulous. Then it had gained in definition. In the beginning, I had had difficulty understanding it, so ambiguous were the words used between us. But today I know that the real difficulty came from our different cultures, from which the words proceeded.

Reestablishing Order

I paid Din a visit. I wanted to question him too on misfortune and its causes. I hoped he would fill in the gaps in my information, in Douala (he spoke no French), and thereby help me find my way out of this everlasting vocabulary morass. He confirmed the essentials of what I had learned from Elimbi's treatment, but he also linked together the two French words *chance* and *malchance*, "good luck" and "bad luck," and connected them with terms in his own language. It was a fine example of how one culture gnaws away at another. In the beginning, vocabulary carries the day. Then, little by little, the philosophy implied in that language supervenes. Only, in this particular case the French words scarcely nibbled into the traditional Douala conception of misfortune at all.

The source of "good luck"—Din and Loe both agreed here—was God. The tree, the ancestors, the *dibandi*, the water spirits, all bestowed a "good luck" that had God as its source. This association of God with "good luck" sounds less jarring in our European languages if we examine the corresponding words in Douala that Loe had used that night at the tree. *Musima* and *bonam*, best translated "grace" and "blessing," are first and foremost the result of a favorable intention, not the fruit of chance. But if we look up "luck" in our own dictionaries, we see that it *is* something due to chance. Thus the distance between this African language and our own is quite striking.

It is not that the Douala is unfamiliar with the concept of chance. It is only that the Douala does not use that concept in daily living. Chance is left to the diviners. They know how to interpret life's fortuitous aspects. Luck, however, is generally believed to be a grace bestowed by God. "I don't think one can add more luck to the luck God has given to each one," Elimbi had said.

The Douala start with a basically optimistic conception of existence: God gives each person their good luck, their own measure of good fortune. If that fortune fails to smile, if it turns bad, then one must either blame oneself or accuse others. Who has disturbed the normal course of events?

Din explained "bad luck" to me as an unnatural reversal. "It is the human being who is evil. Take the banana tree. You don't plant a banana tree upside down. If you plant it upside down, it won't grow. Now, if you plant properly what God has created on earth, it'll grow. And that's why I say it's the human being who's evil. God made everything there is. A human being knows very well that such and such an herb or bark that he shoots at you [*angwe*—that he casts at you as bad luck] will give you *malchance* [Din used the French word for "bad luck"]. It was not God's idea. He tells human beings: "Do what you want, but be responsible (*mbong*) for it."

Bad luck comes from the perversion of relationships among human beings. I think the most enlightening thing I ever heard Din say was: "If someone is out of luck, it's because of bad blood (*maya ma bobe*). If somebody has bad blood, he's out of luck (*musima*). And if you look closely, you'll see that somebody has made him fall into this bad luck. Somebody tripped him up, did him evil, and ruined his blood in this way. That's how it is. Bad luck comes from the relationship between you and me (*mbeu'a nyolo nya wa nde na oa na mba*). If I get mad at you, I give you bad luck. If I like you, I give you good luck, as you do me. It's the same with an evil-doer (*mot'a bobe*)—that's somebody who must be trying to do evil to you. Do you understand?"

Both expressions translated by "bad luck" here have an organic meaning. *Mbeu'a nyolo* literally means "bad state of the body." *Maya ma bobe* literally means "bad blood," and reminds us of our expression, "There was bad blood between them." When Loe performed the pricking upon Elimbi, or another patient, droplets of blood seeped out onto the skin. Merely by the color of someone's blood Loe claimed to be able to follow the progress of a disease or the effectiveness of a treatment. Whatever the value of his or her anatomical knowledge, a *nganga* places physical symptoms in the category of misfortune.

When Loe declared that bad luck was a disease, he meant a disease accompanied by organic complications. Some Europeans would be inclined to range this notorious ill luck in the category of "personality disorders" and consider it a matter for psychiatry. I never heard Din or Loe make a distinction between diseases of the mind and those of the body. They were encouraged here by the tendency of patients to complain of some physical manifestation of anxiety or confusion. These somatic reactions, doubtless stronger with Africans than with Europeans, are the reflection of an important element in the African's philosophical background—namely, that the human being is a single whole. Recall that the primary distinction within a human being is not between body and soul—the physical and the psychic—but between the visible and the invisible.

This is where the *nganga*s come in. Their function consists in removing the unnatural ill luck that has been "cast" upon their patients as an evil turn, and restoring them to a state of "luck," a state of grace. This action of effectuating the return of good luck was well expressed by a marvelous statement made by Loe in French after he had treated his son: "Good luck, I tell you, is the will of God. If I take bad luck away from you, I put you back the way you were." "*Je vous remets au bon poids,*" he said, "I restore you to your proper weight."

Whatever be their physical, psychosomatic, or social dimensions, all these forms of imbalance—evil, misfortune, or disease—are considered foreign bodies to be got rid of, or uncleanness to be washed away, in order to restore someone's original integrity and cleanliness. I once heard this very clear description: "If you are hurting, if you have a headache or a bellyache, I pull out (*na duta*) all these pains, I put them together in one place (*na kotele ni sese nyese o wuma iwo*), I make cuts on that spot (*na ma sasa yi wuma*), and the blood flows and washes out the evil (*ma maya ma ma buse, ma ma busane di diboa*)."

Restoring a lost order—this, I think, is the primary work of the *nganga*s. But I was encouraged to hear from both my masters, Din and Loe, that the objective of the treatment—finding a trade for Elimbi, for example—would not be attained automatically. There were still steps to be taken, things to do, employment offices to visit. "You can't find work if you don't look. It says, 'Knock and it shall be opened to you,' or else, 'Seek and you shall find,' " Din concluded, citing the gospel. There is no magic in these matters. This aspect of the problem—personal effort or skill, which I would be inclined to consider as primary, was doubtless in no better than second place in the logic of my interlocutors. This was their particular emphasis. But it helps to remember that it does have importance in their eyes. Ceremonies such as the ones I have attempted to describe are in danger of being instantly classified as magical procedures by those who come from another culture, and hence looked upon as naive.

When a Douala student fails to obtain a diploma and says "bad luck!" or when someone who is unemployed fails to find work and, again, cites ill fortune, it is not easy to determine the cultural context of these expressions of disappointment, nor is it easy to say just what they mean. In school it is taught that misfortune is often due to unfavorable circumstances. At home, however, misfortune springs from a complex network of intentions and interventions beyond the control of any one individual. From God down to an employer or the person grading an examination, a great number of persons are involved in determining failure or success! Thus there are two cultural poles, and the Douala who says "It was bad luck" does not opt for one or the other, and cannot. The exclamation refers to both chance and sorcery. But if the misfortune persists, and fever, loss of appetite, and general deterioration of health set in, the family will interpret these symptoms in a special way. It will take the victim to a *nganga*, for this misfortune is a disease.

Elimbi's luck, his grace, was his father the *nganga*, who did not wait until things were as bad as all this. After his treatment, Elimbi began to look for a job, and he found one, in a bar. Later he found more stable employment in a cement works in Douala.

Chapter 7

The Trial

> Your sorcerer is pegged to your
> body.
> —Douala proverb

Din's wife had always been too proper to venture to come to my house to see me. But one day she knocked on my door in the Batignolles. I had a feeling something had happened. I was not mistaken. Two days before, the police had taken Din away. They had also taken the drum used in the evening séances, the precious elephant talisman that had been the gift of the Pygmies, the stones, the cloths, the barks, even some of the clasps—everything they could find that might help prove beyond the shadow of a doubt what Din's activities were.

It had been his landlord, Ekwala, whom he had helped in so many ways who had accused him of practicing sorcery. Nor had Ekwala been satisfied with merely reporting him, but had brought to the police station a number of compromising items he claimed to have found in Din's courtyard, things he said Din had buried there.

Din's wife related these things in a detached tone, as if she were reporting some neutral event she had seen in the neighborhood. I was deeply touched by this colorless voice of hers. It was a voice that sounded as if it were being played on a record, the record of resignation.

What was to be done? I had had to be content with merely lamenting the lot of the old village *nganga* who, they said, had become a sorcerer, because there was nothing I could have done to defend him. But with Din, I felt like going into action. I could not simply sit back and watch. My relationship with him was more personal than with Loe. Rarely had a week passed without my paying him a visit. I had attended numerous séances of his. Little by little, the interest I had in his medicine, and the ready will with which he had explained all things to me, had changed our relationship. He had begun to come to visit me. We would talk about whatever

84

entered our heads, as I had made a great deal of progress with my Douala.

I had asked Din for knowledge—and had gradually come to perceive that he desired to communicate experience. Ever since I had understood that, I no longer had the feeling that he was making fun of me when he talked about initiating me into his art. What did that mean for me, in view of the immense cultural chasm between us? But that was precisely the key to the answer: what is generally understood by "cultural" was completely foreign to his concepts. If I desired to "know," in his eyes this could only mean I wanted to work something out existentially. And this is what he sought to "initiate" me into.

It is easy to understand, then, why my reaction to his arrest could not be neutral. I had a personal need to share in his rescue. But first I must give a more detailed account of Din, and of my relationship with him up to that time.

Din's Story

I became acquainted with Din and Ekwala, his denouncer, at the same moment, the first night I went to Din's house. At that time their two families lived together, and indeed I needed several visits before I could tell the families apart. I have already described the ties between them at the time when Engome was treated and the *nyungu* pursued. I had noticed no signs of deterioration in their relationship since. To be sure, I sometimes heard voices raised in the kitchen or the back rooms, but these disputes were no longer or more violent than those of my neighbors in the quarter.

Din and Ekwala themselves were the stabilizing elements. I had never seen them quarrel. It is true that Din had recently moved, with his whole family, from Ekwala's house, and taken up residence in a little house he had just built. But what could be more natural? And now Ekwala was accusing his old guest of sorcery. There must have been hidden reasons.

One day, in a particularly confidential tone, Din had told me the story of how he had become a *nganga*, and what had made him leave his village and his fishing nets for the cruel city. He had told me this story in a prosaic style quite different from the epic and marvelous accounts ordinarily given by *nganga*s to emphasize the exceptional side of their calling. It is true that Din had told me enough amazing things not to have to convince me any further verbally of the importance of his task. Further, a number of persons in his village had also vouched for the accuracy of his words.

Din was the native of a small island called Malimba, situated at the mouth of Cameroon's largest river, the Sanaga, more than a hundred kilometers from Douala "as the crow flies." (And a trip by pirogue through the inextricable tangle of mangroves was not along the route the crow flies!) The riverbanks belong to those who came there merely two centuries ago. The rain forest has been the Pygmies' homeland for thousands of years. Relationships between the two groups are tense, and contacts rare. The story of Din's adoption by the Pygmies, then, is an unusual one.

"I was a student in the Catholic mission school at Marienberg," Din began, naming a town some fifteen kilometers, by river, from the island of Malimba". My father and mother had sent me there. One Saturday, a friend and I had gone to cut wood in the forest, but we were unfamiliar with this forest and became lost. It was about six o'clock in the evening when the Pygmies saw us. They captured us and took us home. We didn't sleep that night—we cried a great deal. They spoke our language a little, and so we were able to make friends with their children. It was they who taught us the Pygmy language.

"In this village there was an old woman, so old she was blind. When the sun shone we would take her out for a walk, and we would scratch her back. So she taught us *mianga* [healing], just the way you'd learn something in school. You could teach me French in the same way, and little by little I would finally understand.

"I grew up out there. I married and had a son, whom I still support. My wife's father continued to show me the work of *mianga* until I knew it. It was he who gave me my elephant talisman. He taught me how to perform all sorts of treatments, and if I took care of you, you'd feel fine. I'm not lying to you. I'm not like Ekwala and the chief [of the quarter]. They told me not to teach you everything. I tell you this because you're my friend and I'm your friend.

"One day I saw one of my brothers, Isaac. I was with Ntonga and Menu Manga that day. (They're Pygmies.) Isaac answered me and came up close in his pirogue. He was amazed. He had thought I was dead! He was going to sell fish in the city. I told him to bring salt, tobacco, and cloth—the Pygmies love that. And I went back to the island of Malimba, where I gathered everyone together. I performed a great treatment, the *salaka* [thanksgiving and food-offering to the water spirits and the ancestors].

"Before, I wanted to go to school. I had no idea at all of doing *mianga*. All that happened because we became lost in the wild. It was the start of many adventures and unexpected happenings.

"I went to Douala because of a war going on in Malimba. I had gone fishing. The sorcerers (*bewusu*) came to fight me over some money. When they came up, we fought a long time, and I knocked them over, but they burned the motor of my pirogue. It was bad luck (*mbeu'a nyolo*). I could say it was 'the death of me.' "

Din's blackened motor was still to be seen in his *dibandi*, lying in pieces in a vegetable sack. The police had not been interested in it.

Din had first met Ekwala at the home of a patient, during one of his quick trips to Douala. After the fight he had lost, he had gone to Ekwala's house and asked hospitality. Ekwala had welcomed him with some surprise, for the rumor was that he had died in battle. So Din moved in with his latest wife, his 17-year-old son Barthélémy ("Bata," the child of a wife who had stayed be-hind in the village), his assistant, and his patients. His Pygmy relatives seem to have been a novelty in Douala. The man who had moved in with Ekwala was already renowned as a grand warrior figure in the spirit world.

Ekwala had always given me the impression of being a peaceful and respectable person, if somewhat ingenuous. He had certain responsibilities in his church and directed a little choir of mixed voices that sang grave, gentle Protestant hymns from German colonial times. He had married but one wife and was the respected father of seven living children. "I've got the blood for children," he often said proudly.

I was surprised that a person of consequence such as Ekwala should have so readily taken in a warrior of Din's mold. But he profited from it. His eldest daughter had been unable to bear children, and Ekwala handed her over to Din for treatment for sterility. The treatment was efficacious, and Ekwala had to admit this, at the height of their quarrel. He asked Din to treat his second daughter, Ewudu, as well, but here all efforts failed—and this was the reason for the breach between Ekwala and Din, as well as for the incidents that were to follow.

All the while that Din lodged with him, Ekwala displayed a boundless admiration for his guest, so much so that I began to feel uneasy. I shall not relate here all the exploits that Ekwala attributed to Din. Din was supposed to have rescued a cousin of Ekwala who had gone mad, in France. In order to achieve this result, Ekwala affirmed, Din had cast a "sleep" upon himself one Saturday evening, and had fallen into that quasi-cataleptic state that comes over a *nganga* and betokens his or her absence. The *nganga* is far away now, waging marvelous battles. A letter, Ekwala declared, confirmed that the moment of his cousin's restoration to health coincided with that of the *nganga*'s intervention.

Ekwala also told me the story of a woman who had been taken to the *nganga* on the point of death, with her legs paralyzed. Din had left the house at once, to find herbs in the thicket, and an hour later the woman was out of danger. And he concluded, "He has the knowledge of the tree of good and evil, the tree of the Book of Genesis."

Meanwhile, however, Din had not made life easy for him. When Din was drunk, he became demanding and subjected those around him to all sorts of caprices. I myself had seen him waken Ekwala at two o'clock in the morning, during a treatment, for really no reason at all. Din had seemed to me to exercise a sort of fascination over Ekwala; I think Din realized this, and encouraged it. One day, when both of them had come to pay me a visit, Din had taken me aside and told me not to speak to Ekwala about what he was teaching me. But this was the attitude that would eventually redound to his disadvantage. Ekwala's veneration gradually turned to dislike.

My Apprenticeship with Din

The evolution of my relationship with Din took place gradually, gropingly. The suddenness with which he had declared himself ready to show me

how he healed, once he had seen my serious interest in his work, had surprised me and made me a bit cautious. What lay behind his ready offer? A
need for money? A desire to impress his clients with a European priest in his
entourage? I could not tell.

At first Din showed he did not entirely trust me. He would have someone
tell me he was not at home, when I knew perfectly well that he was. In my
lodgings, as I have mentioned, he once discreetly slipped a little object in his
glass, as an "armoring," and just as discreetly recovered it once the glass
was empty—not a remarkable demonstration of confidence in me.

I returned his diffidence in kind. In fact, one fine morning my uneasiness
turned into real anxiety. On rising, I immediately felt dizzy. Everything was
spinning in my room in Batignolles, so much so that I was unable to cross
the street to go to church to say Mass. A preposterous thought crossed my
mind . . . could Din have managed to get me to swallow something—
frankly, some poison? I would soon know! It was a transitory fear, and I
spoke of it to no one. As it turned out, I was having trouble with a cervical
vertebra.

In the meantime, Din made me an associate in his work, sometimes asking me to help massage his patients and never refusing to answer my requests for an explanation. "I want you to understand. During the treatment
you must observe, every moment. You saw that this leg wouldn't walk.
Now you see it's started walking!"

One day I brought him a bottle of whiskey. It was the wrong moment.
"You brought that bottle? Why? If that's the way you want to see with me,
I have nothing to tell you. Just look, that's all. But there's nothing to discover that way. If you really want to *see*, then we have to understand each
other."

Once he was settled in his new dwelling, Din undertook to familiarize me
even more with his universe. I was teaching some courses at the Libermann
School, and it was here that he managed to find me one day and extend to
me an official invitation to visit him the following evening. He proposed to
hold a ceremony of protection on my behalf. I was surprised that he had
come all the way over to the college, with its atmosphere so different from
his own, its discipline, its areas for "faculty only," its office hours, with
French as its language, a language that Din did not know. I took this remarkable gesture very seriously. "When I got here," Din said, "I found
other whites. But I asked only for you. It was a white who told the person at
the door that I wanted you. He told me which way I wasn't allowed to go.
Even in the school, you eat one another. In every place there's evil."

I went to Din's house as invited, at six o'clock in the evening, the special
time for individual rites—the beginning of the night and its anxieties. His
new plank dwelling had been built with an eye to economy and was no different in outward style from any of the other houses in this workers' quarter. But it had the advantage of an interior design suited to the practice of
traditional medicine. In the middle of the house was a room with neither

window nor door to the outside, and this was Din's new *dibandi*. I did not
see the impressive paraphernalia that Loe had gradually set up in his house.
Here, the objects and work instruments had been placed right on the floor,
or in pots covered with pieces of red cloth. You don't set up a *dibandi* in a
matter of a few weeks.

We were alone. He had me sit facing him on a chair. This was the only
piece of furniture in the room except for three little benches and a curious
kind of clock hanging from the partition. The clock was not running. I saw
that, once more, Din was slow to begin the ceremony. Din could remain
perfectly motionless a good quarter of an hour, seated on his camp stool,
waiting for some sort of sign, following an unknown route to the beginning
of his ritual. I liked these perfectly quiet moments, which gave me the opportunity of bringing my rhythm in phase with his—and sometimes of making him smile.

I would watch his eyes. Even in repose they kept their gleam of anxiety,
which was accentuated by their color, a tawny brown, with the whites all
bloodshot from alcohol. But the smile would not begin there—it would
begin in the right crease of his mouth, then move up along a wrinkle in his
nganga "mask," before anything else in his face would show any expression. Suddenly something seemed to weigh on his thick lower lip—which
was always inclined to droop—and now perhaps a laugh would burst forth.
No, Din was trying to smile at me, but not yet. Then he finally managed to
do so, and with finesse, by a feat of control over the lower muscles of his
face. I restrained myself from applauding the success of this smile. It was
the outcome of a *nganga*'s victorious battle with a physiognomy marked by
a life of tragedy.

Finally he called for his massive, black cooking stone, with which I had
often seen him strip, trim, and crush herbs and barks to prepare his famous
remedies, his *mianga*. It looked like a stone from the seashore, rounded and
polished by the patient washing of the waves. He had covered it with the red
fabric of medicine and battle. Several of the proofs of his power lay at his
side—the clasps and the elephant talisman. He instructed me to remove my
shoes and place my feet back under my chair. He sat facing me in the same
position.

The stone was one of great power. "This stone is the water spirits' stone,
the ancestors' stone, and also the stone that crushes bark," Din told me
later, after the completion of the rite. "It bears three powers within its mass
(*Le mambo malalo bodila bwao*). It is made for driving sorcerers away, for
keeping a sorcerer from eating you. We can take the example of a drink that
has had poison poured into it. Even if I am drunk, the glass will break.
Why? Because of this stone's blood. (*Onyola na maya ma di dale*)."

"It crushes medicines (*mianga*), good ones and evil ones. If there are
medicines (*mianga*) that you don't eat, but that you use for incisions, it's
still this stone that crushes them. The force of this stone joins together the
ancestors, the water spirits, the barks, and the herbs. There, that's its

power. This stone is what you must depend on for its power to penetrate your body (*nginya nyingeye oa o nyolo*)."[32]

To begin the ceremony, Din prepared two little mouthfuls of a mixture of yellow buds of *ndonga balemba*, "*nganga*'s spice," *ngando*, a black powder composed of several powerful barks. He sprinkled the mixture with a perfume and wrapped each portion in a piece of thick *dibokuboku la wonja* leaf. Then he summoned his grown daughter and asked her to place one of these little balls in each of our mouths, his and mine. I swallowed mine. A moment passed. "If I die from this food, you die too," Din warned. Then he made up a second pair, in the same way, but this time it was too strong for me to swallow and burned my mouth.

"Why did you call your daughter?" I asked.

"She gave you to eat as she gave me to eat as well. It has to be a virgin, or a boy who has not known evil (*nu si bi bobe*). If she knew evil, she wouldn't have served you. I had you swallow those mouthfuls (*matam*) and now inform you that you are as my brother. If anyone seeks to harm you, you won't get hurt. If someone gives you poison, it won't do anything to you. If somebody tries to hurt you in *ndimsi*, nothing will happen to you. You shall escape death by water, and death by car accident, if it comes from the will of a human, but not if it comes from God."

I offered Din a drink, which he accepted, and I left a token offering. Then I got up to go, but Din told me to wait a little, for the food to penetrate me better.

Life and death, evil and virginity—these essential values were all in this ceremony. Din and his family were sincere when they bestowed upon me, before I left the house, gestures of care and protection that evidently had great meaning for them. As for myself, I was esthetically touched by the grandeur of the words, and by a certain beauty the objects held in their extreme simplicity, even if they were a little soiled. I was touched by the budding friendship this ceremony betokened, and my respect and admiration had grown a great deal. But I have to admit that the ceremony itself had no real meaning for me personally. I had made sure I did what I was told, and followed the rites correctly, but I had remained perfectly neutral. Was it because I was on the defensive and therefore it was impossible for me to enter this world that was opening up to me?

Din ordered me to return before the end of the ninth day following the ceremony. "On that day, we shall buy a chicken," he said. "The *dindo* [the same ritual meal as we had shared at the termination of Engome's treatment] will be for only you and for me. On that day we shall eat the *dindo* together, to make you understand that we love your blood, for you have peaceful blood (*maya ma musango*). You are as a brother. If I have something good, my brother gets some too, and eats it. I don't want to make you pay. It's you yourself who will make a gesture (*eyembilan*), and I'll be satisfied. Beginning today I am going to purify my heart, to prepare myself to treat you. Here it is two years that we have known each other, but I haven't had you eat here yet. So you shall know that *ngangas* (*bato ba mianga*) are something real.''

Ordinarily the *nganga* does not share the ritual meal of those undergoing treatment. But Din had reminded me several times in the course of the intimate little ceremony of that evening that he would be taking part in the meal. ''This *dindo* will be to keep us from having bad luck (*mbeu'a nyolo*). I shall eat it myself—it's for you as well as for me.''

The *ngando* powder was definitely very important. When the evening of the *dindo* came, we took some more, mixed with whiskey, the drink of solemn libations. This time it was a great-aunt whose task it was to prepare the meal, composed of a chicken, rice, and various herbs. She poured the rest of the *ngando* in the dish as well, and the immediate family came to partake of it after us. The great-aunt's action was accompanied by her explanation:

''With Esomawuta [one of Din's titles: 'The One Who Reveals What Is Hidden'], we moved out of Ekwala's over there and moved in here. If anyone wishes Esomawuta ill, may it return against him. He wishes evil on no one. But if someone wishes evil on him, may it return against him. The same thing for all his patients. When they are on a journey, if they are looked upon with meanness, may that return against the wishers. The patients and that man have to get well. May he have money, and may he dwell in peace.''

''Why is it your aunt, and not your daughter, who has served the meal this time?'' I asked Din.

''Because there was no prohibition (*ye titi mbenda*). Whereas what both of us ate the other time, that had to be served by a virgin. It's a law. Learn that.''

There is a close relationship between sexual abstinence and the sacred. I found this confirmed in the *nganga* lifestyle. Polygamists though they were, Din and Loe abstained from sexual relations during the period of a major treatment. They would offer no justification other than ''the law,'' and the risk of failure if they violated the law. When I pursued the matter further, however, they gave the prohibition a more positive meaning: their strength was supposed to be directed entirely toward the success of the treatment.

It often happened that a *nganga*, or someone in a *nganga*'s entourage, would ask me in their own turn why I did not marry. I used their own argument, saying that I had consecrated myself to God for life. I was not satisfied myself with this rather terse explanation, correct though it be as far as it goes, but for the moment I could think of no other to give that they could grasp. In any case it seemed to satisfy them, for they stopped asking me about it.

After the *dindo* was over, just when we were licking our fingers—and our lips too, as far as our tongues could reach, lest a single particle of this salutary, sacred food be lost—Din received a visit that had to do with the events that were to provoke his arrest. The wife of Din's old landlord and future accuser Ekwala, together with one of their daughters, Ewudu, seventeen years old, entered the room. I understood none of the conversation, so rapidly did they speak. But when I returned to my lodgings I wrote in my notebook:

Mrs. Ekwala and her daughter came in, suddenly and unexpectedly. Ewudu, all dressed in white, obviously beside herself. Ewudu returning a white pebble, which she handed Din. She sat down next to him, and they said something to each other.

Din took back his little white stone, and mother and daughter disappeared into the night. As I knew nothing of any recent disputes between Din and Ekwala, I was interested only in the stone. It was round, like a large marble. I had already seen it, in Din's *dibandi*. "This stone is God's bullet [*ngad'a Loba*, a meteorite]," Din told me. "If it's thrown at you, it destroys your house or kills you. So we have something to counter it. If it's thrown where this 'counter-object' is, it falls somewhere else. It's my foster parents, the Pygmies, who give out these stones. When God's bullet falls somewhere, they dig until they find it. God's bullet makes a sound like thunder. I keep this stone. It can't disappear or explode. It's a way of 'armoring' (*londa*) yourself."

I had no idea of the reason why Din had wished to protect or arm Ewudu by lending her his stone. He gave me an explanation, and I had no wish to check on it. The young student, he said, was expecting a child, and some of her relatives wanted her to have an abortion. So she had come to Din for help. "That's the heart of the matter," he told me.

After these twilight rites, Din began to try to help me with a problem. I traveled too much, he told me, and had to guard against the dangers I would meet on the way. Just going from the Deïdo quarter to the Libermann School was a journey, to his way of thinking. What was to be said, then, of my trips to the bush and the surrounding countryside that had won me the honors of suspicion and rumor? I had told him everything and, as a friend, he decided to arm me. The procedure consisted in making me see in dreams—that is, for him, in reality—what my social behavior really was all about and what risks I ran.

I may have been indifferent to Din's visible rites, but I was shaken by my dreams. In fact, as I look back today, I may have been affected by them even more than I thought. Din made up a little packet, with two pieces of bark and some dried herbs, all wrapped up in paper and bound with a string.[33] I was to place this packet under my pillow, three or four nights in a row, and pay attention to what would be given to me to see. I reported to Din my first dream, which I made sure to note down on paper when I awoke from it in the middle of the night:

I saw an assembly of *nganga's*, in pairs, probably masters and disciples. I didn't care for the dream very much, and I was glad to wake up from it.

Din's reaction was to tell me, "That's the way you start to see—bit by bit, right up to the moment of treatment—so that when you're up against a disease, you first see during the night how you have to treat it, and in the morning you set to work and you cure it. That's why I want you to see."

Now Din gave me another packet of *mianga*, with the same directions for use, and I saw this, in a twilight sleep:

> I was walking through a strange, but somehow familiar, village, with a group of friends, all Africans, all armed with sticks, but I couldn't see who any of them were. They were going ahead of me to meet another group, a threatening and noisy group. Had reassuring impression my friends were stronger.

Din commented: "No, this is not a stupid dream. I'm giving you this bark so you'll begin to see. If these are good persons you see, you're walking along with them. That's the way you start seeing in *ndimsi*. The moment will come when, in broad daylight, if somebody bad comes up to you, you'll know it. Whether it's a white or a black, you'll know it. I can't do this to anybody but you. No, my assistant doesn't see. I only show him the herbs, not directly *ndimsi*, because he's still a child. Later, when he knows *ndimsi*, he'll fight me."

This time, besides the obligatory bark, Din gave me a little piece of whale gristle (*njonji*). I carefully recorded the following dream at four o'clock in the morning:

> Ceremony, outdoors, alongside some dwellings. No treatment, but getting ready for something. With someone who knows and who keeps me close to him. Can't ask questions. But trust him. Seems as if this ceremony has already been tried and broken off. Lasts only short while. Rather many persons but only slightly interested in me. All Africans. Can't exactly recognize anybody.
>
> I'm like somebody who doesn't know, trying to understand and see the most I can. Reasons for ceremony unknown to me. Don't feel like laughing. Am like a novice. Lots of excitement, but don't know reason—something important seems to be going to start, but doesn't have anything to do with me. Can't make out gestures. Laughter at something I don't understand. A ceremony where something's starting. Would have continued if I hadn't awakened. Transfer of what I see with Din?

Din was pleased. These dreams presented their hero in good company, never isolated and alone. Dreams that reveal a spell isolate the victim, presenting him or her as confronting a group of aggressors—whose faces the victim does not see—all alone. Nor did the disturbing symbols appear here—there was no rope, no chain, and I was not dragged to the river.[34]

Din's arrest halted my apprenticeship in its early stages. I felt called to his side to defend him.

Din in Prison

I waited a few days to see whether anything else would eventuate, then I went to the police station. The precinct captain received me politely, and I declared to him that Din was no charlatan, and that I could prove that he healed in the traditional manner. The captain was unimpressed and informed me that Din could incur a heavy penalty under article 251 of the Penal Code, on the suppression of sorcery:

Two to ten years in prison and a fine of 5,000 to 100,000 francs: anyone given to practices of sorcery, magic, or divination tending to disturb public order and tranquility or cause harm to the person, goods, or fortune of another by way of retribution [Chapter 2, Disturbing the Peace, Penal Code of 1967].

For the precinct captain the case was clear. Din was accused of having cast a spell on Ewudu, Ekwala's daughter, on the pretext of enabling her to obtain her diploma. He was said to have given her a magic ballpoint pen, for a large sum, and was alleged to have attempted to molest her. I remembered the scene with the little pebble. Seeing that Ewudu had failed to obtain her diploma, we were dealing with a matter of sorcery compounded by fraud. To boot, Din had no license to practice the trade of a *nganga*. The case was clear. Din claimed he battled the sorcerers and "armored" persons against them; therefore he must himself be an expert in sorcery. But to do battle, I retorted to the captain, one must know one's arms and one's adversaries. But his mind was made up. Besides, Din had confessed to everything.

I asked to be allowed to speak with Din for a moment. A few minutes later there he was, coming toward me by way of the prisoners' door. His habitual grin was gone. I read panic in his eyes. He was ill-shaven (but when was he ever clean-shaven?), he wore a ragged jacket over his bare skin, and a baggy pair of pants that were much too large for him. By the way he came up—hunched over, staggering—I could see he must have been beaten. I could have sworn on the spot that he had been victimized by a calumnious accusation of sorcery, like the old *nganga* in the village. I could not help being reminded of the suffering of another man, unjustly accused, and beaten in a guardroom, two thousand years before. The similarity intensified my emotion, and I could not speak a single word to him.

In a weak, soft voice, by fits and starts, Din told me the essentials. All the stories being told about him were false, he told me. He had confessed, after severe abuse. He admitted only ownership of the clasps. But he had had the utmost difficulty in making himself understood by the precinct captain, who spoke no Douala. And the interpreter was none other than Ekwala! I remonstrated with the captain, who promised to find another interpreter. I recalled Din's prophetic words on the subject of *ndimsi*: "*ndimsi*," he had said, "is just like what you see in broad daylight: at the police station, there are prisoners tied up, and others beaten. It's the same in *ndimsi*."

In consternation, I went to demand an accounting of Ekwala. He began with a speech on his old friend's ingratitude for having been lodged and fed four and a half years without charge—in fact, with Ekwala giving him money—and then, without a word, going and building his own house three hundred yards away! This was a man of evil life, I now heard, who abused some of his female patients! Ekwala had asked Din to help his daughter Ewudu with her exams. His intervention had been successful in the early years of her secondary education, but disappointing thereafter, when it came time to receive her diploma—two failures in two years. This was too much. Din must have switched allegiance, Ekwala went on, and must be systematically seeking to use Ewudu to harm his whole family. Ah, now we were at the heart of the matter. It had to do with intangibles—charges you couldn't substantiate in a courtroom or police station.

"Din moved out of my house," Ekwala went on. "Din is ruining my daughter's health and future. Din has been bought, by a clan of my father's family, which is in league against me."

Now everything started to make sense. I asked, "Look, why would Din want to hurt you?"

"For money," Ekwala replied. Members of Ekwala's family were seeking to prevent him from acquiring greater prestige in the quarter and had struck a bargain with Din to reduce him to naught. Later, the chief of the quarter was to tell me that there was a great deal of tension between Ekwala and his father's family on a matter of the ownership of some property. The real grievance he had against Din, then, went beyond his daughter and her affairs. Ekwala was accusing Din of trying to exterminate his whole family, and he repeated this to me in a frenzy. But later, in the police station and in court, he never mentioned this "conspiracy."

I reminded Ekwala of his former friendship, and even admiration, for Din. Was not his eldest daughter the mother of a family thanks to Din?

"Don't meddle in our personal affairs!" I was told. However, Ekwala recognized my right to help Din. He raised no objection when I told him of my intention of testifying to the public prosecutor in favor of the authenticity of his medical practice.

The Story Told by Ernest

Ekwala told me how a young diviner he called Ernest had enabled him to find pieces of "evidence" in his garden and how he, Ekwala, had taken these to the police station. This relatively secondary element was what Ekwala counted on as his principal evidence in obtaining Din's conviction. As it turned out, however, it would betray the quantum difference between a *nganga* (Din) and a petty magician (Ernest).

I had the opportunity to meet Ernest practically at *le Grand Fromager* itself, at the house of the chief of the quarter, who had encouraged him to tell me the whole story and let me record it—how he had met Ewudu, and how his gift of divination had enabled him to find the exhibits buried in Ekwala's garden. The boy gave me a lively account, for a price, in a most matter-of-fact way. He recounted the circumstances of the arrest as well. As he spoke with me, the dice of *ludo* players were clicking endlessly under the window.

"How did you learn about all this?" I began.

"Well," Ernest replied, in French, "I live in the firehouse—right in the barracks, first building. I'm there with a friend of mine who works at city hall. So this girl called Ewudu came over. She comes there to play handball. She ran into me and asked me to buy her some aspirins when I went to get some of my own medicine."

"Are you sick?" I asked her.

"I'm often sick, and I see somebody, but I don't know if this 'somebody' is giving me the right treatment. . . . So I told her, 'Sure, if you want, I can do that for you.' "

Ernest, as it happens, is a native of the island of Malimba, where Din, too, had been born. I had to listen to a long account of the sources of his knowledge: he had learned about the water spirits in Nigeria, the Koran in the Sahara, and had visited nearly every city and town in Cameroon, or so he said. The personal histories of these latter-day magicians have to include stories of long, long journeys, as far away as Egypt or India—the modern counterpart of the miracle accounts in the old mythical narratives.

"I picked up a little book I had in Arabic," Ernest went on. "I read in it, and then I said, 'Yes, my girl, you are ill. There was a magician who stopped to see you—am I not telling the truth?'

'No!' she said.

'Well, then, he lived in your house—right?'

'Yes!' she said.

'Well, this magician has been filling your head with too many things. Your head is disturbed. First you failed your diploma. Then this man killed you [made you fail again].'

"Din gave her a ballpoint pen to take her exams with, and she doesn't know how she lost it. It disappeared in the classroom. She just put it down, said something to somebody, and suddenly it was gone. Din took it back!

"Then she took me to see her papa and mama. I told them, 'I can do something about what's going on here.' They accepted the offer. I said, 'I don't take any money for myself. Just get 3,000 francs in slugs and tokens [small change] and give me a bottle of whiskey.' And I went and tossed it all in the water, for the fairies [the *miengu*, the water spirits]. When I came back, I said, 'There. Now I'm going to take things out of your head.' I can do that really well. First I pulled out some scrolls, then a snake."

"This must have been at Ekwala's. Was it daytime or nighttime?" I asked Ernest.

"Daytime."

"In front of everybody?"

"In front of everbody. I took a silk kerchief and tied it around this girl's head. Then I just read that book for a moment. Everybody was sitting down. Then I said, 'Cough a bit. Lift your arms up in the air. Good. Untie the kerchief now. Touch the book again.' And out fell the snake."

"Was it alive? Was the snake alive?"

"Yes."

"What kind was it?"

"It was a green snake like they have around here—called *jembu* in Douala. Everbody ran like the blazes. I told them, 'Wait! Don't be afraid!' I caught the snake, and then I killed it. I told this girl, 'Turn your head a little.' She didn't feel anything now [she was in a trance]. Usually in class she'd take a book, look at it, and her head would get heavy and fall on the book. 'Move your head. Try to run.' She ran. 'Do you feel all right?' She said she did. 'Wait, it's not over, there are still a few little things to do.' There were still this glass, some pins, and a mirror. 'There is still a lot of work to do in your house,' I said. 'There are also some things buried here, some closed clasps, all kinds of things.' "

"What did you find buried in the garden?"

"Under the mango I found a chain, with some clasps. It was raining. I was pulling on the chain, but the chain was pulling me down. The ground was slippery. Something down there kept pulling me. There was a rope tied to the chain, with a human bone and a bottle tied to it, and in the bottle there were pieces of paper with the name of the girl and the names of all the members of Ekwala's family. Din's name was on the back of the paper. Finally I pulled everything up, and Ekwala went to file a complaint with the police."

Then Ernest told me what he had seen at the police station, where he went with Ekwala: "The captain asked Din, 'Do you recognize all these things?' Din said, 'No!' And the captain said, 'Fine, spank him a bit.' And they put Din on his belly and a policeman hit him with a club."

"On the head?"

"On his butt. Finally Din said, 'Yes, I recognize all those things.' They said, 'And the chain too?' Din said, 'I don't recognize the chain. I'd rather be killed.' So they told him, 'Better think it over then. You're going to get hit.' So Din went out, then he came back. 'Yes, I recognize the chain,' he said. 'I gave it to an apprentice to bury somewhere, but I don't remember where.' They said, 'Tell us where you buried the chain.' He said, 'Under the mango.' Then the captain told him, 'You put yourself to a lot of trouble. You should have told us the truth the first time.'

"Then Din said to the captain, 'I know that guy [Ernest]. He's a magician. He can make silk handkerchiefs appear. He can make anything disappear.' And the captain answered, 'That's a skill. That's not against the law. But you, you kill. Who are your associates?' "

"What associates?" I asked Ernest.

"His associates—well, that means his pals in black sorcery. Then the captain asked, 'Din, do you know sorcery?' and Din said, 'No, I know how to treat for healing.' Then the captain said, 'What? You know how to treat sorcery victims, and you don't know sorcery?' And Din said, 'I know sorcery, but I don't know how to kill.' Then the captain said, 'And that girl, what did you want to do to her, good or evil?' And Din said he wanted to do her good. 'Tell the truth. All right, get the club, he's going to tell the truth.' Then the captain told him, 'Fine, that's it, now get your things, you're going to jail.' "

It was a disconcerting story, and told with complete ease and confidence. Did Ernest think I was easy to fool? Or had he been fooled himself? Was he practicing his speech for the trial? If I accepted his story, would this not encourage him to expect the judge to be convinced as well?

No, he seemed to me to be one of the innumerable unemployed persons in Douala who had found—because he could find nothing else—a social rationale in petty divination, and was clinging to it desperately. Was he taken seriously? From my experience with rumor, I was inclined to think it more likely he was being used. Credulity and malice go together somehow.

I informed Ernest, as well as the chief of the quarter, who had been sitting right there, impassively listening to all this, that I would testify on Din's behalf, because I saw no resemblance between him and the picture Ernest painted of him.

"Your Sorcerer Is Your Bodyguard"

As he waited for his trial to take place, Din managed to get out of jail and go home, four days after I had interceded for him. I do not know whether my intervention had been the determining factor. He was released in order to let him go to the hospital, for his sojourn at the police station and in jail had been very hard on him.

Din came to Batignolles and explained some things to me in such a way that I was reassured somewhat. I had begun to wonder whether some of the accusations lodged against him might contain a basis in fact, even setting aside the naivety of poor old Ekwala and the humbug of Ernest. Delicate points were in the balance here, and Din gave me his version.

"At the police station," Din began, "Ekwala said, 'Those are the clasps that are killing me—me and my whole family.' The captain believed this was the truth, and they began to lash me. I was lashed maybe a dozen times, till I vomited blood. They asked me to tell them that I recognized the other *mianga*. I said no, and they kept beating me. It was horrible. When it started to hurt too much, I admitted anything they wanted, and they started writing down anything they wanted. But I admitted only that the clasps were mine: white persons' clasps *(dal 'a mukala),* there's nothing wrong with them. It's just proof the work got done *(le nde mbong ebolo).* You know, during an important treatment, if somebody wants to get well, he has to bring a goat. You put the goat's head in the ground, everybody sees that. If it's not a serious sickness, you just have to bring a set of clasps, and that gets put in the *dibandi.*"

"Did you help Ekwala's daughter with her exams?" I asked.

"No! His daughter had dizzy spells, and she couldn't see very well. She couldn't read very well. That's what I treated her for. Her hand shook every time she held the ballpoint [*esao,* "pen"]. So I was working just so her hand would quit shaking, that's all. It wasn't to give her an exam."

"What about the ballpoint?"

"I only made her this pen so she'd have the strength to keep her hand from shaking.[35] Pretty soon her hand didn't shake any more. Her eyes didn't turn any more [no more dizziness]. So I finished my work; I don't know what else they want!"

"You told me Ekwala didn't get along with his family," I prodded.

"I know what's going on with him because I stayed there four and a half years. I found out they don't like him because he says bad things. He says I've plotted with his cousins to 'kill' his daughter. It's amazing. . . . I stayed there four and a half years and never saw his cousins. I didn't want to have to be afraid they'd accuse me of conspiracy—you know, Ekwala doesn't get along with them. He wanted me to build my house just behind him and nowhere else. But I'm an important person. I've got wives and children. Better I should build somewhere else; usually children and wives [of different families] always have trouble when they live next door to each other. I built where I am now, and Ekwala thought I had some sort of understanding with his cousins."

To Ekwala's view, Din was only an intermediary—though a dangerous one, to be sure, because of his powers. Ekwala's principal adversary had to be a member of his own family. There is no sorcery without the complicity, if not the initiative, of at least one relative. That cousin Din mysteriously saw on the road, when he had had his motorbike accident, has for years been the prime suspect in Ekwala's eyes. Now he even told me how he has discovered it was he.

Once when the family was celebrating a holiday, one of Ekwala's relatives had pointed to another family member, to all appearances someone quite friendly, and had told Ekwala that he was his worst enemy. I asked Ekwala what their exact relationship was. He said he was his eldest cousin on his father's side. Ekwala's uncle, someone Ekwala had disliked, had died, and his son, this young cousin, had fallen heir to Ekwala's animosity toward the father.

Sorcery finds its preferred terrain in the form of certain family relationships—the ones most likely to involve tension. One of these is that between a paternal uncle and his eldest nephew, following the laws of inheritance. (In the case of Elimbi, readers will recall, suspicion spontaneously fell on the lad's paternal uncle, Loe's elder brother.) Everything conspires to instigate conflict between the two. They have the same title to a deceased father's wealth and lands. There is more than average likelihood they will have the same name. When an uncle dies, his rights—and his enemies—pass to his son. Now the battle is between cousins. As the chief of the quarter put it, competition begets jealousy, jealousy begets sorcery, and one's children become the vehicles.

Any adverse circumstance in which members of his family might find themselves confirmed Ekwala in the notion that this cousin on his father's side had undertaken to wipe out his whole family, through Din as intermediary. I suggested to the chief that *he* would be the most likely mediator between the two antagonists.

No, the chief told me, Ekwala had found the chain, along with all the things it had been "tied" to. The chief had seen the little pieces of paper, too, although he had made no attempt to read what was written on them. An official complaint had been lodged, and now it was a matter for the civil authorities.

Ekwala, however, told me that the chief had simply not wished to intervene. Whom to believe? But then, after all, how could this minor chief, stripped of his authority in his own quarter, caught up in perpetual squabbles over property, and in conflict with the high chief, have settled this dispute? This particular chief was someone who had become orientated to modern life, which cut him off from the sages and other notables who would have been his mainstay in such a situation. And yet he was himself an expert in the occult sciences (and to boot, a Rosicrucian, of several years' standing). But these practices were of no help to him. The world of sorcery weighed on him, and he was not the one to rise to the challenge.

The intervention of a respected chief can be efficacious. I had seen such a chief in action and seen him succeed: Caïn Dibunje Tukuru, the man of the roadblock. It had been a matter of reconciling a family divided by sorcery: two sisters and a brother had just lost their elder brother, and the sisters were accusing the surviving brother of being the agent of the other's death. The chief had decided to use the rite called *male,* "alliance." I had a car available, and Caïn Dibunje Tukuru asked me to drive him to the ceremony. He arrived unannounced, so that no one could slip away under one pretext or another. It was he who must resolve this, he told me, for "it is for men to command, not women."

The chief had already conducted his investigation. Before the assembled family, he declared to the two sisters that there was no evidence against their brother. The two women retorted that he had moved out and had obtained *mianga* to bury on his brother's property, thus causing his death. But the chief had ceased to address them.

Now he washed the face of each of the three in a liquor, which had been purchased in a store. Despite the sisters' hesitancy, he made all three drink from the same glass. Then he drew the remaining alcohol into his mouth, and blew it mightily into their faces, pronouncing the ritual words. Thus was alliance struck anew among brother, sisters, and two family heads. The procedure had been undertaken suddenly and spontaneously, but its effect had so far been lasting.

Alas, in Din's case the like would not be seen. Adequate traditional structures were not available here. He must go to trial.

In Court

Father Essombe, Deïdo's parish priest and a relative of Din, convinced of the defendant's innocence, had followed the affair with concern from the very start. He advised Din to engage an attorney. He could foresee that Din, a total stranger in the precincts of the Palace of Justice, that impressive monument with its high-ceilinged rooms and enormous central staircase, would be like a poor, wounded bird, incapable of defending himself against those whom the masses called the "Great Ones." Din complied, and the lawyer he hired called me in the day before the trial to ask me if I were prepared to testify as a character witness. My task would be to demonstrate, on the basis of the documents I had compiled, the genuineness and authenticity of Din the *nganga*.

It was December 1972. The police court sat on Tuesdays. Eighty-nine cases, no less, awaited adjudication on a single day—accidental injury, abandonment, fraud, bad checks, contraband alcohol, and so on. Three charges of sorcery, including the one against Din, were on the docket. A rapid glance at the schedules and decisions posted in the entrance hall convinced me that the case was not a rare one in the Douala police court.

I ascended the wide staircase leading to the courtroom and stood in the rear, with my back to the sculpted, varnished door, knowing that I would soon be called to the stand. It would still have been possible to find a place to sit on the crowded benches, given the infinite compressibility and limitless patience of the people, but to get up and get out once I was seated seemed to me unlikely. I had made the right choice: Din's trial was about to begin.

I could see Din from behind, on the defendants' bench, slightly hunched over, swimming in his best dark jacket (original color uncertain), the only spot of sadness in a great room strangely pervaded by a festive atmosphere. Ekwala, sitting in the same row, but on the other side of the center aisle, held his head high.

The Attorney General of the Republic and Din's lawyer, the two principals in the contest, were young, dynamic Cameroonian attorneys, attired, nevertheless, in the traditional black robe of a French court of law. By way of exordium, the attorney general declared that Din's case looked altogether clear to him—the dossiers were complete, and the whole matter should not take longer than a quarter of an hour. Actually, it would take an hour and a half.

On the presiding bench, perspiring beneath his ermine, the judge followed the brilliant opening joust between his juniors with amusement. The prosecution was mocking, the defense heartrending. The translator shouted himself hoarse, scampering from language to language, repeating all the attorney general's orders, half an octave higher, for the benefit of the witnesses or the crowd that was packed in the rear of the room. A certain popular atmosphere lent a humane air to the artifice and solemnity of the place.

The attorney for the defense was banking on his surprise witness. He asked that, in my capacity as an expert, I be admitted to testify to the professional conduct of his client. I was a teacher in the Libermann School, he told the court, and studied traditional medical practices. "What can this contribute?" objected the attorney general. But the judge found it useful to "have the information." I was motioned to approach the bench, along with Din's wife and the witnesses for the prosecution—Ekwala's wife and her right-hand man Ernest. Ewudu was detained in school.

We identified ourselves, and then were sequestered while the court heard the plaintiff and the defendant themselves. Thus I was not present for this part of the trial, but was later told by René Roi, a Jesuit teacher at the Libermann School, that the debate turned on the diploma and the ballpoint pen, each of the adversaries systematically denying whatever was asserted by the other. I had noted what Din's lawyer had said: "Ordinarily we analyze, we scrutinize such matters in all detail. But I am not interested in Ekwala. We have to approach the basic problem—not only on the juridical level, but on the social."

The judge had me summoned and I took the stand. I began by saying I had no testimony to give on the matter of contention between the two men, because they had not informed me of their dispute until official procedures were already under way. As I spoke, I realized how incompetent this tribunal was to treat the matter in its true scope: the familiar story of family hatred maintained and abetted by sorcery. Official language, it seemed to me, was not attuned to the convictions that gave this trial its real meaning to the spectators. Could I really tell the "whole truth and nothing but the truth"?

The judge opened with a seemingly harmless question, but one that could have been very dangerous for the defendant. "Professor, what do you know about the herbal treatments?" A direct answer would have involved me in the distinction between everyday herbal medicine and occultism, which of course would arouse suspicion. But I did not actually admit this distinction myself. So at the risk of being called to order, I replied that knowledge of herbs and barks was neither the only nor the best remedy at a genuine *nganga*'s disposal—and I proceeded to speak at length on the therapeutic value of the nocturnal séances, in which natural medicinal products—fine for daytime therapy—would have been out of place, but in the course of which patients rediscover the taste for life and health.

When it came the attorney general's turn, he asked me why I was particularly interested in Din. I seized the opportunity of making the distinction between a true *nganga* and a petty charlatan—the distinction on which the case would hang. I said I was interested in Din because he could pass the test to which the people of a city subjected their *nganga* before they would seek his services: Had he stayed in the same quarter for a long time? Was he recognized as a *nganga* by the people of his native village? And finally, did his cures last? Here the presiding judge interrupted to ask me whether I had assisted at any of Din's healing séances, and I guaranteed him, perhaps somewhat too confidently, that I had followed and studied several successful treatments of his.

"Thank you, Father," the judge concluded. He had just learned that I was a priest, and had suddenly grown more cordial. "Do you have any knowledge of the loan of the ballpoint pen? Have Din or Ekwala spoken to you about it?"

That question took me by surprise. I had already admitted that what I knew was by hearsay. But the question was logical: what real connection could there be, after all, between the practice of medicine and success in exams? I answered that a *nganga* observes the spirit of tradition in calming the anxiety of students whose principal concern is an examination. After all, these students ask us priests for our prayers!

The attorney general was not giving up. "Father," he pressed, "sorcerers promise a diploma. Then if the students who have paid them don't get their diplomas, isn't this fraud?"

Din's attorney rose to object: "Father has made a distinction between a sorcerer and a *nganga*. One is a person of evil, the other a person of good. I beg to observe that the court has not yet taken cognizance of this distinction."

I intervened to respond to the attorney general's question. It would scarcely be reasonable, I averred, to blame a *nganga* for being self-confident, when a client's trust in the *nganga* depends on the *nganga*'s own self-assurance, and the client's success largely depends in turn on his or her trust in the *nganga*.[36]

After my testimony the court heard the other witnesses, briefly, both those for the prosecution and those for the defense. Ernest became the star witness, once he had recounted a part of the story I have recorded above.

"There's your magician!" cried the attorney for the defense.

The attorney general and the judge objected.

"Are you a sorcerer?" asked the attorney general.

"I am a practitioner of herbal medicine," Ernest replied.

"You must know who buried the clasps."

"No."

"There you are," concluded the attorney general, as if to canonize the strategic logic of Ernest's response.

Din's wife spoke with great dignity: "My husband was arrested because he practiced his profession." Din and Ekwala continued to dispute the same key points: whether Din had given Ewudu the ballpoint pen or not, whether he had seduced her or not, whether he had demanded a large sum of money from her or not.

The attorney general interrupted to observe that, basically, this whole affair was owing to Ekwala's resentment over his daughter's alleged seduction. Both Ekwala and Din objected, even though Din had not understood the attorney general, because he was speaking in French. (He thought he understood, as when someone learning a foreign language tries to follow a conversation on the basis of the few words they manage to catch. I know this situation and its pitfalls very well myself.)

In his summation, the attorney general declared that Din was under a double accusation: that of fraud, and that of sorcery. As for the fraud, there was no proof. But there certainly was proof of sorcery, for what Din had done was called sorcery in the law, and we had assembled to apply the law. Even the defense had affirmed, and itself supplied the proof, that Din had been doing this for years, without authorization or license. The penal code provided a penalty of two years imprisonment and a maximum fine of 100,000 francs. Here the attorney general paused. Then he went on to list the attenuating circumstances cited by Din's defense—his ignorance of French, his poor adaptation to city life. To my great relief, he asked only for a suspended jail sentence of three months, and a fine of 25,000 francs.

Din's attorney now presented his summation, which I can report from memory:

What have we come to in our country when a person of the healing profession is thrown in jail without trial and beaten by the police? Here are the medical reports obtained by my client during his convalescence. [Documents were received in evidence.][37]

At the police station, who served as interpreter between the precinct captain and my client? The plaintiff himself! Here is the official report of those proceedings. [More documents were received in evidence.] This defendant is a sick man. He could collapse before your eyes any moment now. . . .

This man is no mountebank. The attorney general himself has shown us that. The mountebank, the charlatan, is Ernest. Now, before the law, sorcery and charlatanry are of a piece. I cite articles 251 and 318. Both articles use the same expressions for sorcery as for fraud: ". . . Anyone given to practices . . . tending to cause harm to . . . [the] fortunes of another. . . ." Where there is no fraud, there is no sorcery.[38] But where, Your Honor, is the law that deals with sorcerer and *nganga* together, without distinction? In our city we find European physicians who have practiced in Indochina, and who on the basis of their experience there find it useful to consult a *nganga*. Our jurisprudence should be reex-

amined in this area. I now offer in evidence the dossier compiled by
Father de Rosny on my client's practice of traditional medicine. [Documents were received in evidence.]

I ask acquittal pure and simple, without penalty or punishment.

The judge thanked the lawyers, deferred judgment to the end of December, and moved on to another matter. The audience in the courtroom had
been on Din's side. On my way out, someone remarked to me, "You won!"
Din would not return to prison. But the conflict between him and Ekwala
had in no way been resolved.

Who Is Din?

Din was acquitted. No charge had been sustained against him other than
the illegal practice of medicine. Inasmuch as the judge had not even alluded
to this charge in his declaration of acquittal, I took it upon myself to advise
Din to resume his practice as a *nganga*. But there would be no license. I had
to resign myself to the fact that it is practically impossible for a *nganga* to
obtain one.[39]

I visited the two adversaries in succession. Their positions remained unchanged. Ekwala refused reconciliation. He repeated a proverb to me until I
knew it by heart: *Nyam'a bwaba e labi te oa oen te ekonkong o ma nya nde
mila*—"let a snake bite you and you'll run from a worm." And Din swore
he would have crushed this person like a worm, had the matter not come
before a court. The heart of the matter had not come to light in the hearing.
As long as Ekwala felt the weight of a threat of a near relative against himself or his children, there would be no reconciliation.

The joy of seeing Din acquitted faded, and deep down inside I was dissatisfied. His attorney and I had managed to have justice done in Din's
regard, but there were dozens of cases like his, if the court schedules were
any indication, and the law, not being adapted to the situation, handled
them absurdly. The magistrates, seemingly so sure of themselves in their
black robes, were singularly hesitant in the internal forum of their conscience. I had been uncomfortable with the court proceeding, and very careful to avoid any clumsy words, which the attorney general would have
seized upon. Hence I had not made as forceful a statement as I could have
wished. And yet the case had certainly called for one.

To make up for this somehow, or to express myself better, I paid a
private visit to the judge who had acquitted Din. He received me in a little
office in the courthouse and let me express my point of view as much as I
wished, interrupting me only to make remarks or give examples in support
of my own arguments. Was this just the experienced professional ear? Or
mere prudence? I decided he really agreed with me.

"There is great confusion in the popular mind, Your Honor," I said.
"There are no sure criteria for distinguishing between a *nganga* and a

charlatan. The fact that magicians go around doing tricks is not a decisive argument. There are *nganga*s who make their rounds with the same skill as magicians.

"I might propose three criteria to you. I only alluded to them during the trial, Your Honor. I should have developed them and illustrated them. They have been suggested to me by persons who frequent these night séances— either accompanying patients, or simply the persons I happened to be sitting next to—who spoke openly with me while the ceremonies were going on, and without any provocation on my part.

"The first guarantee of a true *nganga* is *stability of residence.* A fortune-teller's abuses will not long go unnoticed in a neighborhood. The wooden houses are as frail as pasteboard boxes. Clients who have been duped will protest, everywhere. Everyone will talk. Mobs will gather. It will not end until the charlatan leaves town.

"The second test of a *nganga's* orthodoxy, and in my opinion the surest, is *acknowledgment by the nganga's* own native village. How do they speak of him or her? Do their own villagers call them a *nganga?* In this matter, you have first of all to be "a prophet in your own country." How did a *nganga* become one? Did a master *nganga* open their eyes after a long apprenticeship? Has a *nganga* in their ancestry appeared to this person in a dream and demanded that they take up the mantle of succession? Or has this person purchased from another *nganga* recipes for the use of medicinal herbs and barks?

"In a village, everyone will know who has taken any one of these three paths. In a city, it will be helpful to find out what is thought of a reputed *nganga* in the village of his or her origin. I have done this in the case of Din and Ernest. Both are from the island of Malimba. Din is a great figure of traditional medicine there. Ernest has never practiced among his own. Only the city has equalized them, so to speak.

"The third criterion, and the only important one for most of those concerned, is evident to the senses. *Does the* nganga *heal?* Of course, verification is not as easy as might appear. How do you measure a cure? Petty magic can effect a transitory alleviation—as Ewudu experienced, when she believed she had been freed of the serpent. My best informants tell me it's a matter of patience. You wait and see if the improvement lasts. A *nganga's* reputation rests on lasting cures."

"It is this third criterion," the judge remarked, "that determined my decision at the trial. But sincerely, Father, in your opinion, does Din effect complete cures?"

I replied in the affirmative. "Din, it seems to me, can pass the triple test. Ernest would fail. His prowess is unknown to the people of the island of Malimba. He moves about, here in Douala, and no cure of his has ever been of any duration."

To my own surprise, I found myself speaking as a lawyer. "And now, Your Honor, what next? Loe, Din, and other *nganga*s are going to be continuing with their work semiclandestinely, with no hope of a license, and thus at the mercy of arbitrary denunciations. Meanwhile, public officials, who belong to the world of those who judge them in the name of the law, will continue to go to them for assistance. Is this not an absurd situation?'' I was thinking of the day I had seen a long, black limousine discreetly parked along the hedge at the approaches to Din's house, the chauffeur sleeping at the wheel. Everyone knew that one of Douala's most important political figures had come to consult Din.

The judge, searching for an immediately applicable solution, suggested that a physician examine the effectiveness of the treatments, and, where appropriate, issue a certificate of successful treatment and discharge for particular clients of Din.

''I do not think this is something that can be done at this time,'' I responded. ''In the present situation, what physician—indeed what *nganga*—would submit to such a procedure? This formula might succeed in a given case, and this would be very well. But it would not suffice to overcome the prejudice. First, attitudes must change; then the spirit of the law; then the law itself! This is a long-term project, and it will depend on the people of Cameroon. The task for the present is a different one: drawing up documents to establish the legitimacy of traditional medicine, in a more systematic fashion than I have been able to do thus far.''

I left the judge's chambers. With my own impromptu speech still ringing in my ears, I was seized with a doubt. I had defended a friend in difficulty, and there was nothing wrong with that. Our relationship demanded my involvement. But was his cause really as just as I had said? Had I really gotten to the bottom of the matter of Din? Had Din perhaps taken advantage of Ewudu's youth? What about all the allusions to an abortion? Had I not perhaps been carried away by my desire to justify the *ngangas,* so that I spoke with too easy an assurance of the universe of *ndimsi?* I thought of Din's patients, who were so confident that he had cured them, and yet who continued to fear him. Were they wrong? Was the distance separating the sorcerer and the *nganga* perhaps shorter than I had asserted it was? Din, Loe, and others had interfered in the internal battles of families. Despite their protestations of neutrality, were they not actually to be ranged in one of the two camps in each case?

Now I was alone, and I asked myself the question every lawyer asks concerning a client. Who was this person Din?

Chapter 8

Those Who Perform Cures in the Night

Were Din and Loe my friends? The differences between us were evident. But, strangely, the differences did not seem to matter. We avoided emphasizing them or otherwise wounding one another's sensibilities in their respect. We were satisfied without punctilious attention to the fact that each of us was unique. Little by little, a pact had arisen among us that was free of cultural conditions and stripped to the basics. They and I were first and foremost desirous of "acknowledging" one another.

I have been warned repeatedly of the fiercely independent *nganga* spirit. Despite these warnings, a few months after Din's acquittal I sought to take things a step further and arrange a meeting of my two masters. I had never seen them together. It shows how desperately I wanted to understand their universe.

And so I asked Din to invite Loe and his disciple Nkongo to the first of the nocturnal séances he would be holding after his acquittal. I suggested that it would enhance the drama. Din acceded so readily that I was not apprehensive in the least degree. Loe professed himself equally interested in such a meeting. On the appointed evening, then, I drove to Loe's compound and brought master and disciple to Din's new house—now at a considerable distance from Ekwala's, but in the same quarter.

Din introduced Loe to the little assembly of regulars, who had gathered in a space of a few dozen square yards, along the side of the new house. The tone of his introduction seemed a bit haughty, though it was polite and complimentary. But when he had finished, Loe, seated at my side, refused to reply. He seemed furious. I saw his little mustache trembling. And yet Din had announced that Loe was a *jengu nganga*, an *esunkan*—that is, one who held his power from the water spirits, the supreme distinction among the Douala. True, he had alluded to his own seniority in the profession; he had been practicing when Loe was still a carpenter. In any case, Loe kept whispering to me, "He's made fun of me."

Later in the evening there was an even greater surprise. A young woman patient, about twenty years old, was to be treated. Din had healed her of a stubborn fever that had afflicted her daily ever since the birth of her first child. Her husband, a mechanic with Citroën, had prepaid the cost of this final treatment, which was to be like Engome's—a long, invisible journey to the place of sorcery, dancing with the victim, now delivered from *ekong*, walking on the fires, now needed no longer, and the closing meal, of which all present would partake.

The ceremony began. Din solemnly invited Loe to conduct the treatment and Nkongo to beat the drum, perhaps as a gesture of politeness. But Loe and Nkongo emphatically refused. "That's not the way we do it," Loe whispered to me, still angry. And so Din left us, and went to lie down on his bed and begin the endless journey.

The hours went by. It was ten o'clock, then eleven o'clock, then midnight. Nothing was happening. I was ready to greet the dawn still sitting on my chair. The three fires had long since gone out of their own accord, the children had left. Only Din's wife still busied herself at the kettle, preparing the *dindo*. My neighbors were all seated, perfectly erect, motionless as mask-bearers who had not been summoned to the dancing. The waiting became so tedious that I decided to do something.

I found Din stretched out on his bed, a little drunk, with his eyes wide open. He gave orders that the *dindo* should begin without him and declared that he would begin working when we had finished. As we squatted around the great kettle, helping ourselves to pieces of goat meat, prepared with plantain in a special sauce, tongues began to loosen. Loe found the dish to be excellent; it had been prepared in accordance with the customary recipes. But the mechanic expressed to me his astonishment. Din had promised him he would "deal the sorcerers a mighty blow," so that his wife could be cured and return home. Now the *dindo* was over and still nothing was happening.

I went to tell Din I had to drive my two guests home. He was still stretched out on his bed, and he said just one thing to me, something I did not grasp *"Ongwane mba son"*—"just help me a bit". Help him? Why? How? What was happening to him? I drove Loe and Nkongo home. They offered not a word of explanation.

The following Saturday, in their absence, Din undertook the final treatment of the mechanic's wife according to the customary formula. What had happened the first time then? Had he suddenly lost his power? Had he been afraid he would disappoint his guests?

But Din was not a beginner. This incident disappointed me very much. I had been visiting him and Loe for more than two years now. Might I stay by their side ten more years and still not understand anything of this? I was at a loss. Perhaps the failure was a very small one, but it deeply affected me. I could explain my overreaction to the incident only by referring to dreams Din had provoked with powders, where I saw myself incompetent and clumsy in the presence of a number of *ngangas*. I had encountered new difficulties in the progress I was making, difficulties I failed to recognize, something like a psychological block.

In order to find a way out of my impasse, I decided to leave my two friends for a while, or at least visit them less frequently. Perhaps I would return to them later, after having met other *ngangas*. To tell the truth, I had not expected this to happen. I had assisted at treatments here and there conducted by their colleagues of the neighborhood. I had studied dreams with Madame Mbu, at the inland end of the Deïdo and quarter, and madness with Kolombo, at Bonabéri. I had assisted at cures by night at the hands of a number of other practitioners.[40] But none of them had impressed me as much as Din and Loe, nor had they modified the lines of approach I had chosen for my research. Still, I decided to leave Douala, with its familiar sphere of influence, and resume the study of traditional medicine with a fresh eye.

Thanks to a school vacation I was able to go two hundred kilometers down the coast, east of Douala, to near the little port of Kribi, where numerous *ngangas* were in practice. With the help of a teacher from the Libermann School, I made several series of slides and recorded a goodly number of chants, in the course of the treatments I observed. I have written a study of some of them.[41] But the vacation was too short for me to be able to cement a relationship with these new *ngangas* and make real progress in my knowledge of them and their ritual. I regretted this very much, for their ceremonial differs from that of Douala *ngangas*, and seemed to me to hold a prodigious richness.

Then something unexpected happened, and it set me off once more on my research in Douala. Ever since I had first begun my work, I had been showing the research that now forms the basis of this book to some friends and had been asking for their criticisms. I participated in a workshop organized by the Jesuits on "Belief and Healing," at Yaoundé, at which I presented my analysis of a treatment I had witnessed at Kribi.[42] After my talk, the others present formed discussion groups. Here is the reaction of one of these groups, in the form of a written summary:

> Our group discussed two series of questions, the first on the position of the foreign researcher, and the second on the written report distributed to us.
>
> We were particularly interested in the researcher's position. It makes itself doubly felt, for in this case the researcher is both a Catholic priest and a foreign white. The distance between the two cultures meeting here is enormous, and the fact that the researcher is a priest surely facilitates contact: being considered neutral, he is not perceived as dangerous, and for this reason secrets and practices will be freely entrusted to him. Still, one must not forget the censorship automatically imposed on spontaneous expression by the dignity of the religious state.
>
> The researcher ought to accord more consideration in his interpretation to the objective disturbance that he introduces by his mere presence.

As to his being white, this, in the balance, is a positive factor, for it inspires deference and, consequently, persons are flattered to be asked to provide him with information.

The second series of questions has to do with the written report. These questions are related to what we have already said concerning the methodology. The researcher is probably right in being spontaneous in not weighing himself down with techniques, and in recording what he sees. But in doing so, it may be that he deprives himself of a basis from which to criticize his own prejudices. He may opt for spontaneity if he so wishes, but he should make the option more explicit.

The tone of these remarks was impersonal and perhaps seemingly blunt. But they were in no way artificial or offensive. This was simply the style my friends and I habitually use when asked to criticize one another's undertakings. Their observations were crisp and objective and calculated to aid me in my research. Every word of this precious critique was burned into my memory with absolute precision.

From the beginning of my research, I had sought to be as impartial as possible. I had reported only events at which I had personally assisted. I was in a position to say to Douala skeptics, "Here's what's going on in your land. Don't say your heritage has disappeared." I had submitted the results of my research to the consideration of Europeans who had little familiarity with their contents, so that they might grasp the cohesiveness of this world so hastily characterized as "irrational."

Some of my friends, then, were now counseling me to renounce my apparent neutrality and let myself "show" more in my writing. They told me my reports would then actually enjoy greater objectivity.

A Douala friend of mine, an engineer in oil refining, a native of the Deïdo quarter where Din practiced and where Loe had been born, had always been vitally attuned to their language of healing. Culturally he was their brother. But he had lived in France for ten years and now doubted *nganga* power, while still being fascinated by it. He was ahead of me in my own Western universe, by reason of his technological knowledge and ability, and yet he had the innate advantage over me of feeling as an African, which enabled him to anticipate the results of my research. But the profusion of his experiences made it impossible for him to cast them into any sort of order. I attached great value to his reactions. He had never had a single criticism to make, however, until the day he came to pay me a visit in Deïdo and said, "I've read your stories. I only have one question to ask you. What do you think of all this yourself?"

He had been even more abrupt than my confreres. He too was calling on me to let myself come out more in my writing.

He explained his question in the following manner. "You are a priest of the Catholic Church. You have inherited the extreme suspicion in which our traditional ceremonies, former beliefs, and the very struggles of the *nganga* with sorcery have been held. What do you think of all this?'' By ''all this'' he meant mainly the practice of traditional medicine.

''Do you think these practices actually work?'' my friend went on. ''What value do they have in comparison with European medicine, Chinese medicine? Do they still have any utility, or chance for survival?

''And what about sorcery? What is its reality? I sit in an air-conditioned office of an oil company doing my work as an engineer, or else I'm out on a derrick platform along the coast. Where I am, the sorcerer's arrow isn't flying day and night. But in the village!—and no African can ever really leave the village!—it stings family relationships to their death. What do you think of all this yourself?''

As a matter of fact, these questions, or this advice, fell in with my personal sentiments. I was prepared to listen. I had already begun to wonder what to think of *ndimsi*, and the *mianga*—in a word, what to think personally about traditional medicine. I had spent most of my time being tossed about like a buoy atop the waves. Not that I had misgivings. After all, this was what I had sought—to be cast adrift in this culture I was discovering. But now I yearned for a change of air. Was it fatigue? Fear of overcommitment? An unconscious resistance of some sort? Resentment at the behavior of Din and Loe that I could not understand? I did not know. But I felt the need to analyze the workings of the traditional machinery, and to break free of its grasp in order to do so.

My own social situation had been, you might say, regularized. This would make it easier to carry out my project. I had begun to teach English at the Libermann School again. I was no longer living alone in Deïdo: we had begun to set up a little Jesuit community there, consisting of two other teachers, the local superior, a Cameroonian—the same three friends who had criticized my research—and me. And of course the fact that a number of us were now living in a popular quarter meant a wish to take part in the life of the people around us. My research had been only one episode in that life. We occupied a new white house, long and narrow, called a ''two -family dwelling,'' large enough for the four of us and the woman who cooked for us. Behind us was the cemetery, and across the street was the maternity clinic. Beyond the cemetery was old Batignolles, where Philippe still sold his ''carry-out'' beer, and the old grandmother still reared her son's progeny.

My decision to leave Din and Loe alone did not prevent me from paying frequent visits to Caïn Dibunje Tukuru. Ever since the ceremony of reconciliation, I had been able to go anywhere in the village I wanted to without any difficulty, although I sometimes seemed to note a certain hesitation on the part of some of the villagers in my regard. But in the chief's residence I felt altogether at home. Mingling with mourners or celebrating feasts, I was part of his great family. He finally even gave me a name, as was customary with adopted foreigners (known as *njan*). He called me ''Dibunje,'' after his own name, to show that he considered me as a son.[43] I would have found it artificial had he proposed I adopt Cameroonian citizenship; I felt nothing of the kind with my new name, and took on my new identity quite naturally.

This village, and its chief in particular, had been, and would continue to be, my tightrope-walker's balancing pole, just as my first neighbors had been, in Deïdo, every moment of my sojourn among them. I shall be referring to my adoptive family but rarely in the rest of this book, because they taught me nothing about traditional medicine, aside from certain information that Tukuru, master of custom, provided me. But from this moment forward I was to share in this family's daily life.

Chapter 9

The Healing of Dieudonné

As I walked out the front door of the Libermann School one day and into the street—it must have been about noon—I found two strangers waiting for me. I judged from their ages that they might be father and son. There amid the blasting of automobile horns and the shouting of the students, the elder spoke up loudly: "I came to ask you to bless my son."

The lad was standing as close by his father's side as he could, to avoid being swept away by the flood of boys and girls jostling us as they rushed past. I drew the pair aside, and the father, having informed me that he was a captain in the police, repeated his request. His son was seventeen years old and was in his last year of high school in another school of the city. But he was troubled by evil spirits, and his grades at school, like his behavior at home, were suffering. Could I not give him a blessing—right here on the spot—and drive these spirits of misfortune away?

I was not surprised by the abruptness and urgency of the request. Priests here were often approached, regardless of time or place, and asked to turn their power of healing to account. Either because they do not believe they have such power, or because they fail to appreciate the nature of the request—to their way of thinking, a request for an act of magic—some of them work their way out of the impasse with a hurried blessing and a few words of encouragement. My own way of worming out of a like confrontation was, as a rule, to refer the person to their pastor.

But in this case, on the basis of my recent experience, I scented a serious matter lurking beneath the innocence of what had been said. Indeed, the captain had added that I had been recommended to him by another priest, in light of my *nganga* research. And so, before acceding to their request, I invited father and son to come and tell me the whole story, calmly and leisurely, in our house in Deïdo.

But the father came first, alone. He had things he wished to tell me out of hearing of his son. The son, Dieudonné, was the next to come. Finally, Dieudonné's younger brother, Gabriel, visited me. Physically Dieudonné was just the opposite of his father, who looked like the typical sawed-off precinct police officer. Gabriel was a scale model of his brother, down a notch in size. The boys had the same intonation in their speech, letting their words and phrases trail off at the end. Both youngsters were lively, and "on the brown side," whereas their father was "on the black side."[44]

None of the three made any objection to my recording the conversations. After all, I had been asked to help, and of course I was doing so by my own methods, which might not look precisely like a rite of blessing. Their versions of the affair matched quite adequately, except in a few details in which they might well have been expected to view things a little differently. Here I shall limit myself to Dieudonné's account, the most complete of the three.

Slouching comfortably in an armchair in our living room with his teenage false ease Dieudonné turned his face in my direction. I interrupted him as little as possible.

"I Don't Feel I'm Myself Any Longer"

"This whole thing . . . it started last year, when we got here," Dieudonné began. "We were new in town. Well, I knew a certain fellow who didn't live in my quarter, but who's from the same village as we are. This fellow, one day, he came to my house and said he was fed up with women, he didn't want any more women. Well, I told him, 'It must be like being a god to have so many women!' And he said, 'Oh, I've got talismans for getting women.' He had some printed material on the subject, with order forms. He was my buddy, so he showed it to me. Right away I could tell it had something to do with magic, stuff about Madame Mylla.[45] He went home, but he left me the papers. I read them again. It was really something. I thought I'd order something. It was the beginning of the school year. But I said to myself, I'll wait and see. I'll go to school first. If I see I'm having trouble, I'll order something. If I see my courses are going all right, I won't order anything. So I had the papers up over the door in my room.

"I didn't even get a seven the first quarter. I wasn't too worried. I told my father, 'Don't worry—I failed last year, so I had all these subjects before; I'll do better the second quarter.' And sure enough, I had a 10.56 average the second quarter and I told my father everything was fine.

"Then I was coming back from class one day and a fellow told me, 'Your little brother ordered some love chains from Europe.' I said, 'What? My little brother ordered love chains?' He said, 'Yes.' Then I got worried. I went and found my little brother right away, and I told him, 'All right, get home. We're going to talk about this with papa and mama.' And I started thinking. Maybe he had found the papers I hid! When papa came home from work, I told him what the other boy had said. We went through my brother's briefcase and we found the address written down that I knew was the same as on the papers I had hid in my room.

"So my sickness comes from that. When papa started asking my little brother questions, and asked him, 'Who?' and 'Why?' and all that, he

didn't say a word for half an hour. He was thinking. Then I went out to
buy something to drink. While I was gone he told papa, 'Father, it's not
my fault. I saw my big brother had these papers. I took them and copied
the address, but I didn't order anything.' So when I got back papa was
waiting for me. 'Mister,' he said, 'it seems you had something to do with
this. Those papers are yours. You had the papers.' So I told him how I got
the papers. And then my little brother went to my room and came back
with the papers. Papa said I could tell the fellow that gave them to me
what he did with them, and—rip—he tore them up. Then he took a match
to light them. I was sitting about ten feet away. He lit a match and it went
out. Then he lit another match and it went out. So it was on the third
match—and when the wad started burning, right away I felt as if somebody had gone off with my body and my soul and then my whole mind. I
started feeling heat climbing up in me. It started down at my feet, it
climbed, and it climbed, and pow!—right to my head. It was like going
crazy. I ran for the door. I wondered what was happening to me. My
mama stopped me. I felt like I was no longer mine, I couldn't even stay in
the house any more. I asked them to take me to the *nganga*. Maybe he
could see where my sickness came from.''

"What did the *nganga* tell you?" I asked.

"He said there were evil spirits chasing us because we burned the papers.
We shouldn't have burned them, he said; we should have thrown them into
a creek or else given them back to the fellow who'd given them to us.

"But ever since then I don't feel like I'm mine. Even at school I don't
seem mine any more. I feel as if I belonged to somebody else. When I try to
read or study, my mind isn't in it. When I come home I don't feel like doing
anything but sleep, that's all. I don't know what's going on."

"Who wanted to go and see the priests about it, you or your father?"

"I did, myself. And what made me go and see them was just because
what I told you was true: I didn't order anything. So I don't understand
why all this happened to me."

I refrained from telling Dieudonné how uncomfortable I was with his
request. I was torn between the desire to see him well again, and a strong
internal resistance. I had no doubt that a blessing, given at an appropriate
time and place, would reassure the boy. But I did not think that it would
deliver him from what was perhaps a full-fledged nervous disorder, and not
just some minor trauma or passing disturbance.

The reason for my hesitation was not medical, but personal. Dieudonné
had placed me in a situation that I would have taken lightly three years
before—before visiting the *nganga*s, before I knew the power of the traditional system and the weight of its influence on the African mind. Today for
the first time, I, in virtue of my status as a priest, had been asked to act in an
area that belonged to the *nganga*. Dieudonné's innocent proposal called for
more personal involvement than had my dealings with any *nganga*, or the
roadblock in the village, or Din's trial. I needed time for reflection, and so I

made an appointment with Dieudonné for a few days later, at home with his parents. Impatient though they might be, the father and his two sons were going to have to wait a little longer for my blessing.

What was this fear of mine, exactly? Basically it rested on the risk of a misunderstanding. Dieudonné had attributed to me a power that I perhaps had, but that I disliked using for fear of misinterpretation. His request had reawakened in me my suspicions about the idea commonly held of the power of the priest—"magic power." This is what I did not want to encourage: the idea of a power attaching to certain persons regardless of their competence or actual intentions, a power coming from outside, automatically efficacious provided the appropriate words were pronounced and gestures performed.

I confided my discomfiture to some of my older students at the Libermann School, both boys and girls, young persons of the same age as Dieudonné. My relationship with my students had changed since the days of my first classes there, sixteen years before, when I had found myself confronted with youngsters who were studious and docile but quite enigmatic to me. My relationship to them was now more direct. The change came especially from my side. Years of teaching had familiarized me with their problems and attitudes, and my association with the *nganga* had opened up to me a great number of the feelings, apprehensions, and emotions that charged their invisible "other world." I felt more at ease with them since I had discovered the masters of the night.

For their part, the students seemed to take account of my development, and now spoke with me frankly and spontaneously. I showed them the slides I had taken at Kribi and we discussed them freely. At least half of the students had attended a treatment séance for a family member, or even undergone treatment themselves. Rare was the boy or girl who claimed to have no knowledge of them.

I played Dieudonné's story for them, in all three versions, his own and those of his father and brother.[46] Carefully safeguarding Dieudonné's anonymity, I was able to gather the opinions of these youngsters, who were of the same age and the same culture as he, and whose family experience was doubtless very similar to his as well. I asked them what power I was expected to have. Their very incisive answers demonstrated the ambiguity of Dieudonné's request and reinforced my hesitancy to grant the blessing. One of the students put his opinion in writing. It is a good summary of the general view of most of the students:

I should like to know why he didn't go to a [Protestant] minister. Probably because the way [Catholic] priests live is a lot different from the way married ministers live. They have more contact with the people, so there's less of an idea that they have magic power. It's different with priests. Priests have something mysterious about them. And that's what he thinks is going to be the thing that will get him well.

"What Are They, Do You Think—These 'Evil Spirits'?"

The day of our meeting at Dieudonné's house came, and I went there determined to use my influence to get the boy to go back to Nombote, the *nganga* he had spoken of in his story. Nombote lived in Deïdo, in a part of the quarter where immigrants were crowding in from the interior of the country. I had found out where he lived, and promised myself I would pay him a visit later. Dieudonné's family, on the other hand, lived in a remote residential quarter, well outside the influence of the Douala people. The father, originally from Nanga-Eboko, a township in the eastern part of the country, had rented the first available house—as a police officer, he had to be ready to move from one place to another on short notice. The houses in this quarter, all rectangular, and built of boards, so resembled one another that I had difficulty finding which one was Dieudonné's.

I arrived at the door, at the time we had set, but I had the feeling I had been awaited for an eternity. I began to realize how much I was being counted on, and I was moved, but not shaken in my resolve. We sat down in the living room where just the right number of chairs had been placed.

I sought to give this first meeting a tone of solemnity, to make an impression on the entire family, because I knew that the illness of one is often the symptom of a collective affliction. As exactly as I can recall, I told them, "You came to the Libermann School to find me because I am a priest and a teacher. I've worked with young persons in this country for seventeen years—ever since Dieudonné was born. I have listened to the father, to Dieudonné himself, and to his younger brother, Gabriel. Well—it's not a priest who can heal him, or even a doctor. It's a *nganga*. Dieudonné has not completed his treatment with Nombote. He should go back there."

The family continued to sit in silence riveting all their attention on me—even the little sister whose eyes are bigger than her nose. I could see how worried they were about Dieudonné's problem.

"So then is he really sick?" the father asked me.

"Yes," I said, "he is. It's not like a broken leg, but it is a disease."

"We were told to take Dieudonné to the native doctor," the father continued. "I don't know that that would do any good. If he gets well, I'll entrust him to you. He'll go to school in your institution."

I listed for Dieudonné the entrance requirements for my school, so that he would not have false hopes. I knew very well that he probably could not meet the scholastic requirements. Then I asked him what he had done, and what he would like to do.

"I went to Nombote," he replied, "and he started telling me crazy things, like that I'd gone and ordered stuff from Madame Mylla. . . . I wanted to see a priest, so he would get rid of the power those papers have on me."

"That's the *nganga*'s domain," I said. "Are you willing to go back to Nombote and trust in him?"

"Yes," Dieudonné said.

"Of course he'll go back!" the father put in.

But Dieudonné's return was a failure. He spent three days at Nombote's, in Deïdo, submitting to various potions, fumigations, and inhalations, without really believing in them. Then suddenly he disappeared. Finally, adding insult to injury, he was caught writing to Madame Mylla.

Clearly, Nombote had lost his credibility. Vexed and irritated—after all, the failure was mine as well—I went to find out what had happened. The house was locked and deserted. Neighbors provided me with information that enabled me to trace down their new address. But the father was living there alone, to be near his work; the rest of the family had hastily left for the village they had come from.

I soon learned, from Dieudonné himself, why the family had changed residence. "Our neighbors told us the house was no good. Even the owner admitted some man had lived there before us and held occult séances. So we were afraid and we ran away. And I'm still sick. So I asked papa to send us back to our village. Maybe I can find the fellow who gave us those papers from Madame Mylla."

"Weren't you satisfied with Nombote?"

"No, I wasn't. When you're in the hospital, at least there's a change from day to day. There, I couldn't see any change. I would tell him I wasn't coming back to myself. He would just say, 'You *have* to come back to yourself.' But I didn't know how I was going to do that. I realized he wasn't any good."

"I was told that you wrote a letter to Madame Mylla. Why did you do that instead of trusting Nombote?"

"There was a fellow in the army there at Nombote's. He told me, 'Why don't you write or phone the Myllas and ask if they aren't the cause of your sickness?' I looked for the telephone number but I couldn't find it. So I wrote a letter. But I didn't sign my name and I didn't use my own pen. I signed the name of the fellow who gave me the papers. I said he was in jail for giving us the papers. I said we burned them and we got sick, and I asked her what the ransom was so we could pay for the paper we burned."

"So you think the papers made you sick?"

"I've asked a lot of persons about that. We shouldn't have burned them. We should have thrown them in the river, or in the toilet, or given them to a priest. Nombote said the evil spirits of those persons in Paris made me sick."

"What are they, do you think—these 'evil spirits'?"[47]

"Well, I think . . . well, I saw a certain movie they made in Brazil, *Black Orpheus*. There was a woman in it who was bothered by evil spirits. She did certain things and kept shouting, 'Oh! Oh!' That's where I saw about evil spirits."

Now I went to see Dieudonné's father, who lived alone in the new house. "Why didn't you make Dieudonné finish his treatment with Nombote? Don't you have any confidence in Nombote?"

"I *had* confidence in him. But when you go to the hospital and they give you penicillin and you don't feel any better, are you going to let them give you more penicillin? Dieudonné still isn't normal. He told me, 'I'll have to go to somebody else.' But I saw that the only thing *ngangas* want around here is money. You said that this sickness shouldn't be treated at the hospital; it should be treated by a *nganga*. So I decided to send Dieudonné back to the village. There are *nganga*s practicing in the village too."

I did not know how the father regarded my eagerness to follow his son's case. He was probably hoping I would give the boy my blessing and then keep him somewhat under my wing afterward as well. As for myself, I sincerely desired to see Dieudonné get well, but I did not intend to intervene, even with a blessing, without knowing how it would be interpreted and what the consequences would be.

Troubled Conscience or Troubled Reason?

Three weeks later, Dieudonné came to see me in our residence in Deïdo. As always, he looked very much the dignified student and eldest son. I could guess what he was coming for, and I felt irritated. It was evident just from his eagerness to greet me. And surely enough, his first words were another request for the blessing.

Then he told me that he had gone with his mother to pay a visit to the old diviner who practiced in his region of the countryside, but he had been unwilling to give an opinion. Then Madame Mylla's reply had come, and she had said, most kindly, that she was incapable of doing evil to anyone.[48] Then he told me that he had received a piece of advice from his uncle: "My uncle in the village told me that my sickness came from a troubled conscience."

"Brought on by what?" I asked him.

"Brought on by fear."

I was surprised by all this new vocabulary. "What does this uncle of yours do?" I asked. "Has he been to school?"

"Primary and secondary."

"What do you think this means—a 'troubled conscience' "?

"He explained it to me. It's like when they're having elections. You've got a piece of paper with a picture of the president of the republic on it. You roll it up and start to make a cigarette. One of the authorities comes by and sees you've got a picture of the president on your cigarette paper, so he says, 'Look out! It's dangerous to burn that paper like that!' So you're afraid. You can go crazy from being afraid like that. That's what they mean by a strangled conscience. That's how I was afraid that day, starting from my feet, and it climbed all the way up to my head."

I said to him, "You know, when we say *conscience* in French, we can mean either of two things. It means your reason, your consciousness, or it can mean the voice of religious consciousness, your conscience. Which do you mean here?"

"I see the difference. Here it pretty much means a troubled reason."

"Ah, now it's all clear," I said. "You think you've changed a lot recently and that you're better now."

"It also happens sometimes, when I'm in bed, that I say to myself that there's something in my head that I'm going to have to look at before I can find myself again."

Dieudonné seemed to be taking a psychological view of his sickness. I recalled what I had heard from one of my older students after I had played Dieudonné's tape. "He doesn't trust the *nganga* any more. It won't do any good for him to see him." And so I told Dieudonné I thought we ought to go see a psychiatrist.

To my great surprise, he told me he had already taken this step—at the very onset of his crisis, even before we had met. But he had not reported to the doctor the cultural context of his drama, for fear of appearing ridiculous and being told, "Don't bother me with all this business about magic! Go see a magician!" Now, however, he seemed resolved to tell a psychiatrist everything, as he had told me. Still, he insisted on having my blessing.

The Cameroonian psychiatrist Dieudonné visited asked him to tell his story in writing. I read his report, and it agreed with the one he had given me of his troubles. The doctor prescribed tranquilizers for him, as well as some medicines to promote the synergy of Dieudonné's own body, to release the pressure of his emotions. He was seeking to help him regain control of himself.

In the course of the second visit, the psychiatrist asked his client to comment freely on certain matters that astonished Dieudonné. I too was astonished, a bit, I must confess. The boy told me what these matters were: his sexual life to date, his views on the role of sexuality, the nature of his relationships with those around him, and the importance of the *nganga*.

"Those questions he asked me—" Dieudonné began, "I didn't understand why. So I told him I haven't anything to tell him about sexual relations, and I explained to him that I'm a minor; I've never had sexual relations. He didn't say anything, and he just took the paper and read what I had written on it."

The psychiatrist's provisional diagnosis was "failure neurosis." But I was convinced that, sooner or later, he would be discussing with Dieudonné the question of his relationship with his father. The various accounts I had received of Dieudonné's difficulties made it clear that the father ran his family like a true police officer. The fact that the papers had been burned by the father—by this person of order, law, and legitimacy—had implicitly suggested that what Dieudonné had done had been something of enormous gravity, and thus could very well have triggered his son's nervous dysfunction. I was surprised that neither Dieudonné nor his contemporaries in my class at the Libermann School had themselves hit on the causal relationship between the father's severity and the son's traumatism.[49] I had to find a way to help Dieudonné discover it.

"How does your father treat you?" I asked.

"He's—he's too strict. When he comes home after work, you know he's going to have something to say, he's going to find something wrong, some job we didn't do right. No, papa doesn't like anything out of line at home. When he comes home he has plenty to say. He gets mad!"

"And mama?"

"Mama—mama too," Dieudonné replied. "She goes according to papa's moods. She tries to imitate him. But since I've had this thing, whatever's bothering me, I don't like it when papa and mama bawl me out. When I'm bawled out, things don't go right any more."

One of my students had warned me, "I think he does a lot of things behind his father's back." However that might be, Dieudonné admitted to me that he hid his current state of mind from his father. This posed a problem so far as buying medicine was concerned, because his father had thought he was cured when he came back from the village, on the word of the uncle, who had said it was simply a matter of a "troubled conscience." There was a latent tension between father and son; it surfaced in their respective accounts of Dieudonné's sickness. Where the father had actually taken the initiative, Dieudonné would claim the decision as his own. He claimed to have chosen the *nganga* Nombote. He claimed to have decided the family would go back to the village. Dieudonné was very conscious of his responsibilities as elder son, the family intellectual. What a set-up for disappointment and, consequently, what a fertile seedbed for emotional trauma!

I made an effort to follow his line of reasoning. If he was not guilty, then how was he to explain what had befallen him? One would have expected others to have suffered it instead—the friend who had given him the dangerous papers, or his younger brother, who had written down Madame Mylla's address, or even his father, who had rashly burned the papers. He himself had only stored the papers, to return them to his friend! And yet it was he who had been struck down. Then who could deliver him from this mysterious force—which for want of a better name would be called fear? Someone with absolute power. A priest.

Dieudonné, now undergoing psychiatric treatment, was asking me for my blessing once again. This time I was on the verge of giving it to him.

"Papa knows I'm well again," said Dieudonné. "I'm beginning to feel better myself since I've been seeing the psychiatrist and taking the medicine. But when the analysis is over, I'd like to ask you to give me a blessing, and a chain, like Catholics wear, to keep me protected."

The edge of my resistance had been blunted. I had tried one last time to encourage the intervention of persons who I thought would be more capable of helping him, but without result.

Finally I decided to prompt him to reflect on something. "Did Jesus heal the sick?" I asked him.

"Of course he did."

"Why did he heal them?"

"Because he took pity on them," Dieudonné began. "And because they asked him to. They came to him to be cured. There was an old woman who'd lost one of her sons—we've got a song about it—so she went out and explained her trouble to Jesus, and Jesus went to her house and told the child to get up. And the child got up by itself. If the woman had stayed home, nothing would have happened. Jesus wouldn't have known that this woman was hurting. When she showed up, Jesus found out about it and went with her."

As long as we had known each other, Dieudonné had not modified his position on the power of priests one iota. His trust was equally intact. So I had to do a little developing myself. It now seemed to me that, after all these attempts of mine to find another way, Dieudonné's final cure would be by this blessing, which he had not ceased to request with his disarming constancy. I no longer saw what Christian consideration authorized me to refuse him his health.

The Blessing

It took a good deal of work to prepare the ritual. I did it with the help of the students I had already consulted. They too, I felt, were torn between belief and criticism—as the casual bluntness of some of their suggestions demonstrates:

You should make believe something, kind of mystical.

Priests' magic is their breviary, so read some prayers.

If I were in your place, I couldn't do it. It would be doing like a bad *nganga*—pretending. It might not heal him.

Unless a priest does *something,* he won't get well.

You're making it too complicated. All he wants is the sign of the cross and be done with it.

Take your breviary and read a prayer, a different kind of one, not just the Our Father or the Hail Mary.

We finally decided that I would combine two rituals. I would use the liturgy of the word and include a blessing, and I would do this in the library of our house in Deïdo, where we sometimes said Mass. But I would combine this with a rite I had seen performed by a remarkable *nganga* named Ntonga in the vicinity of Kribi. I had attended a departure ceremony conducted by him for one of his patients, to celebrate the latter's cure, by the side of the

road, and certain elements of the liturgy of the word seemed to fit in well
with this ceremony.

I showed my students pictures of Ntonga's ceremony. Ntonga was a
short man, almost a dwarf. He would cover his great gnome's head with a
red cowl, don a white alb that was too long for him and, thus attired,
shoot hither and yon among his patients, jumping up and down about
them and miming a savage battle with the powers of evil—striking out
with his fists, baring his teeth, and grasping his patients' throats as if he
had been a strangler. (I had no intention of doing this with Dieudonné!)
The secret of his effectiveness, apart from the herbs and barks, lay in his
mighty symbolic gestures, his reputation, and his own sense of conviction.
He would conclude a treatment with the declaration, charged with his
contagious confidence, that his client had now been healed. Then he
would initiate with that person a roundabout dialogue that would finally
lead to the client's own formal acknowledgment, right out loud in the
midst of the general festivity, that he or she was healed indeed. My purpose, then, would be to lead Dieudonné himself to state that he was
healed, during a closing dialogue conducted in the same spirit (but in the
hushed atmosphere of our library). Dieudonné arrived on the day appointed, accompanied by his brother Gabriel, and a friend of Gabriel's
who was a Catholic. I had suggested to him he might bring along anyone
he wished to the ceremony of the healing. As I awaited their arrival, I
prepared the library of our house in Deïdo, covering the table with a cloth,
and placing a candle to the right and a vessel of water and a hyssop on the
left.

When the three boys arrived, I assigned them places on either side of the
table, and lit the candle. (My first match sputtered and went out, so did the
second. Strange coincidence. Dieudonné gave me a knowing look. Now I
took my time. Just as his father had, I finally succeeded on the third attempt.)

Then I addressed him: "Dieudonné, you came to see me the first time in
order to be healed, is this not true?"

"Yes."

"Dieudonné, you were sick, were you not?"

"Yes."

"And you expect all God's healing, do you not?"

"Yes."

"Let us pray. Lord, look upon these three young men with favor . . . ."

After this introductory dialogue, I read two short selections from the
New Testament, commenting on each as I concluded. The first was from
Saint John, chapter 9, telling how Jesus restored the sight of the person
born blind. The second was from the Acts of the Apostles, chapter 14, nar-
rating the cure of a crippled person, together with Paul's protest when the
crowd had paid him the honor due to a god. I had chosen this text to recall
that it was God, and not the priest, who should be thanked for a cure.

Dieudonné followed the reading with concentration and seriousness. Gabriel had a difficult time to keep from laughing, but I knew that this feeling of wanting to laugh often conceals a certain emotionalism and a sense of excitement.

Then I moved on to the rite of the water, explaining to the boys that blessing with water symbolized their baptism, by which they had become the brothers of him who is victor over the powers of darkness. Then I sprinkled them with the hyssop dipped in water.

"Let us pray. Lord, you heal . . . ."

Finally, I imposed hands on Dieudonné, declaring: "Dieudonné, you are healed." And I paused for a moment.

Then I said, after the fashion of a *nganga*: "Dieudonné, you *are* healed, aren't you?"

He answered me crisply and surely: "Yes." (A laugh came from Gabriel.)

After the ceremony, as we were enjoying a drink together to celebrate the return to health, Dieudonné asked me, "What about the medal—when shall I come for that?"

I had discussed the medal with my students, and we had decided to de-emphasize the importance of this object, because Dieudonné was inclined to exaggerate it.

"Whenever you like," I replied. "But you don't have to have it. It's not a 'necessary and sufficient condition,' as we say in math."

"Not a *conditio sine qua non*, then," he responded in the same tone.

There was silence for a moment. Then Dieudonné, who had obviously awaited this particular moment to say what he had in his heart, asked this question: "How long does it take to change over?"

"Change over?"

"Yes, become a Catholic."

I thought for a moment. Then I asked, "Why do you want to become a Catholic?"

"There are some things they have better. I see they can receive communion often. I see they can go to confession. Actually I've already taken communion, and I've gone to confession."

"Why go to communion and confession in a Catholic church if you're a Protestant? And if you became a Catholic, what would your family say?"

"As far as they're concerned, I already am a Catholic." (Gabriel laughed in disagreement.) "They consider me a Catholic. I go to Mass every Sunday at Saint Paul's."

"How long have you been doing that?"

"Since I came back from the village."

"I would be glad to have you become a Catholic," I said, "but we have to know why you want to."

I noted down this conversation, and reported it to my students. They were very hesitant, as the following samples of their responses indicate:

It's not his idea to become a Catholic. His father probably told him, "If he heals you, he gets you!"

He wants to become a Catholic to look out for himself, to protect himself against a relapse.

Before the missionaries got here, we had rites more like Catholics than like the Protestants.

But one pupil observed, "In the New Testament, Jesus would cure the sick and convert them; there's nothing wrong with that."

I tended to take my students' opinions with a grain of salt. They tend to shoot from the hip at that age, and criticize everything. But they were helpful.

Dieudonné and I decided to meet once a week. If he persisted in his request, I would give him instructions to become a Catholic. I would prepare him for his "change-over."

It was not to be an easy matter. The main difficulty, and the one from which all others sprang—a particular concept of religious power—had perhaps remained unchanged in Dieudonné's mind. For example, I advised him to continue taking the medicines the psychiatrist had prescribed, in the name of our Christian faith. After all, we should use all the means God has placed at our disposal to prevent relapses. I asked him to repeat what I had said, because I wanted to make sure he had understood correctly. But instead of repeating what I had said, he filtered it through his own mind-set: "God wants us to believe in him—otherwise you can do anything you want, and that's no good."

I counterattacked. "Everything depends on you, because everything is a gift of God, as your name indicates, Dieudonné ['given by God']! This may look like a contradiction, but it isn't; it's far from absurd, if you know that God's greatest glory is a human being fully alive!"

Dieudonné looked totally crushed. I suddenly realized what a distance there was between us, measured in terms of religion, and not just culture. This realization hit me hard, and made me more circumspect, almost timid. It even affected my Sunday preaching: I started to be afraid that some in the congregation might misinterpret my words, just as Dieudonné had done.

This first session of ours reminded me of a maxim attributed to Ignatius Loyola, which I decided to take as the guideline for my catechesis. If Dieudonné ever came to understand it, we would be on the same religious wave length. It is almost untranslatable, so completely and precisely does it manage to interweave human effort and God's contribution. "Trust God," Loyola was said to have written, "as if the outcome depended entirely on you, and in no way on God; yet strive to act in all things as if God alone were doing everything, and you nothing."[50]

The tale of Dieudonné's cure is as much the tale of my resistance to giving him the blessing as it is of his determination to have it.

Dieudonné graduated from high school and gave me the credit for it. A few days later he announced that he was to leave Douala, following a brawl in one of the quarters, to go with his father on a new assignment. They moved to Yaoundé. Dieudonné wrote to me nearly every week. He had the idea that I could get him a scholarship and that he would go to France to study, once he had his secondary-school certificate. His attempts to find another priest, a local one, who would prepare him for entry into the Catholic Church were hesitant. In other words, he was still overattached to me, in my opinion, and I did not answer him as frequently as I heard from him. Now that he was past his crisis, he had to recover his autonomy, it seemed to me, and reestablish a healthy relationship with his father. I wrote this to him, and he seemed to understand. His letters became less frequent, and his request for support grew more discreet and eventually ceased. Now I could understand why Din and Loe kept a certain distance from their patients, speaking with them only rarely. Once they had been treated, they returned to their families and did not remain too attached to their *nganga*.

With the passing of time, I have come to see that my resistance to Dieudonné's request, like my final capitulation, and then my concern to regain my independence once his healing had been achieved, are not to be explained solely in terms of medical strategy. Dieudonné had the luck (or misfortune) to meet me at the point along my journey when I was most hesitant with regard to indigenous tradition and practices.

Chapter 10

"Your Sister Is a Sorceress!"

The following account is not a continuation of the preceeding, although the two overlap. Most of the things I am about to relate did occur during the period of the various attempts to heal Dieudonné. But I thought it best to keep the two reports separate, both to avoid confusion and because the two series of events did actually transpire independently. Still, I must acknowledge the influence of this second adventure on my behavior toward Dieudonné. I would not have offered him such stiff resistance had it not been for this other occurrence.

The only persons to appear in both narratives are Nombote and myself. The house I lived in was located in the part of the Douala quarter that once had been that of the servants and serfs, at a distance from the neighborhood in which the nobility lived, on the river bank. Nombote lived still further back in the Deïdo quarter, where the open country began, in a zone around the city that was inhabited by newcomers, and where new houses were begun every day. His *nganga* precincts were thus halfway between Din's, which were in the upper-class part of this Douala quarter, and Loe's at Bepanda. I often passed Nombote's house.

Douala was not the only language used in this part of town. There was a pidgin English as well, which had been spoken along the coast for two hundred years, and was understood by everyone. Bamiléké was spoken too, along with Ewondo, Dieudonné's native tongue.

I went to visit Nombote one evening, in the hope of finding Dieudonné there. But just at that time, despite my advice, Dieudonné had decided to leave him. I did not find him, then. But I decided to stay a while, and immerse myself in the comforting atmosphere of the healing ceremonies of the quarter. Then I lost track of the time. . . .

"Fly, Eagle, Fly!"

It was midnight. The quarter was wrapped in sleep. The lanes were deserted and totally dark, except for reflected light from far away in the city.

The only island of life and light was this courtyard, where the *nganga* was working. One hundred fifty persons had not gone to bed and now formed as wide a circle as they could in this little enclosure—sitting, squatting, crowded together in several rows, facing the healing area, forming the first rampart against the exterior darkness. The curious, one by one, had discreetly slipped away. Only the patients' families or close friends and acquaintances remained. They were not spectators; they were participants in a liturgy of healing.

Nestling on the benches in the center of the yard, each draped in a sheet, waiting their turn, were the patients of the night. There were fourteen of them—attentive, docile, and not looking sick at all at first glance, except for a special stillness and the fixity of their gaze. They were not a homogeneous group. There were old as well as young, some of them practically children, both boys and girls. The two *nganga*s, Nombote and his colleague Tokoto, who had come to assist him for the night, were as bustling and busy as the large, tightly packed audience was peaceful. Both manifested a dynamism that seemed a little forced. They were dressed in red—the color of blood, the color of combat with sorcerers. Several storm lamps, in place of a brazier, shot long, wild shadows racing out into the dark.

I was seated next to a certain Oyono, whom I had known when he was a student, and who was now employed by Cameroon Airlines. His comely, solicitous face, his white shirt, and his dark, well-tailored trousers gave him the look of a steward. He was not a follower of the *nganga*s, but, like all the young persons of his generation, he had not succeeded in detaching himself from belief in "those things," as he called them with studied ambiguity.

Oyono had come with a family, friends of his, one of whose members was seated in the group of patients. He introduced me to each of the persons around us, so that I made the acquaintance of those who will figure in this narrative. This was not the first time I formed bonds of friendship in this manner, thanks to the warm, dramatic atmosphere reigning at a night séance, simply upon being introduced. There in the half-light, then, were nine members of the same family, grouped about the handsome Oyono: his friend Nkoa, an employee of the Department of Public Works, his wife Dorette, and their five children, all sleeping curled up at their feet. Then there was the grandfather, seated a couple of steps away. Next Oyono pointed out to me his friend Nkoa's younger brother Bruno, whom I could just make out in the group of patients in the center of the courtyard.

By bits and pieces, I learned how Bruno's illness had made its appearance. Psychiatry did not find it easy to identify the symptoms that that illness manifested, but they were easily recognizable in the traditional code: sore throat, high fever each evening, a great sense of fatigue, an occasional generalized trembling, pains in the left side of the head, and a prickly feeling in the eyes. All this was accompanied by nightmares: the victim dreamt that he had just been arrested and he was unable to recognize his attackers' faces. What else could it be but *ekong* sorcery?

Nombote later gave me a spare description of this disorder, which could have different symptoms. "He's been sold," he told me. "Those who've been sold can't tell exactly what ails them."

"But they suffer in particular parts of their bodies," I interrupted.

"No. It's not a precise disease. They can't even say if they hurt exactly here or there. When all the symptoms are gone, they're cured."

Finally it was Bruno's turn. Like the others, he was wrapped head to foot in a sheet. Now I could make out his face—the hooded visage of a beaten boxer. He resembled his elder brother Nkoa—the same thick lips, a receding chin like his, and a broad, flat nose. That big face was not made to be sick, and this made the look of him all the more pathetic.

Nombote and his colleague Tokoto had already begun a series of rites of protection, strength, and deliverance with their clients. Oyono whispered in my ear, "What's surprising is that not everybody has the same illness, but they all get the same treatment!" His observation was inexact, but I shall not delay here on these complex rites. They deserve a detailed study of their own.

I was especially interested in the rite of accusation, the crucial moment in the treatment. I believed I understood the procedure. If Bruno was the victim of sorcery, he was going to have to denounce the guilty party, who would inevitably be a member of the family circle. As the Douala proverb has it, the saying Din had taught me, *Mulemb'ango e nde mot'ango nya nyolo*—"Your sorcerer is your bodyguard." The question that raced about in my head that night was this: Were the search for, and identification of, the guilty party indispensable for the healing, or were they merely ancillary? I went back over a number of dubious accusations in my mind—the one lodged against the old *nganga* suspected of practicing *ekong,* the one lodged against me, the one that dragged Din before the bar of justice. I recalled the terrible anguish of Dieudonné, in search of someone who could be responsible for his trouble.

Even more than the magical mentality, as with Dieudonné's petty magic, the problem for me was the principle of accusation accepted as a technique. Ever since I had begun to frequent the *nganga* world, I had been shocked by the generalized use of accusation. I wanted to know more about it.

Nombote made a sign to the grandfather, the head of the family sitting beside us, that he should rise and take his place in the very center of the courtyard, facing his son Bruno. Nombote and the grandfather now engaged in a terse dialogue, interrupted by refrains, as if they had been conducting a ritual joust. *Bela bio bio,* sang the onlookers—"Fly, eagle, fly!" Nombote's intention was obvious. He was seeking to induce the old man to second the accusation he was about to make against his eldest daughter, the only family member absent this evening. But the old man was resisting all the *nganga*'s onslaughts:

Nombote (in pidgin English): You have daughter. She not in this part of Cameroon, she in the west. Is not true?

The Grandfather (in Ewondo): Yes, it is true.

Nombote: Gimme just two hours and you gonna learn that she dead out there. You know why? Because the way I am, I love sorcerers. . . . Your daughter a sorceress. She bothering you all. And me, I here for good of your family, and I not let people put off payments. Your daughter, if she bother me, I'm gonna bother her. Bruno not brought here to get cured?

Grandfather: I say I don't know if she's a sorceress.

Nombote: Other great seers already say you your daughter practice sorcery. I telling you, eh? You gotta choose. Either you love your daughter, or you love all this family you brought. I not gonna talk like minister or priest, I gotta have answer.

Grandfather: I love everybody.

Nombote: If you sick in eye, other eye hurt too. Better lose this eye than let other hurt. Proverb. You love her who want cast spell on you?

Grandfather: Yes, I love her.

Nombote: Fine! There two things, in front of you. Gimme one.

Grandfather: I'm not giving either one.

Nombote: Then you gonna leave [killed by his daughter], and you gonna abandon your children.

Grandfather: I'd rather die and leave my children.

Nombote: So. You love sorceress more than yourself! Your daughter give two boys. Where they now? You know. You not hide truth from me [an allusion to the two children of this woman, who had died, in her absence, in strange circumstances]. That bad man who let self be killed and who let his family be done all away! That bad man. You want everybody die, just for your daughter? If you say leave in peace her that wipe out your family, she must be most important one for you. She your queen.

Oyono was shaken for the first time. And yet he had said he was a "skeptic by nature and by training." He had done his technical studies, had he not? But now he told me that Nombote was the second *nganga* to accuse his friend's elder sister of sorcery. The first practiced in the Eton country, three hundred kilometers from Douala. No connivance between the two had been possible.

The night wore on, and still to be begun were the treatments of the other patients, who had waited, mute and docile, so long. Bruno's illness so absorbed me that I had no interest in the other cases. Each was a whole unto itself, and I scarcely had the time to grasp even the generalities of each, as the *nganga* "unveiled" them with his allusions and sallies. Later Nombote came back to Bruno and concluded his work by obliging the grandfather solemnly to declare, according to the traditional rite called *esa* in Douala, that he pledged his family's lives that his daughter was not a sorceress. And he muttered to him the formulas of blessing he had to pronounce as he washed the face of each of his children and grandchildren present with the waters of ablution and the leaf of peace *(dibokuboku la wonja)*.

"Say this," Nombote whispered. "If I am on the side of those who seek the misfortune of my family, may this evil fall upon me instead. If this evil comes from another, let this evil turn back on him. If my daughter seeks to bear the evil to another family, may this evil turn back against her."

The old man, uneasy, took liberties with the ritual imposed, managing to avoid unambiguously accusing his daughter: "I have not fathered my children to bury them. Since I have arrived in Douala, none has died. I would prefer to die myself, and be buried by my children, rather than the other way around. If I know anything of my child's sickness, I say: 'May he be healed this very night!' If my children do any *mengang* [practices of sorcery], that is their business. If it is somebody else, even one of my children, even my daughter, who wishes ill to my family . . . it is still their business. I wish, by God, for my children to be healthy, and to prosper. I have no other support but them. So I can't wish evil on my children."

It was five o'clock in the morning. We could see the first faint glimmer of the new day—the slight paleness in the east, barely discernible on the roof-tops, the street lights seeming to dim a little, a commotion in a neighbor's chicken coop. A feeling of accomplishment came over the assembly. Nombote led the patients to their rooms and dismissed us.

Countershock

Toward noon, I returned to Nombote's to seek news of Dieudonné and happened to meet Nkoa's father coming around the corner at the *nganga's* enclosure. He said only a few words, in pidgin mixed with French, but he seemed happy to confide his thoughts to me. When he had left, I noted down the essentials: "I don't say anything. My daughter Clara is good to her brother, she's not the one. . . . I think it's Dorette, Nkoa's wife. She and Clara didn't get along. . . . I'm afraid to talk. That'd only start something. Afterward they'd say I'm the one responsible for all this."

This was the only confidence with which the old man would ever entrust me. We would never be alone in our later meetings. What he revealed to me, then, was that there was a family conflict of which I had been ignorant—between Clara, the absent daughter, who had been accused, and Dorette, his daughter-in-law, who had attended the treatment that night with her five children. Perhaps, then, he had given me the key to the mystery.

That day I asked Tokoto, Nombote's associate, the reason why it was the old man who had been harassed.

"Because he's the one who fathered that whole family," Tokoto replied. "So he has to tell us if we have to make a return shock on his daughter, the sorceress who wants to wipe out his family."

" 'Return shock'? I don't understand."

"Making a return shock means armoring the family. Then, if the sorceress leaves home to come and attack someone in the family. . . ."

"She receives a countershock."

"That's it. So we need the agreement of the grandfather."

"And he's not giving it."

"No, he'd rather die than be the cause of his daughter's death," said Tokoto. "As for us, there's nothing we can do without his agreement."

"So the treatment has failed?"

"The treatment has succeeded. But the goal [the neutralization of the sorceress] has not been attained. You know, in these cases it's better to drop the accusation, otherwise instead of saying we want to save the family, he'll say we're trying to bewitch it, then. . . ."

It was rather surprising to hear these confidences, and to be allowed to record them. And my main confidants were themselves principals in the affair—the two friends, Oyono and Nkoa, once members of the Christian Student and Working Youth, who understood the importance of what I was asking myself because they were asking the same dramatic questions.

Tokoto was a Douala *nganga* who practiced nearby. I paid him a visit from time to time to ask about something and to stay in contact. But I had not had the opportunity to see him at work. We had spent hours in discussion. He understood my objectives in his own way, and once even told Nombote in my presence, "He does theology with all this stuff."

My relations with Nombote, the principal *nganga* of the night, were different and more delicate. I had to admit I felt ill at ease with him. He posed. He manifested an excessive politeness toward me, and gave me looks of infinite tenderness that ill accorded with the brutality he showed his patients. My dealings with Din and Loe had not prepared me for such contrasts. By day, he wore dark glasses, makeup, and perfume. He was less than thirty years old.

Nombote was typical of a rather disquieting type of new-generation, big-city *nganga*s, of whom I had met several, both in Douala and in suburban districts. He collected magical and astrological products, and shoddy European, Egyptian, and Indian curios. His brochures were entitled, "Herb Doctor, Seer, Representing India in Cameroon." His little billboard, erected opposite the door of a private school of the city, gave the same flattering description. Enthroned on his central table was a beautiful edition of the Bible, surrounded by various versions of those modern apocrypha that contain a thousand "efficacious prayers," under the patronage of some medieval pope. All these heterogeneous texts, in turn, were accompanied by the instruments of traditional divination.

In his office, which also served as his *dibandi,* you could see the termite hills representing death, assorted horns crammed with objects endowed with power, the water basin with various shellfish marinating, symbolizing the water spirits, the mirror, the cowries, the barks and feathers, the pangolin scales[51]—in short, all the things you find among the paraphernalia of an orthodox *nganga*. All was mightily redolent of oil lamps. This helter-skelter ensemble of things was the symbol, at once vulgar and mystical, of the two worlds. Clients, instead of seeming startled, as I was the first time, looked fascinated and confident.

This was the cosmopolitan, eclectic *nganga,* who had so resoundingly denounced Clara, the old man's eldest daughter, right in front of me and everyone else. Din and Loe, in their own night séances, acted with more tact and discretion, making full use of a consummate sense of suggestion. They made an effort to bring it about that everyone's suspicions converge on one person, but without naming that person. Their strategy was more professional. But was not the principle of accusation itself the same for them as for Nombote?

"You Can't Take Her Skin Off"

In the afternoon of the following day, when I went to visit Nombote, I was thrown into consternation by what he had to tell me. The sister had left the west and arrived that very morning to visit her younger brother, Bruno, in the very precincts where she had been publicly accused of sorcery. According to Nombote she was aware of the accusation. What was more, she was to spend the night at her father's house—that is, with Nkoa; the son and his family lived with the father. Later I learned that she would be staying there for a longer period of time.

I asked Nombote the reason for this. He replied, "Because you can't take her skin off." In other words, she belonged to the family, so what could one do?*

On Sunday evening, February 10, 1974, the two colleagues, Nombote and Tokoto, who scarcely wanted for clients, decided to treat more patients. Repaying the other's hospitality, it was Tokoto this time who invited Nombote to his own enclosure, only a few hundred yards away. There, to my great surprise, I found Nkoa, his wife, and their five children! I decided not to let this evening pass without interviewing Nkoa on the subject of his sis-

*A reminder:

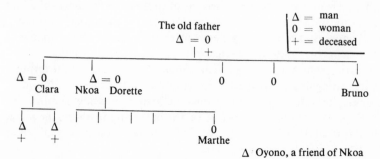

ter's visit, and on the means remaining to him to prevent the violent collapse of the family.

I had my opportunity at the very beginning of the treatments. Tokoto was having the aged father of one of his clients say a prayer, as was sometimes done at the beginning of a treatment. There in the semidarkness, this old man resembled another, whom I had seen stand up to a *nganga* a whole night long. Their dialogue:

> *Tokoto (in pidgin):* You Christian?
> *The Old Man:* Yes.
> *Tokoto:* What church you belong?
> *Old Man:* Catholic Christian.
> *Tokoto:* Now, if I want do something bad to somebody who try kill your son, what you say?
> *Old Man:* Evil for evil. If you do evil, you receive evil.
> *Tokoto:* Now say prayer, so God, who give us so much, also give me power to cure your son.

And the man recited the Our Father, in Ewondo, along with all his family. Then he and Tokoto clasped hands nine times over the sick child.

I was not interested in the rest of the treatment, and I drew Nkoa aside. Nombote saw us, and motioned to us to come and sit down with him in Tokoto's *dibandi*. Was he mistrustful of the influence I might have on Nkoa? The room was a simple one, with a table, three chairs, and a heap of such things as one can count on finding in a *nganga* sanctuary. I knew the special scent well now—an inextricable mixture of the odors of oil lamps, musk, incense, wax, and musty leaves.

The treatments were still going on, and the chants and beating of drums obliged us to speak in a loud voice. I questioned both Nombote and Nkoa on the words we had just heard. Was there not a flagrant contradiction, I asked, between an appeal for vengeance and the willingness to pardon—between rendering evil for evil, and the words of the Our Father, "Forgive us our trespasses, as we forgive those who trespass against us"? My intention was to prepare Nkoa to stand up like a Christian when the formidable family confrontation, which seemed inevitable now, would finally occur. The presence of Nombote, his sister's main accuser, raised the stakes in the discussion, and did not make it easy. We spoke in French.

"You see," Nombote began, "it's a matter of belief. Tokoto has to ask the papa, 'Do you really believe in God?' After all, God's the one who created us. Then the papa prayed for his son's healing. What do you find wrong with that? That's our custom."

"But they could have chosen another prayer," I replied. "They picked a prayer that said precisely that we are to forgive, two seconds after having spoken about revenge!"

"You have to go through the Son to get to the Father," said Nombote. "Jesus is the Son of God."

"But the words of the Our Father!" I cried. "We ask God to help us *heal* the sick. Very well, Jesus healed the sick. But Jesus also said we were to love our enemies!"

"I love sorcerers," replied Nombote.

"Would you mind telling me just how?"

"I repeat, I love sorcerers—if they admit their sins."

"And until they have," I said, pursuing my line of argument, "is it so dangerous to go and see them?"

"As far as I'm concerned, yes. At least you mustn't love a person who can kill."

I did not feel the time was right to handle "fraternal correction," and charity in general, in the presence of Nombote, who was being so ironical. I decided to come to grips with the problem concretely instead. "The sister has come. So what's to be done?"

"That's the same question I'm asking," Nkoa put in.

"There," I added, "there's the real problem."

"Well, now they're face to face," Nombote replied.

"Is she staying in the house?" I asked.

"Yes," Nkoa said. That's why I brought all the children here. It makes me afraid to have her home. Tonight when we go home I'm going to have to stay up. My wife won't like it if I go to sleep.

"Ask him if his sister isn't a sorceress," Nombote said to me. Then he addressed Nkoa: "I am Dr. Nombote and I am asking you a question. Is your sister, who has come from the west, not a sorceress?"

"Yes," I added, "this is an important question to ask."

"I wouldn't know anything about it," responded Nkoa, prudently. "I only know her as one who was born of the same parents."

I said, "Speak truly, straight from your heart."

"It's hard, Father," Nkoa began. "Saying something doesn't prove it to be true. I could tell you she's a sorceress, but deep down inside I'm not convinced. It's possible that she's a sorceress. Because she's at Kumba [a city in the west], I don't know her circumstances or situation. If it is true [that she has become a sorceress], well, that's what I'd consider her to be."

Nombote pressed his point: "Hasn't some teacher already told you she's a sorceress? Do we have to call your wife in and have her repeat that?"

"He didn't say her exactly. He just said I had a near relative who was a sorcerer, somebody with the same father and mother as I have."

"Where was that said?" asked Nombote.

"Near Saa [in Eton country, a region of Yaoundé]. A long way from here."

"Didn't the *nganga* accuse precisely your sister?" Nombote continued.

"No," replied Nkoa. "That's just who the family thinks it must be. My big sister lost her two children. The reason I suspect her is that I've been told she was the one who killed them. I suppose she's the one, then. But that's just on the outside. I still have an idea she wasn't the one."

"Was she there when they died?" Nombote now moved into the old accusation.

"I'd been transferred up north at that time."

"Were you told she was there?" asked Nombote.

"No, I heard she wasn't there when they died. She got there two days after the burial."

"The burial of her own children?"

"Yes, it's strange. The burial was over, and all of a sudden there was my sister."

In order to understand this conversation—which I could see tore Nkoa very much in two directions—the reader must know that a sorceress responsible for someone's death does not dare to assist at that person's burial, nor even see the corpse: if she does, she herself will die the following month. By absenting herself from her own children's burial, Clara indicted herself. This is the somber and singular history that was at the origin of the suspicion surrounding her in her family.

According to Nombote, Clara was what was called a "city sorceress." That is, she was not a born sorceress—an *ewusu*—but one become such in accordance with her own wish, or under someone else's influence. Even if the power to harm had been imposed on her against her will, at all events she acquired a taste for it—whereas the born sorceress does not always realize that she conducts such activities in the night, and that her double takes her place while she is asleep. The "city sorceress" was the *ekong* professional.

On Wednesday, February 13, I visited Nkoa at his place of employment, confident that I should not find Nombote there. His assignment with the Department of Public Works was to take soil samples from little piles of earth ranging from black to brick red, and send them to be studied before building a road. I watched him for a moment—the technician now, and yet the same person I had met a few days before in an altogether different cultural context—before approaching him. He told me that things were tense at home. His sister Clara was living with them in their father's medium-sized house. The father had asked Nkoa not to make the accusation public, lest his sister leave and never be seen again. For his own part, Nkoa encouraged his children to speak to their aunt, but his wife, Dorette, continued to maintain a very aggressive attitude. The animosity between the two sisters-in-law went back several months—to the moment of Clara's opposition to Nkoa's marriage, to be exact. It seemed she had even proposed another bride for Nkoa.

Nkoa also told me that Clara had given him 1,000 francs for the cost of Bruno's treatment, but that, when Nkoa had communicated the offer to Dorette, she had refused to accept it. Now I realized the intensity of the conflict between the two women.

On Saturday morning, February 16, on my way to see Nombote, I met Clara, with her brother Bruno, at the gate of Nombote's enclosure. I could not believe my eyes. The sorceress, the banished daughter, dared appear alongside her presumed victim—and at the home of the person accusing her! I concealed my surprise, and Bruno informed me that he had received permission to go out for a walk with Clara in the quarter, on condition that he not remove his red belt or the two ribbons that encircled his wrists. These, evidently, were to protect him against his sister's sorcery. I asked to be allowed to accompany the two on their slow perambulation. I looked at Clara. She was young, yet her face already wore a tired look. She had on a skirt and blouse, like most women in Douala. I saw no sign of emancipation about her except her hair, which was limp and oily instead of kinky.

Clara gave me her version of the story, which I noted down as soon as I returned home. It included an explanation of her strange absence when her two children had died. Her father, she told me, had sent someone to Kumba, a town in the west, to inform her that Bruno was ill. She was accused of trying to kill him, her little brother Bruno! And yet it was she who had taken on the task of rearing the child after the death of their mother. Why would she seek to kill him now?

She knew, of course, that she already stood accused of all the family calamities, including that of being the murderer of her two children! But the first had been killed in Douala, when she was in Yaoundé. He was watching the Canadian Circus leave the station in Douala, when he was struck by a train. The news had reached her only after much delay, and by the time she reached Douala the child had already been buried. The second died in Yaoundé, in the home of the family with whom he was staying. She was to have been informed by a radio announcement, but she was in Douala that day and did not listen to the radio. Again she arrived too late for the burial. Since that time she had been accused of everything that went wrong.

According to Clara the guilty one was Dorette, Nkoa's wife, who did not like her. It was she who had plotted the whole affair, in connivance with Nombote. "God must not be looking; if he were, surely he would intervene."

The young woman seemed sincerely crushed and bewildered. She added that I was scarcely helping things along. On the contrary, I was enhancing Nombote's credibility by my very presence. In her view every *nganga* was a charlatan. Her little brother ought to leave at once, before the final treatment. I remarked to her that she would be blamed for this, too, and that I thought it would be wiser for him to finish with Nombote, in view of the fact that Bruno himself felt that he was now on the way to being healed. I felt a special fellow feeling for her. Had I, too, not been caught one day in the treacherous pitfalls of *ekong?* I elicited her promise that she would arrange a meeting at which I would be given the opportunity to speak. Was I doing the right thing, to meddle in this family affair, when I had such difficulty understanding what went on between the lines? I did not know. But it was too late now to withdraw.

Saturday, February 16. This was the night Bruno was to receive his final treatment. I arrived at Nombote's at nine in the evening to attend the séance. I found Bruno there, but neither his brother nor Nombote. Bruno informed me that they had gone to the family dwelling to "armor" the house. He told me how surprised he was that his sister had been accused. She had always been so good to him, and had reared him until he was seventeen years old.

At ten o'clock, Nombote arrived, accompanied by a police inspector in civilian clothes, and Nkoa, who was obviously drunk. It had not taken many glasses to get the better of him in his present state of fatigue and discouragement. The police inspector, a friend of Nombote's, was there to make sure that Nkoa did not make a scene.

The inevitable had happened. After the rites of protection, performed in each room of the house, Nkoa had brought out two liters of wine, and called his wife, his sister, and his father. Almost at once, brother and sister had come to blows. Nkoa had beaten Clara severely, and she had run to the nearest police station to file a complaint, declaring that her brother had brought a sorcerer into the house, in the person of Nombote, with the intention of killing her. Nombote and the inspector had dragged Nkoa out of the house and brought him here.

Nkoa told me that there was now no doubt that his sister was a sorceress. Twice, she had taken his wife's footprints—at least, according to Dorette, she had—and had called his attention to the fact that she was wearing Turkish slippers, a remark that had considerable meaning in the circumstances. Anything personal taken from someone, were it only a footprint, could be interpreted as an indication of the intent to cast a spell on that person. The séance was cancelled.

Faci

Sunday, February 17. Nkoa came to our house while I was out and left a message that his little daughter Marthe had fallen seriously ill. I did not go to see him; I did not take the news very seriously. Events of the last days had left me somewhat jaded.

Monday, February 18. Returning to our house around noon, I found Oyono and Nkoa waiting for me. With that singular tone of detachment that goes with terrible news, they announced that little Marthe was dead. The youngest of Nkoa's and Dorette's five children, she died that morning at the hospital where they had taken her. Oyono and Nkoa showed me her death certificate. Under "cause of death" the physician had noted "FACI." The pair asked me what this stood for, but I did not know. Later I learned it meant that the baby had died of a *fiévre á cause indéterminée*, a "fever of undetermined cause." I took special care to conceal this from the family, lest it strengthen their suspicions. This was a notation generally used when symptoms indicated malaria but the diagnosis had not been confirmed. Had those doctors any notion of the effect such a vague suggestion could have had on the minds of a family in the state of Nkoa's?

Nkoa and Oyono had come to ask me to preside at the child's funeral. The two left before I could find it within me to speak a single meaningful word. I could only grasp their hands and tell them I would be there. Once more I was overwhelmed. It was not so much the disappearance of the child. What had left me speechless was the tragic coincidence of her death in the midst of a family conflict of precisely this nature.

I had had a similar feeling—or absence of feeling—in other circumstances, once upon a time, and it suddenly all came back to me. It had happened in Algeria, on one of our routine patrols. Riding along in the back of our truck, the better to be able to see all around, my fellow riflemen and I unexpectedly came upon a trio of corpses, stretched out next to one another by the side of the road. There was a strange detail about the scene—strange in this place, at any rate. They were all wearing factory workers' blue coveralls. Who were they? Who had killed them, our side or the fellahs? Why had they been left there? There were no answers to these questions, and so our truck started slowly on its way once more. A strange death, in a strange land. We rode on in silence, and the feeling we had then was like the feeling I had now.

On my way to visit the family, I went first to inform the pastor of the parish, then to Nombote's house to have someone show me the way to where the family lived, because I had not yet been there. Seeing me in my cassock, Nombote grasped what must have happened, and issued a terse warning: "Don't follow [don't make any connection with] the ceremony we had the other day, you see? Today it's a private matter."

I understood. He was advising me against making any allusions during the liturgy to the accusation against the sister. And he added simply, "The child died. Of course, after what happened Saturday."

Naturally everyone would make the connection anyway. The "evidence" against Clara had mounted to overpowering proportions. But I told Nombote that, in the circumstances, I had no right to keep silent—that my objective, however utopian, would be reconciliation.

In the room where little Marthe lay, on a white bed, and decked out like the Infant Jesus of Prague, I found I could not say what I had intended, because of the persons there in the room. Then the body was carried outside, as custom prescribed when there were other children at home, and placed in its tiny casket. Dorette, the mother, outwardly calm, took a seat with her back to the casket while it was being closed, then left hastily and did not return. Here again, it was custom that ruled.

When the moment arrived to leave for the cemetery, which was near the airport, I noticed that Clara was missing! It scarcely seemed to serve any good purpose to encourage suspicions in this fashion, I thought to myself, so I asked Nkoa to send for her.

"Why doesn't my big sister get out here?" Nkoa cried out to those grouped about. "She's a bit of trouble, that one!"

When Clara arrived, I took her, the old father, and Oyono in my car; Nkoa and his wife rode with the little casket. Thus the adversaries found themselves separated.

At the Strangers' Cemetery, all run down and overgrown with weeds, without paths, and looking more like an abandoned field than a last resting place, the ceremony for little Marthe was very simple. I merely recited the Our Father in French. I managed to conceal the great emotion I felt overcoming me, lest I precipitate some outburst from the family. After a brief silence, then, the little coffin was lowered into the grave, and we sprinkled it with holy water. Dorette, Clara, the old father, and Nkoa, stood side by side, impassive. As had been agreed upon beforehand, no one addressed the group.

On the way back in the car, Clara told me what I already knew: "Nkoa beat me and said I was a murderer. I cried all night for that little one."

Rarely have I felt such a desire to keep silent, and such a need to speak. Now or never, I had to do what little lay in my power, before Clara fled the family house for good. When everyone was seated, in the part of the house reserved for the old father, I gave them the following little talk. I had it memorized word for word, and Oyono translated it phrase by phrase:[52]

Here we are, then, all together—the grandfather, Nkoa and his wife Dorette, Clara, his eldest sister, and his two younger sisters, come for the mourning, and Bruno, their brother, and Oyono, your friend and mine.

I venture to speak to you after the funeral, because you are Catholics, and I am a priest. If I were only a European, I could not do what I am doing now. But I am a priest. That is, I am an intermediary between God and you. And I dare to speak to you because it is God who speaks to you by my mouth.

The problem in your family, just now, is disunity. This lamp is hanging from the ceiling by a wire. [Over our heads, a light bulb hung, without a shade, by a cord that was dangerously corroded.] If the cord breaks, the lamp will crash down and go out. Your family unity is hanging by a cord like this one—a very worn cord. Either you wait till it breaks, or you get a new one. The danger now is that Clara may leave and never come back to her family, for too many words have been spoken. When persons are hurting, they often are too ready to listen to anybody at all, and repeat any tale at all, without proof.

At the cemetery, we said the Our Father. And in the Our Father, we prayed these serious words: "Forgive us our trespasses as we forgive those who trespass against us." Your father has been trespassed against. Nkoa has been trespassed against. Clara has been trespassed against. And Dorette, too, has been trespassed against. God sees that. He does not ask you to forgive at once. Perhaps you will forgive in a year, or five years, or even ten years.

All of you are wounded. All God asks of you is not to destroy anything beyond repair this evening. If you do not, then the day may come when your family will be united once more. Be careful what you say. Be careful what you do. Do not say or do anything that might be impossible ever to repair.

When I had finished speaking, all kept silence, as I had expected. Precipitancy never had a place in these almost ritual celebrations of the word. I did not dare look at their faces, for fear some one of them might feel challenged.

Finally the grandfather coughed, thanked me, and to my surprise, began to tell a story, in his language. Oyono translated it for me, phrase by phrase. For me, until today, stories had only been a more or less educational amusement for children. Now I felt, for the first time, the appeasing, persuasive power it could have for adults.

It was the story of a hunter who had caught an animal in a trap. Instead of carrying it back to the village, and he skinned it and kept only its hide. But on the way home he thought to himself that he would surely be the laughingstock of the whole village, and retraced his steps. When he had finally managed to catch the animal once more—for it was still alive, and scampering about without its skin—he said to it: "If you go home like that, without your skin, everyone will make fun of you! So lie down for a moment." And the hunter, without further ado, killed the animal and carried it back to the village.

I needed to grasp the moral of the story, so I asked the grandfather to explain it in clear terms. He told me that he had left his village for Douala alone, once upon a time, before he had a wife and children. If he were to return now with just part of his family—that is, without his eldest daughter—how would he be received?

When it was Bruno's turn to speak, he observed that I had not asked for an immediate response. He reserved the right to give his later. He understood that, this evening, it was best to say nothing.

The grandfather encouraged Clara to speak, but she declared simply, "I have nothing to say." Perhaps she had expected me to come right out and say that she had been accused unjustly. But the tension among the family members since that morning had been such that a bomb of that sort would either have sputtered and failed to go off, because it would have been alleged to have been hurled by a European who knew nothing of African sorcery, or else it would have exploded and provoked a brand-new battle.

It was extremely clear to me at this moment what effect a belief—any belief—shared by a collectivity can have on the interpretation of facts and the determination of a judgment.

I had had a similar experience in Kribi, during a treatment that I was photographing. The circumstances were less dramatic, and I was far enough removed from the action to be able to analyze the machinery of belief without the risk of interfering with it myself. That evening we were seated in a circle around the treatment area, and the *nganga*, lance in hand, was making ready to deal his patients his miraculous blows, so as to kill the invisible worm the sorcerers had cast down within their insides—when suddenly a huge lizard crept out into the middle of the path and stopped, wagging its head from side to side. For a moment the *nganga* stood rigid with shock. Then he transfixed it with his lance. Finally he trussed the beast up like a roasting pig, grilled it, and put it aside, to make a medicine later. I considered the incident finished, and inconsequential. But at daybreak we learned that someone in the neighborhood had died. "We expected that," the *nganga* told me. The appearance of this particular lizard, called an *ewedi*, was a presage of death.

Belief, then, feeds on events, little and great, which are selected and interpreted in terms of a guiding idea that has already had its proofs.

During this family meeting, so soon after the burial of a child, I felt incapable of helping persons so convinced of the reality of sorcery, and so recently confirmed in their belief, to put the necessary distance between themselves and what had happened. Nkoa, me and Nombote, soon informed that notwithstanding Clara's charges of *nganga* charlatanism, she had paid 1,000 francs to a disciple of Nombote's for protective medicines—for "armor." The young woman was no exception, then. But I wanted to wait to speak with Nkoa about sorcery, without anyone else present, and I promised myself I would speak my mind on the ambiguity of the pretexts for the accusations lodged against his sister.

The opportunity came the day after the funeral. On Wednesday, February 20, Nkoa and I had a quiet conversation in my home. He told me of things that had happened earlier—things that enabled me to understand the entrenched positions, and things that lent strength to Nkoa's convictions.

My own position—and that was what I sought to help Nkoa to come to see—was that sorcery was not the only plausible interpretation of sickness and death. There were other systems of explanation—that of modern medicine, for instance. Hence one could not—without the risk of being wrong—accuse Clara of responsibility for the death of little Marthe. My objective may seem to have been modest, and my argumentation timid, but I discerned no chink in the solid wall of the logic of sorcery. I had seen this often enough, and at my own cost. Clever indeed was the one who could concede the premises and yet the fallacy. And so I contented myself with suggesting to Nkoa that the existence of other attitudes in the face of the problem of evil might make his own a relative one, and consequently uncertain. Here is some of our conversation.

"How long have your wife and sister not been getting along?" I asked.

"Say, eleven years—since we were married. My mother knew she was going to die. She'd told me, 'Now I'm going to give you advice on a woman to marry. That way you'll think of me all the time.' I was very obedient, so I finally went to see that woman. It was Dorette. Less than six months later my mother died. Dorette was still very young.

"My big sister ran around quite a bit; she had even gone to the Mozart quarter [with its red-light district]. She had left her husband and become a prostitute. I don't know what she was thinking of. She introduced me to other girls. She would say, 'At least they would keep house properly!' It's true my wife didn't know how to do anything at first. I said, 'I want a wife who can speak and understand French!' I gave Dorette lessons. Now she can do a letter for you, except for the mistakes in grammar. . . .

"But just two years ago my big sister sent a girl from Kumba, where she is right now, for me to marry, so I would get rid of Dorette. . . .' "

"All right, your sister might be a woman of loose morals," I said, "but I have to say honestly that I don't think she'd be capable of killing her own children, or Bruno either. In all this sorcery business, there's one part imagination. Yes, of course, there are those who try to use sorcery against others. They take advantage of other persons' beliefs. They scare them to death. But I don't believe Clara killed her own children. She's not a monster. She didn't try to hurt Bruno."

"Father, you surprise me."

"Your sister couldn't have killed her own children!" I repeated, vehemently. "Look, every single accusation against her rests on the fact that she wasn't at the funerals of her two children. I know about that—when somebody has sold a family member, they can't be at the funeral."

"Right, if they look at the corpse they die."

"I'm saying that you can explain why Clara wasn't at the funerals in another way! The first child died in Yaoundé when she was in Douala. The second died later, in Douala, when she was in Yaoundé. Is this true or isn't it?"

"Yes, yes," Nkoa admitted.

"Fine. She was supposed to hear it on the radio. But she didn't have to be always listening to the radio. And you—you told me the other day you had doubts, yourself. Don't forget that, Nkoa. At first you had doubts."

"That she could do such a thing?"

"They said she was responsible for Bruno's illness because she had already shown what kind of person she was. You see, everything is based on her two children's death."

"How about little Marthe? She died too."

"As for Marthe, I asked a doctor. It's called 'FACI'. It's a fever like malaria. A child at that age can die in two days from this fever."

"Then why . . . why did this thing happen to occur just when I wasn't home?" (Nkoa had been away when his little girl had been carried off by the fever.) "My children take Nivaquine every other day! I've even got Quiniforme! I was a medic myself before going to Public Works. I only call the doc when it's really bad."

"But the child's death can be explained medically! True, it's a terrible coincidence."

"I believe you. I don't want to be like [the doubting] Thomas. Nobody's infallible. But there are lots of strange goings-on here."

"Nombote made an impression on you," I said. "Don't forget that the first *nganga*, out where you lived before, had said it was one of your brothers or sisters, not necessarily Clara. Then all of a sudden we started hearing about a second *nganga* accusing Clara!"

Nkoa went home. I sat a little while longer, wondering what the chances were that I had shaken him in his convictions. Not the slightest, I decided.

On Saturday, March 2, Nkoa stopped by the house to let me know that Clara had gone back to Kumba. He also invited me to share the ninth-day repast with his extended Eton family. The ninth-day was the observance at which the last meal was served to the deceased child—theoretically, nine days after death. Where she lived now, her playmates in the land of death were reproaching her for not yet having invited them to dine with her. Nkoa smiled as he gave me this explanation, but he submitted to custom. The women would cook up a bit of everything today—meat, fish, peanut butter, herbs, and vegetables.

To begin, some morsels were cast here and there inside the house, then outside, so that the ancestors and the dead child could have their portions. The house had not been swept since the day of her death. Next, the children of the neighborhood, Bamiléké, Eton, or Bassa, whoever had known little Marthe, were invited to come and eat something. Finally, the adults took their turn—mostly Eton, and a few guests. No one might carry any of this food away. It had to be partaken of right here.

As I mingled with this family during the ninth-day repast, I reflected on their moral stamina. It seemed extraordinary to me that they could have been able to live for several days and nights with a person who, they were convinced, had plotted the death of family members! European nerves could not have stood it. Sorcery, then, which involved murder, was both something tragic and something relatively well tolerated. The death ceremonies, of which the ninth-day was only one phase, was part of a response to it. Belief and ritual affect the interpenetration of the world of the dead and the world of the living. In the period following death, the trauma of those who saw rigor mortis transform a familiar body was immediately engulfed in the obligations of funeral and family ritual, and was conjured away, as it were. It took on a vital meaning. Death became more bearable—and death's fomenters less fearsome.

I had already had occasion to appreciate the importance of funeral rites several years before, in Yaoundé, where I was a chaplain at the university. A student had suddenly and unexpectedly died during an operation for appendicitis. An ambulance had transported his body to his place of residence—the university campus—but where was it to be left? The ambulance personnel had not found a better place than simply in the gymnasium, on a ping-pong table.

Later I understood why his companions had been so traumatized, even though the body was later transported to the village and the funeral was celebrated in accordance with custom. Even long after, several of them recalled the shock they had felt, and how their conception of death had been shaken. Life had completely ceased, they said. I reminded them that their traditions and Christianity were of a mind here—it was life that won out. But no, they had seen their comrade's corpse, profaned, lying on a table meant for play. Death, deprived of both its traditional and its Christian apparatus and symbols, had appeared to them in all its radical starkness.

All belief, including belief in sorcery, allows societies to assimilate the phenomenon of death and softens the fear that flows from it.

The ninth-day repast slowly came to an end. There were a few remonstrances addressed to Nkoa, by a delegate of the Eton youth and by the chief, concerning his irregular attendance at family meetings. Oyono, who had been my invaluable intermediary throughout this drama, translated for me what was said and enlightened me as to what was being suggested by innuendo—namely, that the cohesiveness of the extended family was what enabled the nuclear family to perdure.

But now the serenity of this ceremony was disturbed by a representative of the family by marriage—Dorette's uncle. He addressed a single question to the chief. Why had little Marthe's paternal grandfather not touched, or looked at, the child's remains? "What?" protested the old man. "Now I too am accused of killing this child!" I asked Oyono whether this sort of thing often went on at ninth-day ceremonies, and he replied in the negative.

I withdrew, all bemused again. The sorcery, it seemed, was transpiring at the point of conjunction of the two families—Nkoa's, and that of the in-laws. Two clans had come into confrontation, the one standing with the victim, the other with the sorcerer. Being in command of a precise knowledge of family structures, experienced diviners or *nganga* know in advance what the points of latent opposition are. Then an affliction occurs, in the form of disease or death, and they know where the Achilles' heel is in the family, and thus whom to accuse.

Nkoa drove me home. "We're going to move out," he said. "The children are having nightmares. The littlest one calls to his sister as if he could see her. But my wife and I will have another child. In a week or two, when I have the money, I'll get both families together again. We'll kill two goats, and I'll tell them what we've decided.

Accusation and *Nganga* Therapy

Bruno looked like a well man. He was back in his brother's home, and Nkoa had found him a job with Public Works. Things had happened so fast that I had been unable to have conversations with him, to form some idea of the psychosomatic nature of his illness. I had to be satisfied with an account couched in traditional categories—how he had been sold by his sister Clara through sorcery? Had his anxiety been basically calmed? That would depend on the impact Nombote's interpretation would have on the inner recesses of the young man's psychology.

Two factors obliged me to regard my prognosis with some hesitation. Bruno had been surprised, of course, to learn that his sister had bewitched him. On the other hand, toward the end of his stay with Nombote, a nightmare had made a great impression on him: he had dreamt that Clara's elder son, his playmate from the days when they were reared together in her house, assaulted him and beat him with his fists. He had told me of this dream, but apparently had said nothing about it to Nombote. Only the future would tell whether the combined efforts of Nombote and a great part of Bruno's family had influenced him sufficiently to convince him that the cause of his affliction had indeed been uncovered. Suppose he had been cured for good—could not the accusation have been dispensed with? Did Bruno's happiness really have to be tied to Clara's unhappiness? Was a sorceress necessary?

Nombote had proceeded no differently from his colleagues. I set myself to recalling to mind the various treatment séances at which I had assisted. I always remembered an accusation. The target was not always a sorcerer. In some cases it was the ancestors who were on the docket—or even the subject, as in the case of Elimbi, Loe's "unlucky son," saddled with the responsibility for his own frustrations. But pointing the accusatory finger at the guilty party always seemed to be part of the therapy. Differences in a *nganga*'s tone derived from circumstances: the practitioner's fear of being reported to the police, fear of reprisals in a village where everyone knew everyone else, a concern not to traumatize the victim. All these considerations contributed to determine the degree of publicity the accusation would have.

The *nganga*'s accusation was part of the therapy, then. Even if he or she did not come right out and name the guilty party, the mere fact of possessing the secret produced a healing effect. I had seen patients arrive in the greatest pain and distress, totally helpless in the arms of a relative, and then recover some of their strength of spirit merely at the sight of the *nganga*. And when the *nganga* ventured to name the guilty one, the family was truly consoled. The veil of anonymity had been lifted. The danger had been circumscribed, delimited.

A therapeutic procedure that makes one person's welfare another's misery will appear altogether inhumane, of course, unless one keeps in mind the socio-cultural context. There are resources available to enable the family to reintegrate the accused person. The structures of reconciliation had not come into play in this particular case, owing to a number of irregularities. Nombote had left Clara no chance at all. He had said she was a sorcerer, explicitly and by name. Other *nganga*s were much more adroit. They manipulated vague allusion, they forestalled confrontations.

Nombote owed his confidence here, as far as I could gather, to statements on the part of Dorette concerning the life and reputation of her enemy

Clara. For her part, Clara had broken the rules of tradition by going to the police instead of to the head of the family—who, after all, lived right there in the quarter. She had insulted custom, where ceremonies of reconciliation play on semiconfession and semisilence to conclude to repentance, and then a goat is sacrificed in place of the accused.

Secondly, the sorcerer, male or female, enjoys a certain immunity. This immunity is not due solely to the modern legal system that protects a sorcerer from family vendetta and abstains from any judgment of its own unless faced with a disturbance of the public order. (We have only to think of Din's trial. Reprisals are rare simply because everyone knows that they may fall under the same accusation themselves one day. Not all family catastrophes are imputed to the same person. Tomorrow it may be Dorette's turn. Extremely complex rules for the interplay of family relationships imposed the burden of evil now on one, now on another, in such wise that sorcerers suffer but relative, provisional isolation. The attitude toward them may be only that of pure politeness, but they continue to mingle with the family, without dramatic confrontation. Definitive exclusion of a family member because of sorcery is, it seems to me, very rare. And never is there a unanimous long-term accusation of one person.

Sorcerers continue to have a place in the family. When all is said and done, they serve a useful function. Clara's exclusion would have involved the risk of having to point the accusing finger at someone else—the day, for example, another of Nkoa's children were to fall gravely ill. The unconscious fear of a greater danger than that of disease explains the patience, indeed the indulgence, the group shows toward its "indicted," despite formidable counts on the indictment. My feeling was that the group, in its ambivalent search for the guilty party, whom it does not really punish, was fortifying itself against an infinitely more disturbing threat: that of its own collapse. The group owed its relative serenity to the rotated assignment of responsibility for trouble to its various members.

The best image of this salutary therapy I had ever seen was provided by Loe one evening, as he completed one of his treatments, back in the days when I used to visit him with such eagerness and regularity. He began flipping burning coals upon his patient, who was dressed in an ample red sash, her battle symbol. She would promptly deflect each coal out toward us, as we stood around watching, by savagely snapping her sash at it. Then we in the entourage would kick them around among ourselves until the fire went out.

I had learned one thing very well indeed. Accusation played an important role in the practice of traditional medicine. As far as I could see, a *nganga* could not forego it without depriving a patient's treatment of a measure of its effectiveness.

Now I really had to face up to the old question that had been gnawing at me ever since the start of my research. How could Christians—and in

Douala country this would include the *nganga*s and their whole clientele—reconcile the practice of accusation with their faith. The seeming off-handedness with which a person was accused of the most heinous crimes, including the murder of their own children, had often shocked me. Of course I understood the reason for these charges better when I situated them in a cohesive cultural context, along with compensatory rites that tempered their effects. Would not the principal contradiction lie rather in the fact that charity seemed nonsensical? For it was, literally, "non-sense" in the eyes of a *nganga*.

Understanding charity in its gospel meaning, as a love extending even to one's enemies, the question arises: Is it possible to love one's sorcerer? On this essential point the answers were all negative. Din, Loe, then Nombote and Tokoto, all agreed: it was not appropriate really to love the one who was practicing sorcery against you. You would risk enhancing their baleful power over you and those around you. Patients told me the same thing. "Sorcerers can't hurt you if you hate them." One could love them halfway, but not altogether. And Clara's story was an example.

I had never heard such a radical objection to love, to charity. Charity can be considered utopian. One can doubt its practical implementation. But here charity is paradoxically held responsible for bringing on hatred! I believe I had discovered here one of the principal sources of the vague uneasiness I felt from the first moment I had entered the *nganga* sphere, and part of the reason for the profound distance between that universe and mine.

Chapter 11

The Mountain *Khamsi*

"Water washes the face;
it does not wash away
misfortune."

I entered the world of the *khamsi*s, the oracles of the Bamiléké mountains, in the same way as I had entered that of Din, Loe, Nombote, and Tokoto—simply by walking up and introducing myself.

I tell the story of this encounter here because this is where it came in my own journey. The events I am about to relate occurred some two hundred kilometers north of Douala, in a specific geographical and cultural context, via a language I did not speak. Discouraged by the sometimes painfully dramatic events I have just recalled, where magic and Christian faith, ancestral beliefs and modern aspirations, inextricably intermingled and a little uneasy as to what to do next, I longed to find a cohesive traditional society that I could feel comfortable with, and that would reconcile me with the *nganga* world.

Having already traversed Bamiléké country from end to end, I knew, as did everyone, that its inhabitants still succeeded in keeping their traditions alive, in the shadow of their great chiefs. Neither modern life, in which they participated en masse—Douala is some 50 percent Bamiléké—nor Islam, nor Christianity, which touched about 30 percent of the population, had enfeebled their customs. I hoped to find a diviner or a *nganga* there who would be worthy of the name.

I chose the territory of the chief of Bamendjou, near the Batié Pass (1500 meters high), because I was on good terms with the pastor there and with the Poor Clare nuns, who had promised to obtain the good offices of Chief Sokoundjou in my behalf. One did not just barge into a chief's residence!

I was well aware that the time I had to spend in these green and red mountains—six weeks all told—would surely be too short for me to be able to situate the *nganga* with precision within the vast cultural and anthropological context of this "jurisdiction"—as a chief's territory might be called.

This trip was but an excursion, a jaunt, away from my usual place of re-search. But fortune smiled, and I was to be able to take advantage of certain favorable circumstances that counterbalanced the disadvantages of such a short sojourn. The country was completely at peace, for the first time in years. The period of the underground resistance was at an end. Several tens of thousands of persons had met their deaths in these regions between 1957 and 1970.[53] The chief had celebrated the restoration of unity with a great feast. A few years earlier, I should not have had any liberty to move about or conduct my research.

I had the feeling of being the beneficiary of a kind of benign conspiracy entered into by the great institutional bodies—the chief's jurisdiction, the state, and the church. Thanks to the mother superior of the Poor Clares, who had received the title of *Mafo*, or Chief's Mother, her French national-ity notwithstanding, I was instructed in the local traditions by the chief's deputy himself, who was a former catechist and a leading personage of the chief's jurisdiction, and I was sent to the *khamsi* by the pastor himself. After all those years of mistrustfulness, looks were friendly once more. In fact, I had the feeling that my presence was a help, amid the general desire of the people to start working together again.

"God's Important Person"

One morning, following directions I had been given by the pastor, I turned off the red-dirt main road leading from the seat of the chief's juris-diction to the Batié Pass, and took a road to the right, cutting sharply down into the valley. This was the little road to the *khamsi*'s dwelling. I drove carefully now, for the grass was high under the wheels, and the road nar-row. Any second I might smack into a stone, and this worry kept me from contemplating, as peacefully or as frequently as I should have liked, the pattern of low, gently sloping mountain ridges. Except for the more sharply contrasting colors here, the landscape was like that of Auvergne. In the rainy season, the dark green of the vegetation encroaches everywhere on the brick red of the lateritic soil.

I had to leave the car on the road. A path, lined by a bamboo fence on one side and white-trunked shrubs on the other, led down to what was ob-viously someone's property. I made my way down this path, and at last found the *khamsi*'s hut, at the very bottom of the valley. I was not surprised at its isolation: every Bamiléké family lives by itself, surrounded by fields. To get to the hut, I had to go through still another fence, as well as a little barrier built to keep goats out. The hut was like all those I had seen along the way—a cube, as high as it was wide, made of fat bricks of red earth, and covered by a sheet-iron roof like a three-cornered hat. I could see the minus-cule windows, one or two on each side, just big enough to stick your head through, and the narrow door. One's social life was well protected here. I noticed nothing else about the surroundings, as I was too caught up in antic-

ipation of the meeting that was about to take place. I knew that everything
depended on the success of the first contact.

I came upon a country woman, seated on a bench at the door, vehemently
expostulating with a young man standing before her. She interrupted her
discourse suddenly at my appearance and looked at me. I remember nothing
of that moment but the look of her eyes. Before the young man had even
noticed I was there, the woman had plumbed the very depths of me with
that gaze. Her astonishingly intense, brown eyes seemed to flood you with
their look. Fascinating eyes they were, as of someone having a hallucination
—yet with a reassuring little gray gleam of mischievousness.

With the young man as my interpreter, I told the *khamsi* of my research. I
made no effort to hide that fact that I was a priest. She "adopted" me on
the spot, I could see, with the sure discernment she had so long practiced
with visitors who came to hear her reveal their secret desires. And indeed I
had come to her without any ulterior motives or preconceived notions. Doc-
umentation on her function was practically nonexistent. The solitary thing I
knew about her was her title, *khamsi*, and its etymology—"God's important person," which meant someone whose task it was to practice divination. I should have to discover everything else by groping in the dark.

As if calling me as a witness somehow—because I was a teacher—the
young man changed the subject. He let it be known what he and his mother
had been battling about. He had gone to accounting school, in Yaoundé,
the capital, for two years now, but money had run out, and he had had to
leave before completing his course. He had come to spend his school vacation with his mother, as always, and now the *khamsi* wanted to keep him
with her two days longer, in order to perform the traditional rites for finding work before sending him back to the city.

I could guess the real reason for his resistance. He simply had no taste for
the traditional rites. After all, this was a young man whose interests cen-
tered on the new way of life, whatever difficulties and unpleasantness might
accompany it. There was no escaping this confrontation of two worlds,
however far I might wander from the great cultural centers!

She seemed so young, with her round face, brick-ocher, her dishevelled
mop of hair, her bulging forehead. One might have taken her for the sister
of this young man stubbornly standing up to her. She fixed him with her
look. She was furious and upset. Everything about the two of them was
different except their apparent similarity in age. She wore the brown tunic
of a country woman, and was barefoot. He was dressed like the man-about-
town, in his fancy shirt, blue jeans, and pointed shoes—all the rage on the
boulevards those days. He stood erect before her, seeming to hesitate between insolence and submission. The rest of the family was doubtless in the
fields, and these two were alone.

What was at stake in their dispute was very clear. I was reminded of a
similar situation in Douala, when Loe had proposed to his son Elimbi that
he undergo treatment for "bad luck"—that Loe treat him so that he might

find work. The young men were of the same age, were in the same year in school, and had the same hesitation regarding a tradition ceremony.

The *khamsi*'s son, whose name was Jean Fotsing, finally decided to submit to her wishes. I asked to be allowed to assist at the rites, very curious to know whether the *khamsi* would proceed with them as Loe had. She promptly accepted and asked me simply to come for her in my car the next afternoon, because the ceremony would take place elsewhere. By way of leave-taking, she took my head between her hands and blew in my ears and nostrils.

The Tomb of the Skull

I spent that night at the convent of the Poor Clares. The following day, at the appointed hour, the *khamsi*, her son Jean, several children, and a paternal aunt of Jean, all climbed into my car. The *khamsi* had me take the road for the next jurisdiction, Bamendjou. The ceremony would take place in a hamlet of the region where the young man had been born, his father's town. We made a short stop there, without getting out of the car. With her unkempt mop of mahogany hair, her superb red ritual robe, and a European at the wheel of the car, the *khamsi* scarcely passed unnoticed! But she was treated with surprise and reserve, and I would later know the reason why.

We left the village and pulled up to the edge of a vast homestead that lay in ruins. I could make out the remains of the buildings in the tall grass, which came up to my chin. There would have been the master's house, flanked by four smaller, cubiform huts for his wives. This must have been a beautiful estate. I could imagine the buildings when they were new—all of large pink bricks, and topped by elegant roofs, thatched in the traditional manner in the form of a conical hat, like a tarboosh. Today sheet iron replaces thatching nearly everywhere.

The *khamsi* walked up to a banana tree in the proximity of one of the fallen-down huts, recollected herself a moment, and then gathered up a handful of earth—that heavy, black volcanic earth that made this such rich farmland. Jean Fotsing, at my side, explained to me that his mother was gathering earth from the place where his father's skull lay buried, or rather from its presumptive location, inasmuch as no one knew exactly where he had died. This gesture referred to a whole history, which it is important to know in order to understand the meaning and subtleties of the liturgy that was about to follow.

The *khamsi*'s husband had died fifteen years before, when Jean Fotsing was still small. The year was 1959, and it was the eve of independence. The guerrillas were on the rampage. "I heard my father was killed because he was rich. He traded in sheep. In this village, the rich were merchants. First they came for the sheep. Then when there were no more sheep they killed my father." You could still make out where the pens had been, over near the houses. The situation was confused at that time, and no one could say whether it was the guerrillas or their adversaries who had dragged the father out of his house and killed him. The *khamsi* had not been present that night, but she was unshakable in her conviction that the villlagers had committed the murder.

There is a chronicle from this same troubled period recounting how a young man named Gabriel Soh had been executed, on the very spot where the Poor Clares would build one day, for having sought to protect the parish priest, Father Fonjo, from being maltreated or killed. This little book about the young man's martyrdom reports that "dissident guerrillas, the 'killer-killers,' were in this region adjacent to Bamendjou. They killed all Cameroonians, without distinction, who refused to join them. . . . Engagements took place between the guerrillas and the 'killer-killers.'"[54]

The location where the *khamsi* had gathered the black earth was called the "tomb of the skull"—*tunösi*.[55] Because no one knew—or at any rate no one wished to tell—exactly where Jean's father had died, the family had had to call on the services of a *sunku*, who located such places by divination. It had taken the *sunku* a long time, but suddenly a frenzy came upon him and he fell down there. Here was the place, then.

Unlike the peoples of the south, who attach the memory of their dead to trees, the Bamiléké consider the skull of their forebears to be the medium of their presence. They perform a ritual of transfer of the skull from outside the house to inside. It is not a matter of effectuating the material presence of the departed, but of maintaining a physical bond with them, without which the dead would no longer have any relationship with the living.

The *khamsi* now moved to the door of the ruined central dwelling. Here is where the ceremony would take place, for it was here the sinister procession was thought to have begun the day her husband was killed. She had the children make a clearing in the weeds. She was still carrying her handful of black earth. She now called for a large, shiny, new ceramic vase, and placed the earth within it. This earth represented Jean Fotsing's father—or, more precisely, *is* Jean Fotsing's father, as would be explained to me. It was something much more important than simply a sign or symbol. As will appear in the rest of the account, it represented the real presence of the person himself.

Next, a red powder called *hwosi* (literally, "God's medicine")—a mixture of mahogany and clay, with which *khamsi*s plastered their hair, face, arms and legs—was mixed with this earth. Then a white dust (*mbö*), which was mostly clay and was a sign of blessing, was added. In addition to the two kinds of sacred powders, the *khamsi* placed a number of *dethum* pods in and around the vase—something never omitted from ceremonies at which she presided, nor indeed from any of the great rites of this jurisdiction. These brown, oblong pods, the size of a thumb, betokened love and reconciliation.[56] Now the vase, called a *tse*, had been filled in the same fashion as the ones containing the actual skulls of forebears and buried in their graves.

What a strange power of transformation! This priestess of the crumbling wall, whose liturgical paraphernalia were a pot, a handful of black dirt, and two kinds of powder, one red and one white, and whose entire congregation consisted of our little group sitting on the ground before her, and never taking our eyes from her for a moment, was so self-assured, her gestures so simple and majestic, and her vestments so sparkling, that, with the complicity of the setting sun, she had truly transformed this little corner of the wild into a holy place. The exaltation and beauty of the scene vanquished me completely.

This ceremony—placing a skull in its vase, or some black earth if the skull is not to be had—ought to have been performed long before. But the villagers, for reasons that would only gradually be clear to me, had always opposed it. And yet, without these customary rites, the departed father would wander forever, unable to return to his homestead, and relationships among the members of his family would never be normal. Jean Fotsing had not succeeded in his studies, nor had he been able to find satisfactory employment. Was this not to be attributed to the fact that his father was dissatisfied, and had not yet given the boy his blessing (*ndo*)? A man did not succeed in life without the approval of his father, dead or alive. I recognized the same motives as had driven Loe to treat his son when he had been unemployed. The prime condition of social balance was for a young man to take his proper place as son in his father's household. In this way he would be better prepared to take on a man's work.

Now that the vase had been prepared, the *khamsi* placed it on the ground upside-down, and asked us to sit in the clearing facing the door of what had been the central dwelling. "He looks like his father," she told me, glancing at Jean and then smiling at me.

Then she produced a kind of bean cake from her breadbasket and invited us to partake of it. Had she been wealthy, she said with a sigh, she would have killed a buck. Carefully and attentively, she distributed pieces of cake to each one among us, then cast the rest to the four winds, in a gesture calculated to represent a gift to the omnipresent God. I learned that she had done her duty to God the evening before, as well, by setting a chicken free in the wild. No one would ever again be able to lay a hand on it. All these gestures, including that of eating the cake, were a way of inviting both living and dead to accept in good part the ceremony that was about to begin, and not to place any obstacle in its way. The *khamsi* touched nothing of what we ate. She was satisfied to nibble little pieces of earth she could gather in her fingers from the brick wall, to recall that she was not a stranger in this place. She smiled meaningfully for my benefit, thinking there must be many elements in this scenario that escaped me.

The aunt, the four children, Jean, and I did the honors as to the cake. One of the little girls was a miniature *khamsi* herself, with her unkempt head of sticky, reddish hair. "She will be a *khamsi* too when she gets big," I was assured. An old friend of the father, who had been passing by, had also joined our group. He was surprised at my presence, and made some remark about my tape recorder.[57] The *khamsi* reassured him that I was from the convent of the Poor Clares.

And now the *khamsi* turned to Jean Fotsing.

"Go get dressed," she said.

"How do you expect me to get into that thing?" answered Jean, in French.

"If you haven't got a knife, cut it with your fingernails," said the mother.

The "thing" was a skirt, made of long, dead banana leaves (*möfet*). Jean was to remove his jeans and put on the skirt. "I should've brought my old jeans along," he grumbled, still in French. When the master of the house dies, his wives and children must all wear skirts of such leaves for seven days of mourning.

"Go get dressed as you're told," the father's friend insisted. "Gird your loins with that. Next it'll be my turn." I encouraged Jean with a little reflection about the value of the traditions, for I feared he might hesitate if I said nothing.

While Jean was changing, one of the little girls brought an earthenware jar full of water from the brook and poured it into the sacred vase. The aunt was content with just collecting a stack of green leaves, whose purpose would soon be evident.

Now the *khamsi* began a monologue, aloud. As spokesperson of her husband, whom she knew to be present, she uttered sentences and phrases incomprehensible to the uninitiated: "May his estate be overgrown with grass as this one! . . . When the war came the villagers were scattered. . . . They came to pick a quarrel with me by the brook." Shortly I would understand the meaning of these sentences, which were quietly translated for me by the father's friend. But first I had to know the dramatic story of the *khamsi*.

Pauline Nkwedum had married wealthy Tampa, owner of these lands, and had borne him, first, two children who died at an early age, and then Jean Fotsing. After Tampa's murder, Pauline had continued to live on the estate for a while, but soon married a neighbor. Then "madness" had seized her (not an "ordinary" madness, I was assured), and her behavior became abnormal. For example, she would be out on the road naked, and utterly unconcerned about it. Later she would accuse her new husband of having spent his money on drink instead of buying medicines for her. But her madness was not simply a medical matter. God had "taken hold" of her to reveal to her knowledge of hidden realities.

"I was suffering," Pauline Nkwedum explained to me, "and so the *khamsi*s sent me out, with one of them, an old man, to sacrifice a buck. We had to carry oil and *dethum* out to a particular place. Then I went down the road to Bafoussam, and on the way an old *khamsi* mother worked on me, gave me some *dethum*. When I got to Bafoussam I went to the house of another *khamsi*, and I immediately started speaking. It was God himself *(Si)* who gave me the authorization."

Khamsis, the "important ones of God"—men or women "grasped" by God—essentially have the function of "speaking," of telling the truth that God whispers to them. Most of them have experienced a crisis like Pauline's in the form of a mental disturbance, but it is always other *khamsis* "who show them the way." These awe-inspiring circumstances give them an incontestable authority.

An amazing therapy indeed. This is how one particular society treats certain forms of emotional illness in its members. It assigns the afflicted one a lofty religious and social function, corresponding in some way to their particular mental imbalance, instead of categorizing them irrevocably as mad or insane.

Now transformed, Pauline Nkwedum, the new *khamsi*, returned to the village, where she began to reveal to everyone the truth about themselves. She had a great deal to say, especially about those who murdered her first husband. She seems to have taken advantage a bit of her freedom of speech: *khamsis* who have the general welfare at heart do not have to tell all they know. And so the villagers did what they could to get her to leave. It was Jean Fotsing's aunt, present at the ceremony, who told me all this. Pauline Nkwedum, on the other hand, would later tell me publicly that she had left the village because God forced her to. "I didn't want to leave. God beat me. He tied my arms and took me to Batié. I shouted, 'No, no, no, I don't want to go there,' but God took me there, and when I got there he untied me."

Still later—without contradicting herself, really, for the mystical explanation continued to hold the primacy—she alluded to the harassments concocted by the villagers to make her life impossible and oblige her to leave of her own accord. The aunt added that the men of the village took turns at the brook to prevent her from carrying out the ritual ablutions. Twice a week, *khamsis* must bathe in running water, out of sight of any living human being, to purify themselves. Thwarted in the exercise of her function, the *khamsi* fled her village to come and live on Batié, with a *nganga* called Fotpa, who took her into his home and married her. It was in the house of this third husband, where she practiced the art of divination, that I met her for the first time, with Jean Fotsing.

"May My Power Work upon My Son"

Now Jean was ready. Stripped to the waist, with plaited thongs of banana leaves wrapped tightly around his body from the waist down, he stood somewhat awkwardly facing the main door, precisely over the spot where the ritual vase had been placed on the ground. His mother placed two smooth, flat little pebbles, which a *khamsi* used for various purposes, in his mouth, and prepared to bathe him by passing over his body bundles of leaves streaming with ritual water.[58]

The water would remove any curses *(ndo)* from him that might be at the root of his stubborn bad luck (*nösot*; in Douala, *mbeu'a nyolo,* "provoked bad luck"). Now the aunt began vigorously rubbing Jean Fotsing all over. "The leaves are falling off! Should we pick them up?" a child asked.

"Of course not!" the *khamsi* replied. "If the leaves are falling, that's proof that the purification is working fast!"

All the while these lustrations were in progress, aunt and mother exchanged reflections, aloud, protesting their innocence. "No, I couldn't help the bad luck that came crashing down on this boy. I have no reason to curse him!"—and the like.

The aunt said, "I'm here with little Jeannette [her daughter, who had fetched the water]. We have the same mouth [we are of one accord], we daughters of the same mother. All of us children of Taba [their ancestor], we are one. We have the same mouth. Fotsing, whatever be the obstacle you find on your road through our fault, may it disappear. If anything lucky happens to you, may you profit by it!"

"May my supreme power [received from God] come forward and work on my son," said the *khamsi* in her turn.[59] "As long as I lived in this dwelling, the one abandoned today, I never deceived anyone. I didn't go to see my husband's daughter when she had a baby, but that was because I was sick. If it was out of meanness, O God, do not bathe *(sok)* my son! The son of the one who killed your father is going to have to be bathed as you are being bathed. And they'll wash his back, without looking at his face. Jean, repeat: 'I have been washed of misfortune *(nösot).*'"[60]

"I have been washed of misfortune," Jean repeated.

"I am here to represent all," said the aunt, "even those who have died. There is nothing from our side that might make you fall behind, none of those evil medicines that work in the night, not even the ones vampires use. If someone seeks to blind you, may that person become a deaf-mute. But don't you try to take another's things by force. There, everything Satan *(Satan)* has done upon this child has been washed away."

"Go throw all these leaves in the water," said the *khamsi* to Jeannette, "and return without looking back." Looking back represented a return to a previous situation.

Then she told Jean, "First drink some of this water. Go take off this belt and put your jeans back on. And don't forget to urinate." The past was to be completely eliminated.

After the ritual bath, the *khamsi* had Jean step back a few paces, and with the help of their friend she began to paint spots all over him, from head to foot, all over his bare torso, even on his legs below the rolled-up cuffs of his jeans, alternating red spots with white ones, made with the powders that lay in the vase—the *hwosi* and the *mbö.* The meaning of the design was strikingly obvious. To enhance the resemblance still further, she gave him two long pods of *dethum* to hold in his teeth, at the corners of his mouth, like two fearsome fangs. Jean was a panther.

It was not the metamorphosis of Jean into the "panther man," that celebrated terror of the villages, nor his introduction into a secret society, such as that of the *khamsis*. It was a rite to conjure him out of the sight of his enemies. It was a rite of protection.[61]

All the while Jean was being painted, the *khamsi* spoke to her departed husband, emotionally and aloud. She reminded him of the circumstances of his death, just as if she were resuming an interrupted conversation. "One day you were sitting over there. I begged you to run away to Baham [the neighboring jurisdiction] with me, and you said no. When I came to the fence, down there in front, I told you, 'Lord Tampa, you are staying here, and it will bring you misfortune. You shall not live.' Then Jikwo [a co-wife] said we couldn't leave the goats and pigs. And yet we had all agreed to go to Baham. That was the last I ever saw of you. Be it a man or a woman who killed you, may misfortune fall on that head, so no curse may come upon me. And whoever be the person who drove me from this place, may that one always wander through the night everywhere, while I find refuge everywhere. May that one's homestead be overgrown even as this one.

"Ah, Jean Fotsing, we're going to spot you like a panther! We'll make your skin panther hide. You're not going to wash off for nine days."

"But Jean wants to leave for Yaoundé the day after tomorrow," put in the aunt.

"If he washes, that's his business," said the *khamsi*. "He can wipe his face, but only his face or I'll be buried on a hill." (To be buried on a hill, a *khïo*, meant to die like a dog, with neither ceremony nor mourning, accompanied only by interior regrets—the death of someone dishonored, someone dying of the ignominious disease of dropsy, for instance.)

When this passage had been translated for me and I finally understood it all, I noticed that the *khamsi* had spoken to her deceased husband not just aloud, but in exactly the same way as she had responded to the questions of the aunt—in the same natural tone, and in the same register. Only her inflection varied, depending on what she felt at the moment. All my life I had heard Christians pray to the saints, and it never surprised me. And I had often addressed God myself without being able to see God. But to observe the same phenomenon in a cultural and religious context other than my own *was* a keen surprise. Others' belief is, we might say . . . "unbelievable."

Shadow, Eggs, and Forehead

The glow of the dying sun was faint on the horizon now, and reached us obliquely, reddened as if by the bricks of the ruined walls and sifted by the tall weeds as if they had been stained glass. A dozen feet from the shadow of her son, the *khamsi* placed seven eggs on the ground, directly opposite that part of his long shadow that must have been his forehead, and broke them, one after the other, right there on that part of the shadow. Jean had regained his confidence, and said to me in French, "All that goes on me, see?" The number seven represents a large quantity—almost as much as nine, that noble figure of plenitude.

The words the mother used in performing the ritual of the eggs were: "May the one who wishes you ill be cursed. What they did to your father was no revenge for an evil he committed. And so it is that misfortune makes you wander, without your father's being the cause."

Shadow, eggs, and the forehead are three symbols all charged with the same meaning. I had seen them all used on the coast as well. The shadow is a human being's invisible double. Throwing something at a person's shadow is the same as throwing it at that person. The egg has a multitude of ritual usages, inasmuch as, first, it is a living being in potency and, secondly, its shell is a protective covering. Most often it is sacrificed in the stead of a person in danger. Finally, the forehead is the part of the head where chance, good and bad luck, is located. Breaking seven eggs on the shadow of someone's forehead, then, is a very rich symbolism. But Jean Fotsing, too, must have a part in this treatment, and so his chest and back were daubed with the egg white, and once again he was forbidden to bathe for nine days.

The *khamsi* seemed to be hurrying to finish her task before nightfall. The aunt had made ready a little package for Jean to take to Yaoundé with him, to slip under his pillow while he slept, so as to prolong the ceremony's effect. The package was called *fefia,* and contained a mixture of the herbs called *dethum si, baksa,* and *zözö,* along with a bit of earth from the homestead, and—of course—seven pods of *dethum.* It was handed him with the left hand, so as to make the difficulties he would encounter as weak as the left hand.

"Here is the *fefia* we are giving you, from the same mouth," the aunt went on. "There is nothing more you need ask for from your friends to make your strength greater. Otherwise you won't be following in the footsteps of your father. He wouldn't take medicine even for a headache. He wouldn't even buy flea powder. Nothing but the *dethum,* and the earth we know.[62] If you try to own anything else [any magical object] you will be doing as your mother, but not as your father!" And the *khamsi* laughed.

While the aunt spoke, the *khamsi* was off a bit to one side, covering the vase with a large leaf—the *mbömbu,* the leaf the Douala call *dibokuboku la wonja.* It served as the cover for a sacred object, or as the hat of a sacred person.[63] Vase and leaf would stay here, then, soon to be protected from view by the grass and weeds that would grow up again. The vase and the leaf would be the only vestiges of this *sok nösot,* the ceremony that washes a person of all ill fortune.

I took the family home, and thought I had done with the misfortunes of Jean Fotsing. I had not deciphered the information I had recorded as yet, and so I did not know that the ceremony had not been completed.[64] Actually, I had assisted only at the first part of the ritual imposed by the father's family, the part essentially devoted to washing Jean Fotsing of any curse. Thus, in a way, it had been only the negative facet of the ceremony. It remained to give Jean Fotsing "positive" luck, good fortune, and the second act was up to the *khamsi* of the mother's side of Jean's family. For this I was invited to Pauline's home, near the Batié Pass, where she practiced divination.

I returned to the Poor Clares' guest house for the night. I could hear their singing, which filled the church at the canonical times—a solid building of black granite, with a low belfry. The sisters were mostly young Cameroonian country women who had dedicated themselves to contemplative prayer and manual labor. They knew I had not come to serve them, but to visit a *khamsi* in the vicinity. I intrigued them, perhaps shocked them. For what reasons might a priest be interested in the work of a *khamsi*? The sisters might wear rough, brown homespun dresses, much like what the village women wore, and use traditional drums in church, but their aspiration was precisely to dissociate themselves from the *khamsi* world. Had they not taken leave of that universe the day they entered the convent? The presence within them of the energies of their heritage, still lurking deep inside them and doubtless intact, disturbed them, and rendered them extremely chary of anything like divination or sorcery, as if they had been new converts.

And so I listened to their singing from my bedroom in the guest house. From the other side of the mountain, I could also hear the sporadic echo of drums beating. I gave thanks to God that I was the friend and guest of both.

Chapter 12

The *Khamsi* Inspiration: Magic or Religion?

The *Tok*

The next morning I left the wide road leading to the Batié Pass and took the path down the slope to the hut of the *khamsi* and her third husband. All along my route, men walking alone, women in groups, and young persons of Fotsing's age were all heading for the house of the oracle. It was nine o'clock, and the visitors who had had to come a long distance were arriving, without a word, seating themselves on tree trunks that footed the trellises that fenced in the little yard. The yard was square. Facing out on it was the red earthen hut where the couple lived with their children. Opposite, a gate had been made in part of the trelliswork; it opened onto the steep path leading down to the brook. In the center of the yard was a small sacred grove, consisting of two bushes—a *gam*, whose leaves served for divination, and a *nkwenkang*, a symbol of peace, called on the coast, where it likewise stands for peace, a *mwandando*, or *mukoko mwa bedimo*. Stones had been placed at the foot of these trees.

"Before I came here, the *khamsi* told me later, "the spirit of these trees drove me to make a place for them in the center of the yard and plant them there. The rocks—I dived into the water, afraid though I was, and brought them up from the bottom to bring back here. This place gives me the words *(nöga)* I am to pronounce. I turn this way to speak." And indeed the *khamsi* always faced the little grove when she pronounced her auguries.

A police lieutenant, who had encouraged the *khamsi* to make predictions and speak revelations "because there is too much sorcery going on in these villages," insisted she keep a notebook on her visitors. The *khamsi* obliged when she had a student there with the patience to write down all the names, from ten o'clock in the morning until nightfall. I counted 480 names in the notebook from February 24 to April 3, 1975. Allowing for two free days a week—the fifth and sixth days of the traditional week—the *khamsi* therefore had twenty visitors a day recorded on this pad, and of course the total number was higher. The dozen mornings I came, bright and early, I would count between thirty and forty persons, sitting quietly and respectfully, awaiting their consultation. The pastor of Bamendjou thought that a large number of his parishioners had been to see her. Her celebrity, however, was no obstacle to the practice of divination by numerous other *khamsis*—some fifty in the jurisdiction of Bamendjou alone, with its population of fifteen thousand.

The *khamsis* permeate the villages and represent a considerable influence. It has been observed that, in societies in which the authority of the chief or head was absolute, secret institutions arise, deriving their authority from the same source as the head, and thus establishing a political balance. Both the chiefs and the *khamsis* drew their power directly from God *(Si)*.

Pauline Nkwedum had no equivalent on the coast. Hers was the precise, limited role of a diviner, in a chief's jurisdiction where institutions had remained surprisingly intact. In Douala country, the *ngangas* were the last remaining functional element in traditional society, alongside the chiefs who had suffered a marked decline in their power. In bygone times on the coast, the function of divination was most often performed by a *ngambi*. Today the *ngambi* has all but vanished, and this role has been assumed by the *ngangas*, who thus concentrate multiple functions in their person and activity: a *nganga* is both a diviner (as is a *khamsi*) and a healer. Formerly, on the coast, the secret *jengu* societies served to counterbalance the power of the chiefs, just as the *khamsis* do in the Bamiléké jurisdiction today. On the coast, it is the *nganga* who is the last remnant of these societies. Thus Loe was an *esunkan*, deriving his power from a mystical relationship with a female *jengu,* or water spirit. Despite these differences, which are to some extent attributable to the disintegrating condition of traditional institutions, a comparison between the mountain *khamsi* and the coastal *nganga* remains very suggestive.

Now it was ten o'clock, and the *khamsi* returned from her ritual bath in the brook. She greeted the silent assembly: "It is God who has told me to speak to you, now at this hour, without haste, lest certain ones misunderstand and then go out and tell falsehoods. Whatever I tell you, it is God who has ordered me to say it. You, bad-luck woman [the *khamsi* fixed her gaze on a woman seated impassively before her], why do you look at your husband with an evil eye? I salute all but thieves, killers, and vampires *(nthum)*, and women who have a child and cannot tolerate others having them [the apex of sorcery]. I listen only to God before speaking to you. If you don't take seriously what I tell you here, too bad for you! Welcome to all."

Now she led all the visitors, along with Jean Fotsing, who was awaiting his treatment, and me, in a slow farandole around the sacred grove, improvising, to stately, majestic melodies, refrains of topical significance— "Who'll go tell the village?" "Welcome to the old papa from Loum," a distant place. "I never sleep, for God has grasped me."[65]

A polyphonic humming sound arose from the choir of visitors parading behind the *khamsi*, but her alto voice dominated them all. Brandishing her maracas (dried gourds with seeds or pebbles inside), with her wild, tangled hair, she was hideous and beautiful at the same time.

The first act of divination consisted in eliminating undesirable elements. Slowly the *khamsi* traversed the tightly packed square of would-be guests, now sitting once more on the tree trunks. In her mouth she held a large, hollow reed. As she came to each of several persons, she blew through the reed. If it made its bellowing sound, the person in question could breathe easily. But if it failed to sound, there was nothing for the person to do but to flee—the sorcerer had been detected. That morning the *khamsi* drove three persons from her enclosure. Off they scurried, sheepish and abashed. "One day I even drove off a priest," she told me later. " Go, go! He deceived the people." The *khamsi* was a fearsome one!

The sisters in the infirmary had told me how they had once been called to her house for an emergency. A woman accused of preventing other women from having children had been so severely beaten that her life was feared for.

One day, as the *khamsi* was walking me back to my car, we came upon an old woman whom she had expelled that morning, and who had remained there, just beyond the *khamsi's* property, waiting for her, for a good many hours. The two women took each other's measure in silence for a long moment. Finally the *khamsi* proceeded on her way. "She can just keep her evil to herself," she told me.

The *khamsi* appreciated the seriousness of her accusation. "I was unjustly accused once," she said. "They said I'd eaten Yawo [a feminine name]. I had to listen to this accusation and make no defense. There was nothing I could do about it. When you're accused unjustly, sometimes it's better to be quiet and keep your distance." Such violence, such total incompatibility between God—whose spokesperson is the *khamsi*—and certain persons is understandable only in a context of sorcery.

The inescapable component of reality represented by sorcery—the reality of evil—has its corporeal seat and sign, the *tok,* a delicate, sensitive organ lodging in certain persons' livers. The *tok* betokens great force and power and is transmitted from generation to generation along the maternal line. The *tok* does not automatically incline its possessor to evil—most of the important personages of that jurisdiction were deemed to have it—but those who have the power to harm have it as well. In Bamendjou the latter are called *nthum,* "vampires," approximately, with the same terrifying overtones as our own word carries. Invisible, the *nthum* sally forth at night, to suck their victims' blood until they kill them. The imprint of their fangs is found on animal carcasses—two little puncture wounds close together. It is asserted that physicians sometimes have confirmed their presence in hospital examinations. This form of sorcery—a form of cannibalism—is very widespread, for women who have the evil *tok* are particularly prolific, and they transmit this "original sin" to their numerous progeny. The expulsion of every woman with the *tok* would be tantamount to the exile of a considerable part of the population of any village, according to the more pessimistic of my informants. Hence one must be content with driving out those who misuse their power.

The *khamsi* played a great role in the detection of these vampires. They never confessed, but her privileged relationship with God rendered their presence intolerable. Her third husband, Jean Fotpa, who was a *nganga*, was more compromising: if there was no way to eliminate the *tok* without killing the person who had it, he would simply calm her—"hypnotize" her, to use the felicitous expression of the local chief. Here, then, was the same system of weights and counterweights to defend society against evil as I found in the south of Cameroon.[66]

Divination

The *khamsi* sent the group, now smaller by three, down to the brook, where each was to bathe while inwardly confessing their faults. She forbade anyone to return before Jean Fotsing's treatment had been completed. Remaining in the little courtyard for the ceremony, then, were the *khamsi* herself, her husband, Fotpa—the *nganga*—Jean Fotsing, Jean's maternal grandmother, a few children (including the little *khamsi* of last evening), and I. I had not met Fotpa before. He was an extremely affable little man, quite reserved, even retiring. He did not seem to me to be of his wife's temperament or mold. He merely observed Jean's treatment: Jean Fotsing was not his son. The presence of the maternal grandmother was not surprising: it was the mother's side that was standing in for the father's family today.

The *khamsi* and her mother now busied themselves with the preparation of the familiar ingredients: the red *hwosi*, the white *mbö*, the *dethum* pods, all placed in a large pot before the main door of the house. There was no more black earth, no funeral vase, nor as many allusions to the father. The two women set aside the banana leaves to be used in Jean's second washing and added something new: seven branches from the *nkwenkang* tree, the tree of peace in the sacred grove. All was in readiness for the second act. But Jean Fotsing—decidedly stubborn—now refused to change out of his jeans into the skirt of dried leaves, on the pretext that the young persons who had gone down to bathe would make fun of him when they returned.

To persuade Jean to obey, his mother employed a tactic the *khamsi*s use. Mother and son agreed to submit the matter to divination. The procedure was simple. Jean Fotsing went to the sacred grove, picked a leaf from the *gam*, the tree of clairvoyance, and tore it in half. Then he mentally assigned one alternative to each half—one part meant he stayed in jeans, the other meant he dressed according to custom. He took the first half, placed it in his mother's lap, and set himself to concentrate on its meaning. If his mother returned it to him, he stayed in jeans. But if she threw it aside, it was the other part of the leaf that had won out, and he would wear the traditional costume. Everything then happened too fast for me to be able to follow the contest. I only saw Jean rise, docile and resigned, and leave for the brush to change his jeans. He donned the banana leaves. He had lost again.

Had the *khamsi* mesmerized her son? "I wanted to argue," he told me, "so she took the two halves of the leaf. She found out I had to wash, and put on the banana leaves. It was the only thing I could do. She plays that game every day of her life, except Sundays, thirty or forty times a session, and she's always right." Despite his somewhat cavalier tone, I had the strong impression that, deep down, Jean Fotsing was not unhappy that the ceremony would proceed as provided by tradition.

The *khamsi*'s divination was not limited to the leaf game, and I have described it here only because it was what she used to resolve the little difference she and her son were having. Actually, this is not really divination, but rather a means of learning which way the will of God inclines. We must remember, she was the sole judge of that will. More often than not, she asked a visitor to open their hand and then spoke without a great deal of attention to the lines on it. I thought I was beginning to understand how she penetrated the lives of her guests—an immensely difficult task if the client was a stranger and kept silent as convention dictated. She used a literary style that is perhaps the standard format for oracles of all time. "Who has twins in your family(?)" she might ask, in the tone of someone saying, "There are twins in your family." These questions, which sounded like statements, were probings. The interrogatory form enabled the *khamsi* to keep the conversation going if the client answered. And if the "question" hit the mark, she scored a point: in virtue of the affirmative tone, she would not be considered to be asking anything but to be revealing something. Little by little, patiently, the *khamsi* delved into the life of her visitors and discovered the reasons that had led them to abandon field or town for a day of meditation.[67]

Pauline's husband Fotpa was both a *nganga (nganekang)* and a diviner *(ntchwonga)*. According to the chief they did not necessarily have the *tok*: the *khamsi*'s power came to her from God, the *nganga*'s from his medicines *(nekang)* and (in his capacity as a diviner) from a trap-door spider *(nga)*. The *khamsi* was held in greater respect than was her husband because of her relationship with the divinity, and because of the success of her consultations. Fotpa did not seem to have much of a following. He possessed—or rather, was in the service of—a trap-door spider, which he kept carefully protected and fed in a field some three hundred meters from the house.

On several occasions, Fotpa and the *khamsi* practiced their art of divination for my benefit. It taught me the difference in their methods. One asks the *khamsi* no questions. It is she who speaks, it is she who takes the initiative. On the other hand, one does interrogate the trap-door spider, which replies, through the mediation of its official devotee, the *nganga*-diviner, to one question asked of it. The two approaches are complementary—and many are those who would like to come to know them in order to be able to set them in contradiction.

Jean Fotsing finally reappeared, clad in banana leaves. "Stay at the door," the *khamsi* ordered him. Then she blew in his nose and ears, as she had done with me the day I had met her. With the grandmother's help, she would now perform a double rite upon him: they would wash him of any stain and curse and strike him with the *nkwenkang* branch. Seven branches, with their leaves still on them, had been laid on the ground for this purpose. The grandmother took hold of them, folded back their ends, and made two knots in each. She worked very earnestly—I could see the wrinkled skin of her old weathered face, like parched earth, contracting in still tighter wrinkles over her short-stemmed pipe clenched in her yellowed teeth. The patient was to be lightly scourged until the knots in the branches came undone. If they stayed tied, it would be proof that some bad thought, some unpardoned fault, some obstacle to family reconciliation, remained.

The knot symbolism is very important. The *khamsi* used it frequently in her incantations. She would say, for example, "If I tell a lie about this person, O God, bind me. But if I tell the truth, unbind me."

Now the grandmother and mother began to pour water over Jean from huge snail shells (called *nkanesot,* in these circumstances), and struck him in concert. Words charged with meaning accompanied the blows. There is no rite without its accompanying incantation.

"O God, yes," the *khamsi* chanted. "If this youth has found no work—and indeed he has found none—it is not because I have deceived anyone, for I act ever in conformity with your word *(nöga).* All the money I give him is the result of my toil. I tell the truth to everyone, and it is to honor me that they give me money. I have never taken a dishonest sou for my son's benefit."

"Yes," put in the grandmother, "I represent all my children here."

The *khamsi* took the opportunity to protest her innocence: "When mama comes here, she can't say about me, 'She's a prostitute,' because she knows very well that I didn't come to her entirely of my own accord."

"Yes, that's right," chanted the grandmother antiphonally, "but I asked you to stay where you were. I never say yes to two men for the same girl."

As on the day before, the *khamsi* was protesting her innocence. But she was no longer addressing her deceased husband. She spoke more of the situation in Jean Fotsing's life in Yaoundé, and even interrupted the ablutions twice to have me told that she certainly counted on my recommending her son to my European friends.

Suddenly a humorous dispute arose between the *khamsi* and her mother. The incident demonstrated the two women's sincerity and total involvement in the ritual action, which was anything but a mere formality.

"The *nkwenkang* knot mama's holding isn't coming undone!" remarked the *khamsi.*

"Yes, you're right," said Fotpa.

"There are two knots that aren't undone!" said the grandmother.

What was not right between the grandmother and her grandson? If the knots resisted, she must have something against him. And so the *khamsi* proposed to Jean Fotsing that he reconcile himself with her, by promising to bring her oil and salt, symbolizing abundance and loyalty. Then the grandmother could only wish him employment with an abundant income, and a marriage that would be a model of stability.

The old woman was not happy about this proposal. And admission of a difference between them would be tantamount to admitting some measure of responsibility in the young man's failure in Yaoundé. This she was not about to admit, not for anything in the world. And so, while continuing to strike Jean and wash him, she began to expatiate bitterly on the subject of the oil and salt.

"Say you're going to buy some oil and salt and you'll bring it to your grandmother tomorrow," said the *khamsi* to her son.

"Do you think God hasn't done it already [given her this gift of oil and salt]?" protested the grandmother. "God has. There's my oil! [She pointed to one of her granddaughters, present for the ceremony.] She's my everything. God's the one I look to for my oil."

"That's true," the *khamsi* admitted. "As far as oil is concerned, mama's had her share."

"I contemplate my granddaughter and I till my field," the grandmother went on, "and that's all I do. Oil and salt are nothing. And I built a house. What I ask from you is not oil and salt, but to build me a roof. Oil and salt are absolutely nothing. If there's too much talk about that, it'll be like a curse on me."

At last the two knots came undone.

Better than any ritual words could ever do, it was the asides that opened up to me the daily life of these persons. I was glad to be able to discover the humor and sensitivity of an old woman through conventions and symbols other than my own—conventions and symbols that are characteristic of all grandmotherhood. When I came to be able to understand homely scenes like these, I had the feeling of finally beginning to achieve my goal, the feeling of really having my feet on the ground of Cameroon.

The *khamsi* had done two things with stones or pebbles that aroused my curiosity. In the course of the first act of the ceremony she had placed two flat pebbles in her son's mouth. Now she took a necklace of porous, hollow stones, which she kept over the doorway of the house, and dropped it nine times on her son's forehead, the seat of good and ill luck, and then on his chest, saying, "Here are my wonder medicines *(nekang)*." And the grandmother added, prosaically, "God *(Si)* has given you these wonder medicines, but me, my wonder medicines are my ten fingers!" The *khamsi*'s seven smooth and nine hollow stones were called "God's stones" *(posi)*. Once the ceremony was over, the *khamsi* favored me with some explanations.

"What is the difference between the smooth pebbles and the ones with holes in them?" I asked.

"There isn't any real difference," she replied. "God gives them to me, in the water or along my path. There are two kinds. The ones I took to hit Fotsing with were so he wouldn't steal money from others, and others wouldn't take his. These flat stones give me the words I have to say."

"Do they stand for anything?"

"The pebble with a protruding corner is God's bullet, to shoot vampires in hiding. This flat, black pebble is the earth. Here is the moon and here is the sun [the two pebbles that she had had her son hold in his mouth the day before]. And this stone, here—the instant it fell I was worried. I picked it up and felt all dizzy. He [probably God] told me to put it in my house, he had a lot of work to do with it. Most of the time, when I come back from the sacred place *(tusi)*, I see pebbles that have been placed at my feet and I pick them up."

That was all I could ever learn about the meaning of these stones, which the *khamsi* used all the time and handled lovingly. It did not seem to me that the names she gave them referred to any cosmological system into which she might have been initiated, for some of the most celebrated *khamsi*s make no use of them. She merely capitalized on their physical resemblance to the heavenly bodies, or to everyday objects, as the case might be.

The last phases of the traditional ritual were now under way. The *khamsi* broke a raw egg against her son's forehead and smeared it over his face and chest. "You shall not bathe for nine days. Yesterday you didn't like it when I told you that. You said you had to leave. Fine, leave, then, and too bad for you! So go down to the brook and wash only your face before you get dressed. Return and don't look back. Don't greet anybody, and when you're back, go to your room and stay there as long as you can."

Here Jean Fotsing turned to his grandmother and asked, "Did you pinch me?"

"Yes, I did," she replied. After a ceremony of regeneration the subject must experience a new sensation. And now, as we came to the end of the rite, it was the grandmother who made the concluding statement, and reaffirmed her position on the gifts of oil and salt. "We have washed away everything, swept away everything today. Absolutely everything. I've bathed Jean Fotsing, who is my real oil and real salt. If anyone has enjoyed them it's certainly me. I had three children. One died. I have two left—my oil and salt. I hope God gives me peace—lets me spend my days and nights in peace."

While we were partaking of a dish of semolina, the visitors received permission to return from the stream and share the dish, and then await the revelation of the hidden reasons for their anxieties.

At eleven o'clock, the *khamsi* took her station on the doorstep, had a campstool set up for herself, and began to peer into the palms and face of the first visitor to be seated. During the next few minutes, those waiting in line would occasionally burst out laughing. Then, an instant later, they would seem astounded and dismayed. And so went the consultation, in front of everyone, with each visitor all in a tither about the situation of each of the others, and chiming in with remarks and bits of advice.

The joy or the sorrow of each of the *khamsi*'s clients was shared by the whole group brought together just for that day. Revelations could be serious: I caught such words as "sorcery," "poisoning," and "misfortune." Or they could be joyous: I heard a few marriages foretold, the birth of twins (a divine blessing in this land), and the like. There were private moments, too, when only those being interviewed learned the truth, and I watched them turn away in silence, pensive and shaking their heads. And so the *khamsi* went on apportioning public revelation and secret divination during the course of these endless interviews, which she presided over with the stamina of a confessor and the easy assurance of a seasoned judge.

The next day I drove Jean Fotsing up to the main road, along the pass. On the way I asked him whether he believed in the effectiveness of the ceremony he had just experienced. His behavior during the rites had betrayed a certain irritation, and I wondered whether he had submitted merely out of loyalty, or out of conviction. "Did your mother treat you so you'd be able to get a job in Yaoundé, or to get rid of your father's curse?" I asked him.

"My father's curse, that was the other day. Yesterday it was so I'd be able to get a job in Yaoundé," he replied.

"Do you believe a treatment like that is really going to help you?"

"Well—I don't know. I'll see when I get there. In Yaoundé I'll see what kind of a job I like, because it depends on me too. When there's a treatment like that, it's not some sort of magic, see, it's a way of getting rid of a curse. They think it might be on account of a curse if somebody can't get a job."

"What do you mean, 'It's not some sort of magic'? What's the difference?" I asked.

"What's the difference? When they do that . . . see . . . maybe you won't get a job for a long time, but when you do get one, it's for sure. With magic you can get a job the very first day."

"Why don't you just practice magic, then?"

"Magic goes bad on you," Jean Fotsing replied.

"But this other business . . . ?"

"This other business. . . . If you get a job, it's because God got it for you, not you. It's more of a sure thing."

Jean's answers seemed clear to me on two points. They reminded me of Dieudonné's responses. Jean Fotsing now felt that he was in a better position to get a job. And yet the ceremony had not been magic for him.

I would have had to agree. He was returning to Yaoundé from his visit to the Batié Pass with the feeling that his father's curse had been lifted. Now he was reassured that no one in the family blamed him for anything: his paternal aunt, and then the next day the maternal grandmother, had spoken in the name of them all. He had satisfied the demands of his mother by submitting to customs that nettled him a bit, but he was leaving for the city in deep tranquility as far as his family situation was concerned. I could not help but feel that the recovery of his balance in this regard would be a real plus for him in his job search.[68]

There is no lasting success without a stable social infrastructure. This is what Jean Fotsing's example illustrates so well. Europeans are surprised that the Bamiléké are so successful in business, and yet remain so attached to the customs of their aboriginal jurisdiction. But this is precisely the secret. I once asked a chief how he himself managed to honor his ancestors' customs and still be open to the modern world. He replied, "The ones who encourage us to hang onto our customs are the most advanced of our people [those who have had the most formal education]. They encourage it themselves." More experienced observers than I are of the opinion that the traditional structures encourage free competition, foster interpersonal relationships, and allow for a certain social mobility, and that these are three reasons for the ability of the Bamiléké to adapt to modern practices.[69]

The ceremony had not involved magic. No claim had been made that the mere performance of certain rites would produce a certain effect. To me it was remarkable that Jean Fotsing had been able to distinguish between magical practices and the ceremony he had just gone through. A number of his expressions showed that he did not think he was excused from personal effort. "Everything depends on me too," he had said. His mother had reinforced this interpretation of the ceremony in her final advice to him: "Don't stay home with your relative. He's not your father. Tenkwitampa owes you money, so take it. And then start working with it. Then we'll see how to make it grow."

Here are realistic attitudes, and yet these attitudes in no way contradicted the notion that it would be God who would grant the outcome. I recognized familiar old categories of Christian theology: principal and instrumental causality. Nor did they entail magic. (Of course, here they were implicit and unspoken.) Neither Jean Fotsing nor his mother saw any contradiction between the scrupulous observance of the rites and recourse to common-sense measures to attain the same objective.

I came to the same conclusion I had come to in Douala, when I had studied Elimbi's treatment.[70] These ceremonies, when conducted by *ngangas* or diviners of the stature of Din, Loe, or the *khamsi*, far from being magical, are essentially religious.[71]

"God Sent Me Spinning"

The best evidence I can offer for the religious authenticity of such a ceremony is the *khamsi*'s own attitude. She made no attempt to justify her behavior by appealing to an obligation to observe a ritual. She appealed to the need to be faithful to a religious experience she had had, a theophanic experience she retained from the dim recesses of her early childhood. I base this conclusion mainly on her own testimony—on what she told me after her son had left us that day. Night was falling by then, deepening the pink and green blanket that covered the hills. The mood was right for confidences. I was the stranger, anxious to depart; the *khamsi* was seeking to delay my departure.

We were seated on a pair of benches that the visitors had not carried out into the courtyard that day—the *khamsi* and her husband on one, and two children and I squeezed onto the other, facing the couple. And now, as if to give me the key to everything she had shown me, the *khamsi* delivered the secret of her life. I did not have to question her. She simply spoke. Her husband translated for me, phrase by phrase, and thus I was able to record an "interlinear tape" on my machine, as I listened to this brief but astounding religious testimonial.

"When I was very young," Pauline began, "at the age when I could talk, I knew I was going to be a *khamsi*. A *khamsi* told my father so one day— and as he was speaking, I knew myself he was right. It wasn't very clear, though.[72] From time to time the'd give me *dethum* pods.

"One evening my parents were out. My brother carried me out in front of the house and put me on the doorstep, so I'd sleep better. I dreamed I saw a huge pile of something in front of me. This pile was like a person.[73] But I didn't know who it was. This person blew in my mouth and ears. It had something in its hand like [she pointed to a sacred stone], and hit me in the head with it every once in a while. Every time, I was afraid. And then it knocked its forehead into mine. After that I saw the same thing, day and night. I still see it now, and my body feels it. When I got sick [her mental illness, after the murder of her first husband], the *khamsi* who took care of me, he had seen the same thing."

"I started to take instructions with the Protestants, but God told me to stay sitting [not continue]."

"I don't see why you can't be a Christian and a *khamsi* at the same time," I observed. "All you're trying to do is tell the truth."

"I wouldn't mind following the teaching, but how are you going to have time," when all these persons keep coming and never give you a moment's rest?"

"Well," I objected "you go to the market, and to burials."

"I'll try; later on. But if God *(Si)* still tells me to keep sitting . . . ."

"Ask God again. God may let you."

"If God lets me, all right. If this big thing lying in front of me lets me, I'll do it.[74] And I'll be glad to do it. I wish for baptism, all the time. But I keep being told to work on the persons who come to me.[75] When God talks to me I don't go asking anybody, not even my mother, I just act. It's my Creator God who's asking me to do it.'"[76]

The *khamsi*'s attitude and behavior, it would seem, then, could only be understood in terms of two basic experiences—the dream she had in early childhood, when God came between her and her relatives, and the manifestation of this vocation to the eyes of others, when the sacred madness seized her in her maturity. The acts and gestures she used with her visitors, especially with her son Jean, came from these two special moments in the history of her relationship with God.

This was particularly apparent in the course of the second part of Jean's treatment, when the *khamsi* took the initiative entirely. On the first day, it was the prerogative of the paternal family to perform the traditional acts and gestures for lifting curses *(sok nösot)*. This first ceremony was not the special prerogative of the *khamsi*. But for the second part of the ceremony, in her own home and "sanctuary," she truly acted as *khamsi*. She had Jean Fotsing take his place on the threshold of her door, just as her brother had carried her to their threshold that day long ago, when she had received her first visitation from God in a dream. She blew into Jean's nostrils and ears, just as that "huge pile of something . . . like a person" had once upon a time blown into her own. She placed pebbles on Jean's forehead, just as she herself, trembling with fear, had once had pebbles thrown at her forehead. But I had not seen her go through, with her son, the act that recalled the vertigo of the time of her visions, whose benefits she passed on to younger boys and girls: "The way you see me spin the children, that's the way God really made me spin."[77]

This analysis enabled me to follow the whole course of the *khamsi*'s spiritual experience, from her first encounter with God, all the way to this concrete case of unemployment. There were no magical practices along the way. There was only a religious conception of existence. The *khamsi*'s son had made no mistake about that.

My sojourn in the mountains with the Bamiléké had reconciled me with traditional medicine—if we may apply this concept broadly enough to include what the *khamsi* did. It was a true time of rest for me, after such difficult times with Dieudonné, Nkoa, Clara, and the "city *ngangas*," Nombote and Tokoto. Convinced anew of the therapeutic value of the great treatment practices, I felt ready to restore contact with my first two initiators, Din and Loe. I owed my pacification to the *khamsi*. Incontestably, a spiritual current had passed between us. Culturally speaking, she had been the furthest removed from me of all the diviners and *ngangas* I had met. Everything seemed to separate us—nationality, language, religion. (She is the only non-Christian *nganga* or diviner studied in this book.) And yet, we had instantly felt a close affinity for each other. Did we not share a mysterious vocation we had discerned in early childhood? Her manner of speaking of God's "spreading out" before her and separating her from the rest of the world of the living—in the exalted language of her religious culture—reminded me at once of the call I had received myself at the age of eleven. To be sure, I could not have managed to formulate my early experience in a symbolic language comparable to hers—owing to my theological training in the years since then, I fear. But, like the *khamsi*, I was convinced that it was this call of my childhood that had given my life its basic orientation. The only time I had sought to express this conviction in words was in a prayer to the Holy Spirit, fervently recited the day I received the sacrament of confirmation, the day I first became aware of my vocation. My mother knew how important it was and had kept it. It was a prayer of Cardinal Mercier:

O Holy Spirit, soul of my soul, I adore you. Enlighten me, guide me, strengthen me, console me, tell me what to do. Give me orders. I promise you that I shall submit to all you desire of me, and that I shall accept all that you permit to happen to me. Only give me to know your will.

The little *khamsi* and I—a thousand leagues apart—had we not had the same sort of mystical experience?

Chapter 13

Order Lost and Restored

Every time I came back down the mountain and reached the outskirts of Douala, by the highway with all the broad-leafed vegetation along it—the macabo, the banana tree, the taro—I always felt as if I were back in our family greenhouse, where I used to love to go with the gardener when I was little. Suddenly my skin was all moist, I was engulfed in heat and humidity, and I found myself once again in the oppressive power of the vegetable kingdom.

I knew it would take me about three days to get used to the tropical climate again. My method was to adopt the slow pace of our old gardener, and try not to think about the heavy atmosphere. Soon my body would be feeling a certain well-being in its warm steam bath, provided the early-afternoon sea breeze came along and tempered things a bit.

After a period of getting used to the weather, then, I felt ready to resume the study of medicine with Din and Loe. To tell the truth, all during my long time away, all during my other experiences with other *nganga*s, I felt I had never really left these two. I had paid them an occasional visit, and sometimes assisted at the start or finish of a night séance, but without any real involvement on my part.

But Din was away from the city, and I went to his door in vain. He rarely appeared in Douala since his trial, as if he had been a wounded vulture, afraid to alight. He would treat a few patients and then disappear. I was told he usually practiced on the island of Malimba, or else in the open country around Douala.

Loe, by contrast, was the very model of presence and stability. I had no doubt I would find him at home, just as I always had. And there they all still were, the *nganga*, two of his wives, his elder brother, his sister-in-law, and a swarm of little ones belonging to one couple or another. Loe, of course, was the chief of them all. Elimbi kept more in the paternal orbit since his treatment, and Nkongo was ever the fervent disciple. Nothing had really changed—and yet there was a distance now between this world and me. It was high time for me to return to it, if I were not to lose it.

My opportunity was not long in coming. Loe had been told of my desire to assist at a whole treatment again, and one day he sent Nkongo to inform me that he would be treating a number of persons the following Saturday evening. It did not occur to me to ask just what type of illness he was preparing to treat or just who his patients would be. After all, who could venture to announce the schedule of a ceremony so dependent on the intervention of water spirits, ancestors, and sorcerers? And yet the preparation was always planned to the minutest detail, and a ceremony followed a plan of attack decided in advance in accordance with fixed norms. Was it a matter of pure convention? I believed it was linked to the conviction that the real actors were always occult forces, hostile or protective, regardless of the competence of the *nganga*.

I gratefully accepted the invitation. Conditions appeared to me to be remarkably favorable for undertaking the study of a major treatment. In Bamiléké country I had had to discover everything all at once. Here, however, in Douala land, I was familiar with the language and the cultural underpinnings. Loe and I had had our adventures together. We were cronies of a sort. The courtyard was familiar, and surely Nkongo would furnish me with all the necessary information.[78]

The Ancestors' Tree

This time I was not admitted to the company of pilgrims who sought out the tree on the outskirts of the city. This night the patients were all female, and "would be ashamed." But I was told by Nkongo that the ceremony of the tree had been no different from the one at which I had assisted the night of Elimbi's treatment.

Selebenge—I had finally learned its name—was a "family " tree. I had never known a sacred tree along this wooded coast not considered to be the dwelling place of ancestors. Nor had I ever assisted at a treatment of any importance to which the dead had not prudently been invited to take their places beside us and participate in the work of healing. But in this region of the world, where backwaters, rivers, and ocean are everywhere the place reserved for the ancestors of the earth tends to be modest in comparison with that for the *miengu*—the water ancestors (for the descendants of noble Douala families, that is; water spirits, merely, for the rest of humankind.) As we shall see later in the course of this night, Loe invoked mainly the latter. Still, he also sought the favor of the dead at the guardian tree.

According to Nkongo, Loe had performed the customary series of rites. He had planted a lighted cigarette in a gash in the bark. He had broken an egg on the tree's roots, where they came up above the ground, had poured out some perfume, and had scattered some coins about. He had spat the *nsote* of good intentions—the *khamsi*'s *dethum*—on the mutilated trunk. The symbolic materials used for these rites were the same I had seen him use myself—water, fire, breath, vegetable matter, animal sacrifice, and money.

But economy of gesture and material is the rule, for *the whole is present in the part.* This was axiomatic, and it was something I had heard often. It was a helpful principle to keep in mind, for a stranger is inclined to find mini-rites insignificant. Each was executed nine times, the number representing totality for the Bantu, to whom the Douala belong, as for the Bamiléké.

In the same spirit of execution of obligatory acts and gestures, Loe had commanded the women to cut off locks of their hair and clip their nails, and bury the hair and the clippings at the foot of the tree. "It's a way of hiding," Nkongo said.

Finally, each of them was directed to rub against the trunk with her whole body, while reciting her misfortunes. This, we recall, was a way of asking the tree, or the earth ancestors, to bestow good fortune and health. "This tree has much power," Nkongo explained to me. "It can give good luck and bad luck. You come to it to talk to it about what's hurting you, what you're looking for. God created this tree before he created human beings. So he gave it more power than he gave us."

Their prayer ended, Loe and his entourage came back up the ravine in silence and returned to the courtyard. No one dared turn around or utter a single word before the master gave permission. A couple of miles away, back in the city, we were awaiting them, beating our bamboo sticks in a rhythm that gradually built up the desired atmosphere of incantation and liturgy. There were about sixty of us—family members, neighbors, my confrere René Roi, who taught at the Libermann School, and I.

The *Esa* Ritual

By ten o'clock Loe was getting himself ready in the *dibandi*, which served as both sanctuary and sacristy. We could hear him muttering and jingling the little bells that summoned the water spirits. Loe never skipped his brief moment in the presence of his formidable pile of bark.

René and I sat waiting, in our assigned places among the men. Facing us, obediently all in a row, were Loe's whole family. To our right, out against the *dibandi*, were the percussionists with their resonant, jarring music.[79] To our left, the neat square was completed by the women, including the patients of that night, who had returned from their pilgrimage to the tree. There were four of them this evening—a girl of twelve, a young woman with a babe-in-arms, Loe's fourth wife, and Kwedi.

It was Kwedi who monopolized Loe's attention. This major séance had been scheduled on her account, and the other three were there only to profit from forces that would be unleashed on this occasion. Loe did not forget the others, however, and showed them too, in the course of the treatment, what gestures they were to make and where they were to place themselves. Each had her own story. Each was in a different stage of healing as this evening approached.

I shall be speaking only of the principal patient of the night, Kwedi.

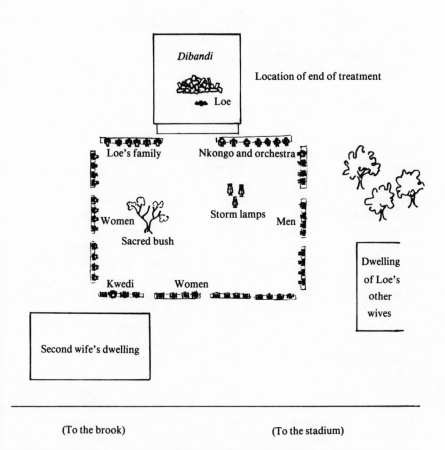

Plan of Loe's Treatment Area

Nkongo had described for me how she had looked and behaved the day she had arrived. Sounding like someone reciting a litany, he told me she had come two and a half months before, "in very serious condition. She kept both eyes closed; she couldn't see. She looked the way persons look when they're going to die. She seemed in another world already. She went on about things we'd never heard of, she called on beings we couldn't see. Sometimes she asked for her mother. She was deaf and blind, and so tired that she didn't even have the energy to sit up. She stayed lying down all the time."

Since then, an assiduous inhalation treatment with herbs and barks , administered morning, noon, and night through all the pores of her flesh, had gotten the better of the disease. This chubby little young woman, sitting in the shadows on her bench to our right, wrapped in a white sheet with only her head appearing, was in perfect health today. Her energy and stamina would shortly have ample opportunity for demonstration in the Spartan treatment she was about to undergo. How could she still be considered a patient?

As we have seen before, *diboa*, "misfortune," "sickness," is a tricky word. "Symptom," probably, would correspond better to what the term suggests in Douala. The manifest signs of physical affliction or mental disorder are never considered independently of the cause *(njom)* that has provoked them—a genuine disease in its own right. The symptoms are taken seriously, and treated with herbs and barks, but what good would it do merely to be rid of the symptoms? They would only return, unless the evil, the disease, is cut off at the root. The evil forces responsible for the symptoms must be unmasked and stopped in their tracks. And one never has far to look for these forces. They will always be found in the network of the victim's personal relationships. "Your sorcerer is your bodyguard. Your attacker is always one of your own."

This is the sense in which Kwedi was still "sick." There would be no cure without the restoration of family harmony. This, it seemed to me, was the reason for the therapeutic efficacy of the *esa* ceremony at which we were assisting.

Loe was shooting spectacular jets of flame all about his *dibandi*, accompanied by great, throaty roars, as if he had been an itinerant fire-eater. Through the little windows, we could see the whole house light up every time he spat fire. Then he unostentatiously emerged on the little terrace that separated the *dibandi* from the first benches. He descended the two steps, came to the center of our square, and carried out a meticulous inspection of all the objects Nkongo had gathered there. All eyes were on him. For Loe, as for any *nganga*, order was sacrosanct. If anything were to be missing, he might decide to postpone the séance. Or perhaps instead he would decide to supply for the lack with an additional rite. "Major treatments almost always go the same way," said Nkongo. "If the ceremony isn't gone through with the sharpest attention, you can skip something and not notice it. You must use a banana cane, or you mustn't; you must toss red-hot coals on the patient's head, or you mustn't. . . . Father Loe gets ready days in advance. He likes to take his time.''

The *nganga* saw that everything was there in the great basin that brimmed with water—different sorts of herbs, barks grated and then sprinkled in the water, a pinch of earth (part of it from the cemetery where Loe's father lay, part from a busy intersection, part from a marketplace, part from under Kwedi's bed, and—very especially—part from the house of her uncle here present), all mixed together. The basin—Kwedi's world in miniature—also contained ashes from the family hearth, nine ten-franc coins, a new plate, and an egg. Each of these things, which Kwedi had had to procure herself (except the herbs and barks, which were the exclusive affair of the *nganga*), said something to her. Unlike me, she had no need of explanation.

"Why the earth?" I asked Loe.

"Because earth has all the power in the world," he replied, a little irritated.

"Why the money?"

"Because money brings luck, and that's what everybody wishes for," he said.

I knew that the plate represented food, and that the egg, which would be sacrificed in place of Kwedi, represented life.

Loe also made sure that the beer, wine, and tobacco were what he had ordered. The goat and three chickens to be sacrificed later were well tied up not far away. Now he could begin the questioning—the dramatic overture of the rite of *esa*, in the very place where he had performed this rite upon his own family and his son Elimbi.

Loe motioned to Kwedi to come forward. She adjusted the white sheet, which covered her like a Roman toga, and advanced majestically toward the center of our square, facing the great basin where, in miniature, the elements of her particular universe bathed. We could see her better now, with her flat face, broad little nose, and slightly protruding eyes. With her perfectly impassive look and light-colored skin she could have been taken for an Asian. Many women in this part of Africa resembled her. She had braided her short hair like a schoolgirl on a holiday—in series of little squares, about an inch on each side and perhaps half an inch high, separated by broad parallel and perpendicular partings. Now Loe summoned the three principal members of her family—the mother, with an identical physiognomy and dressed in her everyday sash, and the two men, her paternal uncle and her elder brother, wearing light-colored shirts and dark dress pants. These three were now the center of everyone's attention, and they took their place at Kwedi's side with their arms dangling a little awkwardly.

Then came the exchange of questions and answers. They were subtle and laconic, and their premises and conventions must be well understood if one is to grasp their import. It was understood by all (or if you doubted, you took care to keep silent about it) that Loe already knew how the matter would end, because he was endowed with double sight *(miso manei)*. His evasive manner of eliciting information about family conflicts, then, was not to be ascribed to ignorance, but to a rhetorical genre that consisted in revealing each person's secret actions and ulterior motives piecemeal and by insinuation. None doubted his capacities as a seer. Only, he knew a good deal more than he told.[80]

Loe had not had to await this interrogation, then, to make up his mind as to who was responsible for what. "It's Kwedi's own fault she's sick," he told me, in French. "As far as she's concerned her family can go to the dickens. And the family isn't happy either—they're always bawling out the mother and the uncle. She tries to boss her brother around. She left her husband and went whoring around with another fellow. It's her own fault if her family made her sick to punish her, and got her bewitched by the *ngango*, the caiman that kills in the water." Loe had even concluded that Kwedi's paternal uncle, present tonight, must be responsible for the sorcerer's spell cast on his niece.

According to Nkongo, Loe had sent Kwedi's sister-in-law, the wife of the elder brother who had come tonight, to the village, the day before the treatment, to go to the uncle's house and gather the pinch of earth that had been placed in the basin. When the uncle had learned of this, he had come to see Loe to ask him whether Loe wished to kill him, and Loe had responded, "It's to save your niece." According to Nkongo, "This was how Father Loe gave him to understand that he was the cause of the sickness."

That Loe could draw such conclusions even before the interrogation was evidence of his knowledge of family structures, knowledge he shared with all genuine *nganga*s. It showed he had not need for confidences to be able to declare that feelings were strained between, for instance, two persons who were in line for the same inheritance. Loe had had Kwedi with him for more than two months. The little he had heard from her was enough for him to be able to accuse the uncle. He knew that the uncle had become head of the family at his brother's death, had married the widow, as custom permitted, and thus become Kwedi's stepfather. Hence the uncle was the main victim of the young woman's antisocial behavior in the family. Then too, he was in direct competition with the children of his deceased brother for the property, and, as he had children of his own, he nurtured a darksome jealousy in their regard. I knew all this to be the case from my few visits to Loe's family during the period I had lived with the Bamiléké.

Loe could not divulge this information during the séance. Sometimes a *nganga*—Nombote, for example—might accuse someone during a séance, but never, to my knowledge, in the presence of the suspect. As Nkongo put it: "Father Loe does not think all truth is good to tell. Not all secrets ought to be revealed. Even if he knows everything about you, he'll tell only part."

There was another reason for Loe to hold his tongue. He sought to get the accumulated family wrongs confessed and acknowledged by their authors themselves, to the end that the rite of the rejection of evil, which closed the *esa*, not be a mere formality, but express a genuine commitment. This treatment seemed to me to constitute an excellent example of what a *nganga* tried to do in such circumstances: stir the members of the family to admit their wrongs, undertake a purpose of amendment, and be reconciled. This was no inconsiderable dimension of the *nganga* profession. It is here, doubtless, that the success of failure of treatment hangs in the balance.

I shall record some extracts from the long period of questioning and answering that accompanied Kwedi's treatment. We shall see Loe moving in every direction, irritating, jostling the relationships among the four key persons: Kwedi, her mother, her brother, and her uncle, all of whom now stood before us. Obviously, all were on their guard, careful not to say anything compromising, and hence attentive to the *nganga*'s insinuations. Loe crouched in a corner of our square, like a cat. From there he approached his prey, to harass them with questions. Suddenly he would simply leave the assembly and be lost in the night, for suspenseful minutes. No one would dare to move. Then he would leap back into our midst and start a song, or send a drum galloping. He would smooth his delicate mustache and throw out an ironic or enigmatic thought- provoking statement, such as, "Each of my questions is a way of speaking directly." Finally he said, "Thanks to this girl, I can save you all"—and he laughed, laughed all by himself, oblivious of all else besides, until he had laughed himself to exhaustion. Then he resumed the interrogation.

Loe (to Kwedi):"Who is this man?"

Kwedi: "My father [stepfather]."

Loe: "And this woman?"

Kwedi: "My mother."

Loe: "And this man?"

Kwedi: "He's my brother."

Loe: "I've told you I'm not trying to reveal anything. I'm afraid that if I told you anything, you'd collapse immediately. And this family of yours . . . do you think they're proud of you?"

Kwedi: "I know they're proud of me."

Loe: "Well, I'm telling you they aren't proud of you. Look, I'm the garbage can. Whether you like it or not, you're going to toss your garbage in the garbage can. Music!"[81]

Now Loe asked the uncle some questions. He posed them in statement form, after the manner of a *khamsi*. And the uncle would reply, very prudently: "Yes, she's stubborn. Well, she's stubborn when she's with girls her own age—not when she waits on me."

Loe (sarcastically): "Oh, come on, now, isn't there any little tiny thing you think's wrong with her?"

Uncle: "There might be something, but I just overlook it."

Loe: "Do you enjoy that?"

Uncle (posing, then circumspectly): " . . . No."

Loe: "Sir, I know this girl belongs to you. My name is *sanakope* [a woody, tropical vine]. If I climb a tree, it'll die." [Beginning a song, which was taken up by the group:] "You drink of the brook, and know not its source." [Approaching the mother, until their bodies were touching:] "This girl . . . who gave birth to her?"

Mother: "I did."

Loe: "You remember the day you slapped your belly and said, 'Am I not the one who gave birth to you?' "[a way of expressing great dissatisfaction with one's child].

Mother: "I never said that."

Loe: "There's plenty to tell you, but I don't want to talk today. If I try to, the boats'll leak [dissension will arise]. I've got fly's feet [I can alight anywhere I choose]. I'm starting to open the package [which you do not wish to open yourselves]. Each of my questions is a way of speaking directly."

Now Loe imitated the voice of a child, and intoned the first notes of a song, *Ekumbulan esoka*, which is about a game: two children take turns trying to guess what the other would like to have to eat at the moment. In other words, Loe was making the family play a guessing game. Then he continued:

Loe (to the brother): "How many other heirs are there to your father's land besides you?"

Brother: "None. I'm the eldest son, so I know there's no rival for my father's land."

Loe: "That's what you say. But I know you're in competition with somebody. Are you on good terms with your family?"

Brother: "As far as I'm concerned, I am. But the person who married my mother after my father died . . . I don't know if he hasn't got some idea of arguing with me about my father's property."

Loe (intoning a chant): " 'He pulled at the elephant till it spoke like a human.'[83] I know Kwedi has lots of bad habits. Do you deny it? Whoever has nothing against Kwedi, raise your hand. [No hands are raised.] Well, look at that! [An immense laugh from Loe. Then, to Kwedi:] Your own mouth condemned you. It's stubborness that condemned you, it's your smugness that condemned you. Everything your family has just said was said lightly, off-handedly. But I know the depths of things. But today I can only keep my mouth shut. I'd have liked to hear you say to your family, 'Yes, I've been a bad girl. I admit it, and I know you're the ones who gave birth to me, too.' [To the other three:] Every one of you has said you have nothing against her. That's what you've said out loud, but the bottom of your heart is black. Now, thanks to this girl, I can save you. I am going to treat her, to show you I know my business. Because I love to work for Jesus my master. [To Kwedi:] But your uncle had better watch out, because his heart is not pure or bright. If he fools around, he'll get hit, right away! Not by me, but by somebody else. He'll know somebody's hitting him, all right" [probably the water ancestors].

Long did Loe continue to assail the two men and the two women with questions, throwing up to the uncle that he had never married before marrying his brother's widow, and couldn't have a child, interrogating the nephew about his younger brothers—did they not perhaps covet their father's estate?—and scolding Kwedi, until he finally decided to start the *esa* rite.

The *esa* rite is not the *nganga*'s monopoly. It is without a doubt the most widely performed ritual in Douala society: it is used whenever any danger threatens group unity. The father of a family can use it with his family. Douala chiefs use it with their entourage, in the annual *ngondo* ceremony, for political reasons (as with the presidential election of 1970), or in times of calamity (as in the cholera epidemic of 1971). It can even be used by someone with a reputation for prearranging the outcome of soccer matches. Din had practiced it with Elimbi, and Nombote had forced it on the old grandfather on account of his grandson Bruno.

The most common procedure involves washing the faces of the persons concerned with a large, broad leaf, the *dibokuboku la wonja*, steeped in water. Then each person must declare their faults and their responsibility for the misfortune in question, before finally casting the evil as far as possible into the brush. The danger of such a ceremony is that it may become formalistic. Loe's long psychological preparation of this family was for the purpose of laying the groundwork for a rite without hypocrisy, one that would truly hold the potential for reconciliation. The intent was clear. Had it succeeded? I thought that it probably had, as far as the mother and brother were concerned. I doubted it in the uncle's case.

There's the pan of water in front of you," Loe said to Kwedi. "That's the water you're going to die in." Loe was alluding to the river sorcery, which I shall describe presently.

Until this moment, Kwedi's uncle, mother, and brother had not moved from their places. They were still standing in a row in the very center of the assembly. Now Loe invited them to go up to Kwedi and wash her face with the leaf. They were still on their guard against this snickering rascal of a *nganga*, who was surely laying a trap for them.

Loe (to the uncle): "Bless your child. Don't you want to see her freed?"

Uncle: "Of course I do."

Loe: "Quick, baptize her."

Uncle: " I want my child to be cured. Everything we've said against her, all the times we got mad, and said this thing was wrong with her or that thing was wrong with her, we toss all that into the brush, don't we?"

Assembly: "Yes!"

Loe: "Amen."

Assembly: "Alleluia!"

Uncle (passing the great leaf steeped in water over Kwedi's face): "O water basin, here I stand before you and wash my child's face. May what I do here be clear and transparent. If I'm the one who's the cause of her sickness, we'll soon find out."

Loe: "What did you say?"

Uncle: "Well, according to you, we got mad at Kwedi."

Loe: "That's what *I* said. But have *you* admitted it?"

Uncle: "To whatever extent we were mad at her, I'm saying that it's all over with from today on."

Mother (taking her turn with the leaf): "All my hope is in my children. I know that they're the ones who'll bury me when I die. I haven't any reason to get mad at them. From today on, I hope everything will be clear. Even you, Kwedi, you slight me. You slight me, and I gave birth to you. . . ." [Loe's volcanic laugh drowns out the final words of her blessing.]

Loe: "What do you mean?"

Mother (embarrassed): "I mean I'm saying that my own daughter, that I gave birth to . . . she may have slighted me till now, but this contempt will stop, from today on."

Loe (satisfied): "Amen."

All: "Alleluia!"

The brother, then each of the other members of the family, now took their turns with the leaf and spoke their blessing.[83]

The Water Spirits

It was midnight. Loe strode forth from his *dibandi* with a red cape over his shoulders, and a scarlet tunic about his body, down to his ankles. He looked like someone modeling priestly vestments in a Fellini film! I was surprised at this pompous, ludicrous demonstration. He did a few dance steps for us, then vanished, and this time he came back draped in a white robe with a red cincture, and a saber in his hand! ("It's a gift from a Hausa he healed," Nkongo explained, "but he has other weapons of war, too.") The time had come to join battle against sorcery.

The *nganga* began to pass back and forth within the square we formed, brandishing three pieces of cloth impaled on his saber tip, one red, one white, and one blue. He cried, "I tell my enemies, 'Do you want the white one? That's peace. Do you want the red one? That's war. Do you want the blue one? That's death.'" Blue, deep sea-blue, was worn by widows. Blood red, to all the *nganga*s I knew, meant that the battle with the sorcerers had begun. White, the modern symbol of peace, was traditionally the color pleasing to the ancestors of the earth or to the water spirits, the *miengu*, here being summoned to the rescue against the sorcerers. Now Loe would fade away, and they would come to the fore.[84] Everything was prescribed by custom. Loe had danced his pavane as a prelude to what was to follow.

The *miengu*, those water genies, as much feared as they were loved, came indeed, nor did they give warning. The very first sign of their arrival was to be read in the faces of a number of the women. They were seated facing us, with nothing to distinguish them from their neighbors, except, now, the sudden grimace of pain that distorted their faces. The stark glow of the storm lamps dramatized their grimaces even more. Soon we beheld these women rocking, rolling to right and to left, without leaving their places, as if someone were pushing them back and forth. The order that had reigned until now was profoundly disturbed. Their neighbors remained alert, and strove to keep the benches upright, while the convulsing women held on to the benches with all their might, grew stiff, then adopted the rigid attitude of manikins, or puppets with joints. Then uncontrollable convulsions seized their bodies, shaking them from head to foot, but without yet managing to hurl them from their benches. It was like the dry phase of a tornado, when the wind alternates its brutal assaults and sudden calms, before the unleashing of the waters. Impressed in spite of myself, I tried to be as inconspicuous as possible, sitting motionless on the men's bench.

Unexpectedly, as if taken with an irresistible urge to dance, Kwedi rose and joined Loe on the path. At first her movements had the elegance and restraint of ordinary dancing. Then a slight trembling seized her. It was no more than a shiver at first. Then it grew before our eyes, until it had subjected Kwedi to regular, jarring convulsions of her whole body, over which she obviously no longer had any control. The sheet had slipped away, and Kwedi now appeared almost in costume, in an ensemble of white undergarments that surely had been selected for just this eventuality. The women in their trance joined her from their bench. Now there were five of them writhing helplessly before us. The drum that had set them moving fell silent a moment, but the possessed continued to tremble and twist in the silence, like palm trees in a flood, shaken by an invisible current.

Besides Kwedi, there were her sister-in-law (the one who had purloined the handful of earth from the uncle's residence), Loe's second wife, his daughter, and a young neighbor. It was not very difficult to distinguish those who were really possessed from those who were forcing themselves to dance frenetically. "The dance is the battle with the enemy," Loe explained to me later. "The dancers are fighting, but they don't know it. The *jengu* is here. They have become *miengu* [the plural of *jengu*]. But the ones just dancing for fun aren't doing anything at all."[85]

The *miengu* were there, all right. In the twinkling of an eye the atmosphere had changed completely. The musicians, who often enough were small-time, blasé entertainers, suddenly grew serious. Now it was they who were overcome by the *jengu* rhythm.[86] Besides, Nkongo had taken the drummers in charge—there was no question of making fun of *miengu*.

If you are of the *miengu* race and descendency, or under their protection, they deliver you from sorcerers, or ensure all manner of success. To women they grant fecundity: one can have intercourse with them. Loe had a *jengu* wife, one Hélène Yambe, whom he would occasionally summon during a treatment by whistling for her familiarly as he did for his visible wives. A woman could have a *jengu* husband. But *jengu* spouses are demanding: they impose their dietary and sexual laws. One cannot, for example, eat certain kinds of fish, or approach one's visible spouse at certain times, without risk of reprisal.

Suddenly Kwedi, still under the sway of the *miengu*, came up to me and seized me by the forearms. She froze there for a few seconds, and I could see her eyes, scarcely four or five inches from my own, rolled back in her head so that they were almost entirely white, and I could feel the regular, pulsating spasms of her body. Then she rejoined her companions and continued spinning around the square. "She was asking you to help her," Loe told me the next day.

Nkongo added, "She mustn't let a foreign strength go unused; or else she was looking for someone with strong blood."

Later I questioned Kwedi. "When you were dancing," I said, "you grasped my arms. Why?"

"I don't remember any more," she replied. "When you dance like that, you aren't aware of anything."

"Well," I said, "I was told you had come to ask for help. I agree to your cure."

It was not surprising that Kwedi remembered nothing. The trance placed its subject in an altered state, resembling that of a sleepwalker. But altered consciousness, or amnesia, did not mean indifference. On the contrary, in a trance, subjects manifest desires that social life otherwise forbids them to express. This was why Loe was so attentive when anyone was in a trance, assuming such a humble, submissive attitude, as befitted the servant of the *miengu*.

As for me, obviously I had to be on my guard—although some thought I overdid it—with the women of the *nganga*'s entourage, because of the uncontrollable flow of rumor. Ever since my adventure with *ekong*, I had begun to pay more attention to my reputation, and tried to see that it was in keeping with my identity as a priest. But when Kwedi—with whom I had exchanged no more than a polite hello until then—fell into a trance and physically seized my arms in the ritualized gesture of a bride, I doubted whether anyone in the assembly had any suspicious thoughts about it. She was asking me to share with her my power as a priest; that was all. In any case I was grateful to her for crossing the social frontier separating the foreigner from the African and the priest from the woman. I offered not the slightest resistance or defense, and sought only to calm her anguish simply by bodily composure.

At two o'clock Loe allowed Kwedi to rest on the bench before the departure for the river, which would be the next step in her treatment. The *miengu* had left the clearing now, and Loe summoned his three other patients to come to the center. He placed his hand upon each of them, questioned their families, and pronounced a few mysterious, oracular words, which were listened to with great attention by the interested parties. There were but preliminary labors, for the great treatment of these women would be held another night.

Nine Saving Plunges

Kwedi's native village was up the Wouri, the river that flows through Douala before joining the sea. Sorcery had gripped her in water, then, and it would be in water that she would be delivered. Loe now designated those who would go down to the river in Kwedi's company. René Roi and I were among them, as were the members of Kwedi's family—except the uncle, who was to remain the whole time with the *nganga*. (The exception was a meaningful one.) We lined up single file behind Kwedi and our leader, Nkongo, who was Din's delegate for this rite. Kwedi had to keep a short of *mukoko mwa bedimo*, the cane of the dead, in her right hand, and in her left, the herb *ngonji*, as well as the *epindepinde*, the little command staff an officer carries when he goes to battle.

Our procession wound along, past houses where everyone was asleep, singing a *jengu* melody ("not a special one for this occasion," Nkongo would later tell me), and finally came to a narrow backwater—called, by some stretch of imagination, a "river." This was all that was left of the sacred stream Mbanya, which in earlier days had watered the roots of the *selebenge* tree where Loe had gone at nightfall. But the city, which had diminished its volume and polluted its water, had not deprived it of its symbolic power.

Nkongo seized the "cane of the dead"[87] and struck the surface of the water a single time, to beg safe passage. Now Kwedi walked forward into the brackish water and squatted in it so that it came up to her breasts. She remained there until Nkongo had spat a purifying blast of fire over her head. Then she had to rise at once and answer *"E,"* "yes," when her name was called. This was done nine times. According to Nkongo, "if sorcery has gotten hold of someone in the water, you dive in nine times, and there's nothing to fear in the water any longer." At one point during the nine plunges someone, inspired by the Bible, cried out, "This is the water the Holy Spirit hovered over! This is the water that wipes away sin. One of our sisters is suffering. May this water heal her!"

Then we went back to the house, singing a joyful melody, for we had "won the war." Kwedi was forbidden to look back under pain of "spoiling all the work." She had endured the trial by water and fire with astonishing endurance and impassivity.

We found the other three patients awaiting us, with Loe. They had profited by the power of the tree as Kwedi had, but had not been allowed to go down to the river. Kwedi was the victim of *ngando (caiman)* sorcery, whereas her companions suffered from other kinds of spells. One had been sold in *ekong*, and the others were to be eaten by the sorcerers *(bewusu)*. These other sorceries required their own treatments.

Later I questioned Kwedi, in Nkongo's presence, as to what she under-stood by *ngando* sorcery.[88] The vigorous, forceful manner in which she answered me made me realize that her docility during the treatment had required a great deal of energy, and by no means betokened any passivity of character.

"My uncle is involved in *ngando*," she began. "That's an organization that grabs its victims in the water. That day I left to go with mama to Tonde [a village on the river], they managed to catch me like that, in the water. I got sick right after that, and they took me to Father Loe."

"Did you recognize those who grabbed you?" I asked.

"No, they closed my eyes, and I suddenly went blind. But now I see well."

Later, Nkongo explained to me: Kwedi had discovered the sign of the spell of sorcery in the water. Something like a wake, or a current that sud-denly swept against her, had terrified her, as if it had been the wake of a caiman that was after her. Thus she thought she had been snapped up by a crocodilian. There is no longer a crocodilian in the Wouri large enough to attack a human being—it must have been a submerged branch, grazed by a passing pirogue, that had caused the current and the wake. But Kwedi must have been so taken up with thoughts about her personal enemies and family disputes, especially her uncle, that the wake on the surface of the water had materialized her fears. She had been seized in *ngando* sorcery.

"What do you know about *ngando*?" I asked. "What do they say in the village?"

And Nkongo added, peering at Kwedi, "You ought to be able to answer that! If anybody knows sorcery it's you! Sorcery's not something in short supply around your place!"

Kwedi was cut to the quick. "As if you Abos [Nkongo's tribe] didn't have any! When they want to get rid of somebody in *ngando*, they have you fall out of a pirogue. They take you away and hide you in a corner somewhere in the brush. That's where they heat water and pour it on you. After that they stick you back in the river. That's why they always say, 'You've been in the water a long time. Your skin is all white.' That's the worst sorcery there is."[89]

In this case, the family knows it would be useless to take the patient to a hospital. The *nganga* is steeped in the cultural milieu in which the disease has been born and bred. Only the *nganga* will be able to perform the rituals and pronounce the words that can save the victim of this sorcery.

Escape from Imprisonment

Now it was four o'clock in the morning. But Kwedi's labors were not over, nor were ours. She still had to flee the hiding place where the caimans, the *nganga* sorcerers, were keeping her until the next Sabbath night, and offer them animal sacrifices in her stead. Then all would be once more in order. A series of extremely trying ceremonies, which she endured with stoicism, was to begin now. Her face remained perfectly impassive. If there was anyone who thought she still was sick, that one must now be convinced of her complete recovery.

During the two hours remaining to them before dawn, and an hour beyond, Loe and Nkongo undertook a series of meticulous, spectacular rites, in an ambiance of fire and bloodshed, calculated to persuade Kwedi that the saving rites had now been accomplished once and for all. To enhance still further the ceremony, which was already wildly colorful and intense, Loe, in the highest excitement himself, now challenged the sorcerers, his adversaries, in a colonial French dialect.

According to the explanations of Loe and Nkongo, a cure depended on the exact repetition of certain actions—the formulas had been passed down from generation to generation—whose therapeutic effects were still verified in our own day. These actions manifestly corresponded to the secret maneuvers of the sorcerers. And so Kwedi would think she saw a battle being waged before her eyes, even if she saw only one camp's tactics—for the sorcerers were there all right, invisible, but active. Only those who enjoyed double sight—Loe, in this case— were deemed to know what fencing-thrusts the paradings of the *nganga* corresponded to.

It was not easy for me to keep in mind that Loe was not play acting. He was convinced that certain practices and gestures thwarted sorcery. There was no doubt on this point. "Those mouthfuls of fire—" I had asked him, "are they a symbol?"

"The fire," he replied—not without exasperation—"*is* my bomb. It isn't a symbol. It's the bomb itself! It's not a symbol, it's direct war! I've been hit too hard by their bombs, and I've fallen on the spot. I've been mourned several times."

Now I knew why so many rites were performed, and so seriously, and why the presence of us Europeans caused so little distraction.

Preparations for an escape are generally made along a side wall of the *dibandi*, the side running along the courtyard. We were invited to go there now. Kwedi herself first had to disappear for a moment, in the company of her mother, to anoint her body with a battle oil that could spare her some terrible burns. She returned girded in a new white sheet, wrapped tightly around her hips like a dress, and sat down on a camp stool, around which the rest of us stood in a protective circle somewhat more open than the one before.

In this posture, we assisted at the slow construction of Kwedi's prison. It could have been completed in ten minutes. It actually took many times longer than that—a time proportioned to the importance of the event being symbolized. (I retain the word "symbol," with all deference to Loe. I assign it a much richer meaning than he would have suspected.) Nkongo could have walled Kwedi up by using the cinder blocks that were lying down at the end of the yard, for example, and doubtless this would have taken less time.

But it would have deceived us as to the nature of her captivity. These ferns, laid on the ground with great care, forming three sides of a square, and the stalks of the "cane of the dead" meticulously placed atop them to represent beams, manifested, better than realistic scenery could ever have done, Kwedi's situation as prisoner of sinister forces.

Three walls out of four had now been symbolically built. Next the floor was laid, of broad banana leaves, which Nkongo slipped under the captive's bare feet. "That's to entice the enemy. That's where they'll wait for him, there's where he'll fall into the trap." A thick taro leaf now teetered on Kwedi's head. Was that the roof? No, I was being too realistic, and the explanation was a surprise: "The leaf makes you invisible, but *you* can still see." Kwedi had the vacant look of someone in prison. Softly she squeezed the command staff, which she had not let fall from her grasp since her trip to the river.

Three walls were complete. The fourth, the rear wall, was open. Now the laborers hung from Kwedi's neck, down along her back, a large leaf from the raffia palm. In order to better represent her situation as a prisoner, they wrapped a long black thread about her, from her feet to her head. Finally, Nkongo traced on the ground the impression of a trench, which totally separated her from the rest of the world, and poured ashes on it, "to blacken it, and so they won't see her."

Two thematic strands, then, ran through the whole ritual of the prison-building: captivity and ruse. Sometimes these were attributed to the sorcerers, and sometimes to the deliverers, and I was not always able to make the distinction. Even as he was building his prison, Nkongo had astutely camouflaged it.

Sorcerers fear nothing so much as light, particularly when it flashes down into the heart of their dark kingdom. And so Nkongo, under the direction of Loe—who hovered over him constantly during this dangerous phase—would not only bombard the prison with his jets of flame, he would also hurl them upon the victim, so that they would lick the very flesh the sorcerers had bewitched. Now Kwedi's head and shoulders were covered with soaking-wet, red fabric, whose purpose was obvious.[90] Then Nkongo grasped a fistful of dry twigs, which he lighted and lifted to the level of his mouth. With the other hand he took hold of a bottle filled with a blend of gasoline and an oily sap. Then in one motion he took a mouthful of the mixture and shot it with all his might through the flame at Kwedi's face. A stupendous blast of fire lit up our night from end to end. The young woman sat there while she was bombarded nine times, then nine more times. She was bathed in fire from the soles of her feet to the hair of her head, yet she uttered not one cry of fear.

As he shot the fire at Kwedi, Nkongo peered at that marvelous taro leaf atop her head and made some quick calculations: "That leaf is going to tell us something. It has two sides. If it falls bottom-side up, the treatment must not be going well. If it falls top-side up, though, everything is going well.

Oh, oh, this time the leaf's fallen upside down. Still—there are leaves that show their back first, then turn over. . . ."

Now Nkongo cried out to Kwedi, commanding her to rise, to throw off all that bound her, to break her bonds—for she had found her freedom once more. Kwedi rose, all docile amid the applause of our little assembly, shook herself so that the threads fell away, along with fabric, herbs, and burned twigs, and seated herself once more on her stool. She manifested no emotion, for the trial was not yet ended.

A wood fire had been lighted, and Loe and Nkongo divided the glowing embers between themselves. Loe placed nine little heaps of them about Kwedi, "to protect her," and Nkongo grasped a machete, upon which he balanced his embers, and used it to hurl them onto the white sheet Kwedi had around her. "Fire to burn the dress she wore when her enemies carried her off," he said. Kwedi parried the hot missiles instantly, by snapping the sheet tight whenever they touched it.

Fire and Blood

After this deluge of fire, a long truce was struck with the night. An extraordinary calm suddenly came upon everything. The contrast was absolute. All, or nearly all, curled up right where they were and went to sleep. I stayed awake. I could not doze off, right on the ground, as they did. I tried to make out Loe, Nkongo, Kwedi, her mother, her uncle, her brother, and the others, there in the dark. They were but dim little shadows now, as if turned to stone, right where there had been so much agitation a few moments before. But this passive interval was the prelude to one last episode in the treatment.

First, two chickens would be killed. This was not a sacrifice, in the proper sense of the word, because the birds were offered neither to God nor to the ancestors. It was the execution of hostages, who must die in the young woman's stead. It was the sop offered to the sorcerers—the uncle and his associates—to placate their hunger. After all, Kwedi would have to continue living with them.

It was a scene of blood, curses, and great ritual violence. René, my confrere, judged it excessive and sadistic, at least there in the heat of the moment. Loe was perhaps putting on an act in a way, but was it not better to replace the actual violence wreaked upon this young woman with a vicarious violence? For me it was enough to observe Kwedi's calm, impassive face to be convinced of this.

Nkongo set to work. He caught the white hen, plunged it into the *esa* basin, passed it over the length of the young woman's body, slit its throat, tore it to pieces in a single deft movement of his hands, and stuffed the bird's raw heart into Kwedi's mouth where it was swallowed at once. Then Loe grouped the family members around the patient, required them to repeat their *esa* declaration of peace, and took the occasion to taunt the uncle cruelly as a "big talker who took his brother's wife and still doesn't have any children," telling him he must henceforth abstain from all conjugal relations with Kwedi's mother. "The man is a serpent," Loe was to tell me later.

The red hen was not as peaceable as the white one had been, and beat her wings and squawked desperately. "Quiet, savage! This is not the chicken who resists me, but the enemy! Never could a chicken so resist! Big talker! Dirty African! Shit!"

The hen was whirled about alive over Kwedi's head, where each of the principals grasped at it, the family from one side, and the *nganga*'s entourage from the other, until someone had a wing, another a foot, and so on. At a prearranged signal, everybody pulled, and the chicken was quickly in chunks. Loe's party had come off with the biggest pieces, so Kwedi was free of the claws of family sorcery.

As for the black hen, the third one, she was reserved for the day Kwedi would leave the *nganga*'s house. The *dindo* would be eaten on that day.

Loe took the egg that had been carried to the tree before being placed in the *esa* basin along with everything else, and plastered it against Kwedi's forehead, smearing it vigorously. "This egg could have been thousands of chicks, Kwedi. Now it loses its life for you. When an egg becomes a chick, it can peck already. May the man who is against you feel the hurt!"

Kwedi showed her approval by responding *"E!"* Gracefully she spread the yolk and the white over her face and in her hair, while Nkongo ground over her head some powerful spices, likewise taken from the *esa* basin, so that a gray dust rained down on her. Then a mouthful of fire.

Without my being aware of it, deeply absorbed as I was in this spectacle of fire and blood, day was breaking. The basin, the cloths, the humans, the beasts—living or dead—everything suddenly converged into a pitiful sight. Was I the only one to feel the disenchantment? Loe, Nkongo, and their companions continued to press forward with the ceremonial, which was seriously behind schedule. Now they would settle the fate of the goat, and, by way of consequence, that of Kwedi.

The rope by which the goat was tied was hitched to Kwedi's hips as to a post. The young woman sat with her back to the beast, because "only a woman who has no wish for a child may look upon a bleeding goat."

The manner of slaughtering a goat varied. In the case of *ekong*, the animal was suffocated by blocking its nose and mouth. In the case of *ewusu* sorcery it was split in half, from tail to head. Inasmuch as this was a matter of river sorcery, the goat had to have its throat slit so quickly it would not have time to bleat.

"If they push you under water, can you talk?" Nkongo was to ask me. "The goat is the animal that lives not in the brush, but among human beings. She is your friend. So Kwedi, who was supposed to depart [die], has given up her friend the goat in sacrifice. The goat dies in her place!"

Two executioners seized the goat, threw it on its side, and held it still while a third pulled its head up with both hands so that the throat was tight, and Nkongo deftly slit its throat.[91]

Kwedi was silent while Nkongo immolated the victim, and it was Loe who spoke up: "Kwedi, if you are present when someone decides to kill another, and you do not go to warn that person of the danger, it is you who shall be pierced. You shall not spill the blood of a human being. I have sworn it."

Kwedi still had the strength to leap nine times over the fire. Then she went to wash behind the wall of the *dibandi*. For nine days she must wash in the *esa* basin, without anyone seeing her, and eat from the plate put there for the evening. During the same period, she could have no sexual relations with a man.

It was seven o'clock Sunday morning. I had just enough time to stop for a quick wash-up before going to the church to preside at the Eucharist. After the ceremony at which I had just assisted, the Mass seemed very serene by comparison. Was this merely the effect of weariness after a sleepless night? In any case I could not help thinking that what had gone on over there in Loe's courtyard was truly about death and life, while the assembly here seemed more concerned with the solemn singing of the choir than with the true sacrifice taking place on the altar.

That evening I ran through in my mind the different sequences in Loe's treatment—which he had prolonged until dawn, contrary to his usual procedure. Two months before, Kwedi had been deaf, blind, and unable to walk. The loss of her means of communication had been the sign of the most complete abandonment. Daily, Loe had administered to her his good medicines, which had put her back on her feet, but which had not healed her definitively. The essential part remained: to reestablish her disturbed relationships with her universe. And the best way to bring about this return to normal was still the effective application of ritual. To this end, Loe culminated the treatment by effectuating the general mobilization of the forces on which Kwedi's life depended. This was the price of healing, and was well worth a full night of toil.

Was it because Christianity is now part of this country's tradition that I seemed to represent a natural zone in the life of this young woman? After all, she had most effectively reminded me that I did. At any rate there had not been a moment during that long night when I had felt out of place, unwelcome, or superfluous. Quite the contrary, I believed I had shared in the work of restoration, convergence, and equilibrium regained, which had given Kwedi back her health.

Chapter 14

Truth and Beliefs

I now considered myself better able to confront the question the Douala engineer had asked me that day: "What do you think of all this?" This sudden question, I could feel, involved a second question, one more vexing for me: "Do *you* believe in it?" And in fact it raised a third, a more delicate question still, and one that betrayed a doubt of his own: "Is all this true?"

The *nganga*s never questioned me in this fashion, nor did anyone in their entourage. To them it seemed evident that I acknowledged the value of the treatments, and that I believed in sorcery and the existence of the *miengu*. My presence and participation showed them that I did. Besides, they believed the evidence of their own eyes, so why should I not? To them, questions like these would have made little sense. But there were other persons for whom these were meaningful questions—some of my Deïdo neighbors, the students at the Libermann School, my network of educated Douala friends, a few Europeans, and, finally, the priests with whom I lived.

Europeans would ask me straight out about the reality of the traditional beliefs and the efficacy of traditional medicine. And yet—innocent as their curiosity might be, just as their sympathy was sincere—my explanations struck no responsive chord at all.

Matters were just the contrary, on both scores, with educated Africans. They projected their hesitations and uneasiness on me, asking me their questions in a general, amorphous manner, as if somehow seeking to avoid being found out. But they listened to my answers with a revealing attention. Most of the time I felt ill at ease in this matter, frustrated at not being able to give an explanation in depth in a way that would be satisfying to them. These questions about the "truth" of the traditional beliefs haunted me as much as they did them.

After having long been satisfied with evasive explanations, I hit upon a reply that, up to a certain point, seemed to me clear and adequate. When I was asked what I thought about "all this," I would respond: "It works." At first my questioners, too, were content. This is all I had said at Din's trial and he had been acquitted. Efficacy was the major argument, the decisive evidence in favor of the truth on the side of all those who could contribute to making a person sick or well: sorcerers, *nganga*s, ancestors, *miengu*. By answering "It works," I had reached my interlocutors' soft spot—their realism. Truth is on the side of what succeeds. When the wild manifestations of the *jengu* trances were in progress before your very eyes, you believed in the authenticity of possession. And that belief preserved family unity. The system was true because it worked. It was as necessary to heal in order to believe, as it was necessary to believe in order to heal.

The Power of the Forest

I had no difficulty in authenticating traditional medicine insofar as it relied on the curative power of herbs and barks. During World War II, French pharmacists in Douala, deprived of medicines from Europe, had successfully employed a number of concoctions made from saps and powders, as told to them by *nganga*s. And the renewed interest being taken in Europe in its own folkloric medicines had contributed to enhance the prestige of the vegetable medicines of the dwellers of the tropics.

Tourists adventuring in the tropical rain forests would have their senses assaulted by the fertile, overflowing abundance of vegetation, in all seasons, the heavy, humid heat, all this luxuriance unknown to the forests of Europe—how could they not believe in the power of the active principles of this miracle of life? As for the Cameroonians themselves, one had only to remind them of their grandmothers' family recipes—to say nothing of the powers of prestigious *nganga*s.

I have not spoken much of the pharmacology of these regions. Orally, anally, nasally, through every pore, by potion, unction, fumigation, or inhalation, *nganga*s penetrate the bodies of their patients with vegetable substances whose secret is theirs. Herbs, fresh leaves, barks, roots, bulbs, sprouts, and fruits are cut, ground, crushed, pureed, or made into a soup for the sufferer's consumption. Nature's health permeates the exhausted organism and repairs it, restores it. The proceedings begin with the first light of day, in the rear courtyards of the houses of healing, and keep their boarding patients busy for a good part of the day. The cure can take months to complete.

I had brought samples of these vital plants to the Libermann School, and had noted down the manner in which each was used. But I had been content to have just a few identified for me, the ones that could be of use to me in my endeavor to comprehend the meaning of some treatment under way at the moment. The relative paucity of my observations must not deceive the reader: to my knowledge, a *nganga* never undertakes a psychosocial treatment without recourse to pharmacology.

I had accompanied Din quite a number of times on his quest for herbs and barks. Forest and fen were all around the city of Douala. But they were

gradually receding, year by year, making the excursion a long and difficult
one. As I have said, Din often found himself obliged to purchase some of
his vegetable products at markets. But he always preferred to obtain them
himself, if he could, right where they grew, in order to be able to use them
while they were still fresh. We would sometimes walk for hours without
gathering anything. Then we would finally come to the humid valley, with
its particularly dense vegetation, that Din had chosen. There he would generally find all he was looking for within a relatively small area.

Din's routine was fascinating. He would put down his sack and his machete on the path, and be lost in a thick copse, which to me looked like a
hundred others we had passed up. There he would stand, on one foot, for a
good many seconds, motionless as a cat eyeing a cornered mouse. He would
look through the grasses with rapt attention. Suddenly he would shoot out
his arm and come up with a bunch of young shoots in his fist. I could hardly
distinguish its features from the innumerable species around it. Then he
would hunt a few meters farther, and grasp another plant, as if he had
finally seized a beast he had been tracking, as it was crouching and ready to
spring into flight.

With trees, Din demonstrated more respect. The ones that interested him
had already been trimmed. Empty bottles lay at their foot, the vestiges of
old libations. He would pour out a cup overflowing with wine, or spit some
spice against its trunk, before cutting away long strips of bark, all the while
speaking softly to the tree to calm it. It would be night when we returned,
loaded with barks and draped in leaves like forest genies.

A systematic study of native pharmacology held only secondary interest
for me in my research because I was but little concerned with organic diseases. The study of the herbal medicine of a region represents years of
work in its own right, and presupposes a herbalist's knowledge, which I do
not possess. Those who have devoted themselves to such investigations
have produced works of great technical quality, but they have not delivered to us the secret of the mentalities of their users. The curative vir-
tues of these vegetable products are practically all known now, thanks to
parallel research conducted in other regions of the globe in the same proximity to the equator as the Douala country. The essences of many of these
medicines, extracted from plants that grow in these countries, are now
sold in the pharmacies of Northern and Western lands.[92] The secret herbs
of the *ngangas*, then, are no longer in competition with remedies purveyed
by Northern pharmacologists, who now have access to substances ori-
ginating all over the world. Even some of the *ngangas'* own clientele purchase modern medicines, despite their exorbitant cost, rather than use the
simple products of the forest.

I do not think the *ngangas* owe their consistent success to their herbs and
barks alone. They owe it rather to their manner of putting together—
recomposing—the totality of the life of their patients. The powers of the
forest concern only one aspect of this existence.

Therapeutic Religion

> "A sick person is sick only in
> reference to a particular notion
> of health."[93]

My daytime interlocutors were open to the "argument from globality." I
had no difficulty in explaining to them, with the help of the examples I have
given all through this book, how *nganga* medicine takes charge of its patients' whole life—their body with so many invigorating herbs and barks,
their tangled skein of social relationships with the liberating liturgy of *esa*,
their cosmic environment with the fire treatments, where the very soul of
things becomes palpable and, finally, their mysterious relationship with
God, the ancestors, and the *miengu*. Of all the treatments I have reported,
perhaps Kwedi's best illustrates the *nganga*s' labor of recapitulation and
reunification, although a number of other cases would have served equally
well had I presented them in the same detail.

In order to understand the success of this holistic medicine, one must
appreciate—either from experience, or, if we have no experience of it,
intellectually—the tremendous mobilizing power of ritual. When I had to
explain my view of ritual, my position was weakened. Speaking about rites
or symbols meant isolating them, looking at them from a distance, and
"demystifying" them somewhat. It was an intellectual, desacralizing exercise, and my friends could see the danger. They had reacted just as Loe had
when I asked him to explain to me the symbolism of the blasts of fire that
came out of his mouth: "The fire is not a symbol, it's the bomb itself, it's
direct war."

The use of the words "rite" and "symbol" involves a tactical with-
drawal, proper to language, which runs the risk of impoverishing the very
meaning of the action they denote. I could tell that Loe and every other
nganga I have known were so hesitant to employ these words because they
feared, rightly, that the words might distort the content of the therapeutic
undertaking. Far from playacting or directing any kind of psychodrama,
the *nganga* claims to be at the heart of reality with his entourage—not
another reality than that of ordinary life, but ordinary reality itself, intensified, concentrated, and unveiled. The *nganga* practice of medicine does not
have its efficacy solely in the use of herbs, as is claimed by those who have
chosen to ignore the religious dimension. It does not even have it simply
from its globality. It has it from its capacity to integrate.

Such a medicinal theory and practice can succeed to such a high degree
only in virtue of its own integration into social life as an especially sensitive
nerve center in that life. We in the West customarily place medicine side by
side with the other liberal professions, like architecture or law. It is not
natural for us to consider it as the actual functioning of life in society. To-

day, as a result of the influence of modern social structures, some *nganga*s seek an official status, like medical technicians or physicians. But in the eyes of the people they are still the regulators of social relationships. Health in the broad sense of the term—well-being, or simply life—is such a common and primordial aspiration in Douala country that the persons called to minister to it have an especially eminent place in society. If we were to distinguish, for the benefit of our theological language, the religions evasively called "traditional" from the Christian or Muslim religions—called "salvation" religions—we would have to call them "therapeutic" religions, so intimate to the heart of social life is their quest for holistic health.

The cult of whole health explains the *nganga*s' success when most of the other functions of traditional society have lost their influence or even disappeared completely. The chiefs have retained a certain prestige, in proportion to the strength of their personalities. But the ritual of young persons' initiation, their social passage to adulthood, has not been practiced in Douala country for years. The degrees of age that governed life in society have practically disappeared as a point of reference, save in the memory of the oldest members of that society. The structures of modern society have been superimposed on those of the past and have smothered them.

A traditional society, called the Ngondo, which has long played the part of a court for the settlement of claims among chiefs, still exists in the city of Douala. (There has never been a single chief of all the Douala, other than the legendary one of the same name.) Today the Ngondo is maintained by intellectuals engaged in a remarkable effort to preserve, in the midst of urban life, the originality and unity of this vigorous tribe of twenty-seven thousand persons—together with the tribes most closely related to the Douala. "Ngondo Day" is still celebrated every year. But the strong central politics of Cameroon has deprived the Ngondo of any political influence, so that its activities have taken a "cultural" turn. It is a matter of "arts and letters" now, and popular life is no longer very much among its concerns. Thus the *nganga* abides.

Paradoxically, the secret of the *nganga*s' power—the ability to integrate—is also their weakness. The *nganga*s fit in so well with the cultural context in which they exercise their activity that their effectiveness comes to depend on this context. This is both an advantage and a disadvantage. As the Cameroonian psychiatrist who treated Dieudonné said to me, "Each culture has the medicine it deserves."

The *nganga*s seem not to realize this inherent limitation of their power. Notions of culture and particularity are foreign to them. They practice as if there were but one system of medicine on earth—theirs. Could they but step back from their cultural sphere and consider it from without—from a Western point of view, for example—they would see how they lock up the phenomena of disease and healing, including their irrational dimensions, in a coherent system of explanation that they persuade their clients to accept.

But then they would cease to be so effective, for a good part of their effectiveness resides in their cultural universalization of a particular approach. Everything is done on the assumption that disease and healing form a closed circle.

The most striking example of this interdependence is in the area of mental disorders. It would never occur to a *nganga* to assign them neutral labels— as the West is accustomed to do, where one hears of madness, paranoia, hypochondria, and so on. The *nganga* sorts out these aberrations according to the particular mischievous personal activities deemed to be their cause— sorcerers' invisible traffic in human beings, cannibalism, the punitive intervention of the water spirits or the ancestors, or the violation of prohibitions. The language itself is not without its effects. Persecution complexes will be more frequent than guilt complexes, because of the inclination of patients to consider themselves victims. Attacks of delirium resembling transitory hallucinations will occur more often than schizophrenic psychoses, doubtless by reason of patients' freedom to take refuge in a universe peopled with mysterious powers. Other examples could be given as well, drawn from the treatment of diseases we call organic.

Ultimately, the *ngangas*' effectiveness in treating their patients will be in proportion to their success in imposing their cultural language on them. But by the same token, the *ngangas* run the risk of finding themselves disarmed the moment a cultural separation intrudes itself and they are no longer understood.

For this reason, the most stubborn cases, the ones most difficult to heal, by the *ngangas*' own admission, are persons like those who asked me, "What do you think of all that?" or "Do you believe it's *true*?" They are the product of the very place where the *nganga* was first called into question—the school. There they learned to believe in nothing that cannot be proved—demonstrated, dismantled. The schools have done more to sap the influence of the *nganga* than all the thunderbolts of law and persecution that have ever been hurled against them, and are still hurled against them. It is told how the Germans, at the time of the first colonization of Cameroon, hanged *ngangas* as sorcerers. But that was less harmful to the cause of traditional medicine than the critical spirit of the schools.

This is not to say that the critical spirit is lacking in traditional circles. Here too are nonconformists and freethinkers, rare though they may be. So, for instance, Medi, the old man of the island of Jebale who had been accused of the death of seventeen persons during the cholera epidemic, took me aside one day and confided to me that, in his view, the *miengu* did not exist. Why? He had gone fishing, he said, since his boyhood, in the place reputed to be frequented by *miengu*, and yet had never seen a single one.

There is one more category of subtle mind that deserves mention: that of manipulators of belief. They lodge an accusation of sorcery against their adversary, sowing terror in the heart of that person's family by "revealing" that "fate is against it." Or they manage to convince someone that, for example, leftovers from a meal have been buried in a cemetery with a view to provoking the death of one of the guests. These cases occur frequently. How is it that these persons—genuine flesh-and-blood sorcerers—are not conscious of their own fraud, when they play on common belief in this manner? Probably they find it impossible to doubt this belief in any radical way because of the service it renders them.

However this may be, the art of doubting, taught in the schools, in likewise the ravager of tradition, because it is considered to be educational and constructive. Those who asked me questions about the "truth" of the traditional beliefs were, to be sure, impregnated with this critical spirit.

Mystery, Science, and Religion

Inevitably, the moment came when honesty, as well as the insistence of my schooled interlocutors, forced me to go beyond the question of effectiveness. Reluctantly I must at last pronounce upon the reality of possession and spells, give my opinion on the existence of witches' Sabbaths celebrated well beyond the limits of ordinary mortal gaze, and say whether the dead or the *miengu* really spoke through the mouths of the possessed. "Are these things imaginary?" my interlocutors would ask. I had tried different kinds of answers, but all had been received with reserve. When I proposed the notion that the physical reality of these fantastic phenomena was of little importance—because the essential thing was their meaning and role in the functioning of society—my response seemed evasive.

Of course, we must not forget that ethnologists from all over the world, including Africans themselves, have scrutinized these phenomena all across the African continent, and written countless pages on these questions, without ever being able to verify the accuracy of the stories about the witches' Sabbaths or the return of the dead. It is a matter of imaginary, secret phenomena, the scientists tell us, kept alive by these societies in order to regulate collective life. To be sure, exception is made for the more plausible parapsychic phenomena, such as certain forms of divination, or communication at a distance—although I must say I have no personal experience of anything unusual in these areas. This type of explanation, inspired by the humane sciences, usually failed to impress my interlocutors, who until this moment had been doing the challenging. They would now counter with endless reports, recounted in the most vivid detail, of wondrous events (which they themselves had not directly witnessed) that seemed to run directly counter to their own skepticism.

I had taken the position that this sort of incomprehension was the fruit of ignorance of the philosophic disciplines, and of the monumental role of the imagination in these particular societies. But then one day I really had to begin to doubt the validity of my own arguments. I was showing my older students slides of major treatments in the Kribi area when an idea occurred to me. I saw how I might bring out the distinction between the explanations the *nganga*s had furnished me, and those provided by the humane sciences. And so I first presented the slides with a commentary based on tradition. Then, a week later, I showed the same slides with a scientific explanation. Total failure. The students emphatically rejected the second version. I simply had not understood what was going on in the pictures, they told me. This reaction to my sociological or psychological explanations sent me back to do more reflection. I decided I had to present the medicine of the *nganga*s in some other fashion.

My pupils' stubbornness—which they shared with most of my schooled interlocutors—in defending the reality of their beliefs, and their repugnance to speak of them in psychological terms, was the product of the irrefutable nature of experience. If they were convinced, rightly or wrongly, that these explanations cast doubt on the authenticity of the great experiences of their life, they closed their minds to such explanations. No rational system can exhaust the mystery of life and death, or health and illness. You cannot deny the existence of sorcerers when experience clearly shows that certain persons have the power to make their neighbor fall ill and die.

In my language, of course, one can obviously detect a tendency here to "rationalize"—to claim to be giving the ultimate explanation for these phenomena while knowing that what is being said is not really the last word. The naive logic of the *nganga* seemed to my interlocutors to be ultimately more respectful of the reality of life, even though they had begun to doubt its haughty self-assurance. They wavered between the evidence of their childhood, and new convictions acquired in school. But when the physical or mental anguish was their own, they hardened in their old positions.

I could not feel that this was something to be smiled at. Like them, I believed in the inability of any scientific, philosophical, or even theological language to take full account of the basic mystery of the human being. It is this incommensurability, in everyone's experience, of language and reality, that is for me a sign of the existence of God. One should be on one's guard from the very outset regarding any school of thought claiming to exhaust truth in words. And so I had to change my manner of responding to my interlocutors' questions about the reality of their twin world, or the effectiveness of their medicine. Now I started with a profession of faith in the unfathomable character of life and death. Then I would try to distinguish among the three languages that my interlocutors employed in discussing these mysteries, languages that they often confused—the languages of tradition, of modern science, and of Christian doctrine. Each of these languages has its own cohesiveness, and represents, on its own level, an attempt to accommodate mystery.

I presented Christian discourse as the language most apt, in my view, to confront the language of science without caving in, and in this respect as a language superior to that of tradition. Jesus Christ was able to manifest a critical spirit because he had created a real rapport between God and the human being, between faith and its understanding. In this sense Christianity constitutes an opportunity for reconciliation, and the reestablishment of equilibrium, between tradition and modernism, for those who find themselves torn between the two.

This schema—the triple distinction, then the rapprochement of Christian and scientific discourse—was impossible to present in a few words without neglecting crucial nuances, hence was without meaning or purpose if my interlocutor wanted a cut-and-dried answer. If so, I preferred not to say anything at all. When I had the time to develop my thought, for those who were ready to listen—in the course of an evening with African friends, for example—I now chose to expound my position in these terms. This way of explaining my position on the matter was always well received by them as it was perceived as an echo of their own feelings.

Chapter 15

"Your Eyes Will Be Opened"

The church has need of genuine
dialogue, stripped of all conde-
scension, in which it will seek at
once to render testimony to the
word it bears (or to the Word
who bears it), and to *read upon
the face of the other the very
thing it must become in order to
be what it is*.
—Pierre-Jean Labarriére[94]

After witnessing Kwedi's treatment I had the feeling of having reached a
new threshold. Had I not completed my tour—at least a first, quick, get-
acquainted tour—of the traditional medicine of the Douala country? When
I considered the prospect of going ahead with my research, I felt divided
between two contradictory sentiments—between a desire to go on, and a
great weariness.

A researcher's lassitude is proportioned first of all to the weight of
thralldom to a project. The servitude weighs light when knowledge makes
strides. But it is heavy when there are no surprises in store. For the first
time, I felt disheartened at the thought of throwing myself into the study of
yet another case only to find it practically a replica of others.

Do nonprofessionals realize the cost of ethnology's little disappointments? Do they know what it feels like to come on time for a treatment, and
then to hear three hours later that it is not to take place because of a missing
herb?(Is this an excuse, or the truth? There is no way of knowing.) Do they
know what it is like to sit perfectly still a part of a night on a straight-backed
chair, which one's doting hosts refuse to replace with a more comfortable
folding stool? To have the crucial moment come and then realize that the
batteries in the tape recorder are dead? To ride home at daybreak on a motorbike in the rain, pursued by a pair of mastiffs?

I threw myself into other activities, just as important in my eyes. I was entrusted with theological training of one hundred fifty candidates for the lay ministry in the parishes of Douala. We launched Christian communities in contexts where they might speak out and exercise responsibilities. I was alert to the implicit references of these new students of mine to their second world, the invisible world of tradition, when they spoke of their faith. All the questions that had appeared in the milieu of the *nganga*s flourished here as well. They came back to my ears like the main theme of a concerto. I no longer felt obliged to continue my research. I felt I already knew enough. And surely there could be no question of dilettantism—of continuing to attend treatments without a serious purpose.

I had assisted at a hundred healing séances, complete or partial, con- ducted by thirty different *nganga*s. After Kwedi's night, I had suddenly realized that I could no longer come and sit down as I should have liked to, on a bench in the crowd, without feeling uncomfortable somehow. It was an uneasiness that had doubtless been present from the very first séance at Din's, only it had been so weak that I overlooked it. But ever since, it had come back again and again, like a thorn in my side, and pricked worse and worse with the passing of time and the degree of my integration into the *nganga* world. Now it jabbed hard.

How might I describe it? I felt as if I had been absorbed by Douala society—or, to employ an image with privileged connotations in this con- text, "devoured" by that society. Rumor had once metamorphosized me into an *ekong* sorcerer, and my uneasiness had become anguish. Today, rehabilitated, and once more on the side of good, of order, and of healing, I suffered this anguish no longer. And yet my basic situation remained the same: for better or for worse, I had been assimilated.

But had I not desired all this? I had been admitted to the company of those who pass the night in the open air, feet flat on the good, hard-packed earth of a courtyard—Christians busily engaged in healing one another, after the manner of their own tradition. And I was one of them, at last. This right had been accorded me without any concession on my part. In fact, I had been urged to retain my identity as a priest and a foreigner. And be- cause I was available, my own useful powers had been employed for heal- ing. Whence, then, this malaise?

My feelings of insecurity were due first of all to doubts welling up within me concerning the real value of the healing that went on here. I had had to redefine "sickness," and "bad luck." Now I had another word to work on. What was the *nganga*'s "healing," really? For me, it was defined by the title I have given to a previous chapter Order Lost and Restored. But this order, to which Elimbi, Bruno, Jean Fotsing, and Kwedi must adhere once again if they wished to continue in good health—was it fully theirs? I found myself asking this question more and more often. Could this traditional universe, whose cohesiveness and equilibrium I had discovered, ever really coincide with the modern urbanized world—my own world, now become the world

of these young Africans? Emerging from her long night, was Kwedi better
equipped to do battle alone now, to join in the competition, to keep up with
the changes of the city without becoming lost? In a word, had the treatment
she had received strengthened her "individuality," besides reinforcing her
group membership? If not, her renewed emotional health might surely collapse all over again, this time under the blows of the new society. In devot-
ing myself to the traditional rites, I was lending support to a cultural system
whose self-sufficiency I had begun to doubt.

I also had to ask myself whether I was not occasioning misunderstanding
in Christian consciences. The majority of the *nganga*s and their patients had
been baptized. I had never found any evidence of idolatry or superstition
among them, and rarely of any magical practices. Accusations to that effect
were made too lightly, and did not stand up to scrutiny. The liturgies of
healing were inspired by a genuine ancestral religion. But did they become
Christian just because they were practiced by Christians? Between God and
living human beings, there was a place for ancestors, but I searched in vain
for Jesus Christ, the great absent one as far as these liturgies were concerned.

I was still asked to use my power as a priest. But were my clients really
after anything more than "good luck"? I could not get over the reservations
I had once had about healing Dieudonné, who had demanded a blessing
that had seemed so much like magic to me, or my consternation at the pitiless accusation lodged against Clara, and my powerlessness to help her.

To concretize the situation in my imagination, I fantasized a great tableau, in the purest *ndimsi* style. I figured in the foreground. Then I would
visualize a double procession, stretching from the *nganga*s' courtyards to
the Catholic and Protestant churches, and back again. With my eyes of
flesh, then, I saw, as everyone did, streams of parishioners, in their Sunday
best, peacefully on their way to Mass or some other service. But with my
"double sight" I could see the "true reality"—a second procession, made
up of the same persons, retracing their steps after the service. I saw them, in
this waking dream of mine, piously bearing religious objects, or vessels of
holy water, from the churches to the *nganga dibandi*s. And I was waiting
for them there, cheerful *ndimsi* volunteer, the phoniest priest in the diocese.

I had these doubts and phantasms more and more often. I was unwilling
to make a distinction between my priestly purpose and my goals as a researcher. Hence I had to consider all the effects of my presence at the treatments. Had the moment not come for me to slip discreetly away, out of the
circle of *nganga*s and sorcerers, and consider my research project complete?

The Sway of the Masters of the Night

What force was driving me to perservere, in the face of so many arguments against it? Was this the same hand that had settled on my shoulder in
my childhood, to lead me away from the family front drive, apart, and

somehow off the property? Or was it simply the spirit of curiosity, the taste for research? Was it stubbornness?

All my life I had felt this impulse to "go all the way." For instance, when I returned from Algeria in 1956, without taking a single day off, I threw myself into the reading of Hegel's *The Phenomenology of Mind.* Then I read it again. The project took me five months. I would rise every day at dawn, and, working with a tutor, read and reread every word of those seven hundred pages of philosophy. Nothing could have prevented me from following my "path of initiation" to the very end. The events of the Algerian war had managed to overthrow so much of what had seemed to me to be self-evident in Western civilization, that, in order to reassure myself of its validity, I had to undertake a systematic verification of its foundations. In this critical light, I traversed the field of knowledge as if I had been back in the Jebel region, at night, an officer of the guard making my rounds of the camp with a flashlight, questioning each sentinel, peering into the deepest corners of the darkness—and when the jackals fell silent, stopping still a moment, nor resuming my circuit until they were whining and yapping once more.

Other secular experiences in my past life, too, came to mind, and strengthened my determination to press forward. In particular, one timely jolt set me tottering, and sent me plunging back into the universe of the *nganga*s. It had often come back to my mind, irritatingly, but right on time, like a flashback in a film. It must have had some meaning. It was something that had happened in group analysis, in Paris, in February 1970, just before I had decided to come back and live in Douala.

I have already described how I had had to leave Yaoundé for a time, in consequence of politico-religious difficulties occasioned by a strike by university students. Group analysis was all the rage in Paris in those days, even in church circles, and I had thought it would be interesting to use this technique to evaluate my "staying power," my reactions in a crisis situation, after what had happened in Yaoundé. (But was this my real motivation?) I shall attempt to describe the main phases of this experience, which now seemed to have a special significance for me.

I had gone into group analysis without preparation, knowing only its theoretical principles, and the names of the animators, who had sent me a sheet to fill out. This was no different from the approach I would later use with the *nganga*s. I would investigate their treatments, too, in this way, without preconceived ideas. I would come as an amateur, almost as if I were happening upon them, but with a strange interest.

One Friday evening in Paris, about six o'clock, a little apprehensive, I rang at the apartment whose address had been given to me. I was led into a little parlor, which had nothing special about it, by a middle-aged woman who introduced me to a man who was a little older. They were the analysts, and I was the only client to arrive so far. The man wore the little ribbon of the Legion of Honor in the lapel of his three-piece suit. We sat down, and waited, saying nothing. Waiting, I was learning to my discomfort, was part of European treatments too. I spent the time observing how the room was arranged. The furniture was limited to six chairs and a table. The wallpaper was a perfectly neutral beige, with a few prints of Japanese dream landscapes hanging on the walls. A less obtrusive furnishing and decor could not have been imagined. I had the feeling that everything had been carefully arranged to avoid any impression, any esthetic sensation, imposed from without.

The doorbell announced the arrival of a second person. She was a young woman of about twenty-five, rather sloppily clad in a long, black dress, very thin, obviously pregnant, and called Marthe. And we sat some more. Then, one after the other, there entered another woman of about the same age, short and plump, dressed I no longer remember how, then a twenty-year-old man wearing a blinding white sheepskin shirt and green felt pants. His hair was long, and he had a thick, bushy beard. His name was Pierre; hers, Jocelyne. Our first names were written on little cards in front of us. Except for ash trays, there was nothing on the table.

The analyst started right out with the rules. All four of us were to say publicly what we felt toward one another, holding nothing back, for two and a half days. The "game" might seem artificial. We did not know one another, and would never see one another again. And yet, decisive, healing words would be spoken. Ten years later, I had no need to look at my notes to remember what those words had been.

The Friday evening session dragged slowly along. Inasmuch as we were permitted to speak neither of the past nor of the future, but only of what was going on in our lives at the present, naturally our various subjects of conversation were each rather quickly exhausted. The analysts offered us no assistance, and sat in silence. In a corner, seated on the floor, was a young man taking notes—a student, no doubt. I asked myself what in the world he could be writing during that long moment of heavy silence. It seems that the minutes of the session helped the analysts prepare their rare intervention. When the time came to adjourn, we did so without any special formalities that I can recall, and went our separate ways.

I telephoned the Jesuit psychoanalyst, who had recommended the experiment to me, to let him know how things had gone. I complained that there had been only four participants, instead of the expected dozen. I was disappointed, I said, and could not imagine what we were going to do with the time. I was lucky, he told me, in effect. People live in fours more often than in twelves. I would learn more this way.

Saturday morning. Same decor, same persons. Tongues began to loosen. Each sought to explain why he or she had come. The reasons were very different. Pierre told us he was a professional actor. He, who should have been the expert in expressing himself, had found himself unable to "speak out" in May 1968, as the others of his generation had done, in the student riots. He felt frustrated, and wanted to know why this had happened.

Marthe was a teacher. I was dumbfounded to hear her say that she would decide, as soon as our meetings were over, whether to have the child or have an abortion. She seemed to mean what she was saying. I remarked that we had not come together to counsel one another on an act of that importance.

Jocelyne's problem was very different. She was a bourgeois Jew, she said, and couldn't stand it. She had an "identity problem."

Finally it came to my turn. I explained that I had been in conflictual situations in Africa that could well recur. How should I behave in such circumstances? I no longer recall the discussions that followed my presentation.

Suddenly, about midmorning, Marthe suddenly declared that I must surely be a priest. I had had no intention of hiding the fact, but I had been awaiting the opportunity to have it come out naturally. How had Marthe known? I would soon learn. There was an oppressive silence. One of the analysts remarked, in a bland tone, that this seemed to be a more meaningful silence than previous ones.

Once the moment of surprise and rumination was past, I was drenched in a flood of sarcasm. Within a few minutes I knew what stood between each of the three and the church. Pierre was an atheist, like his father and his grandfather before him. Marthe, who was from Brittany, had stopped practicing religion after her first communion. Jocelyne was Jewish. I wish I could play back the ensuing diatribes on my tape recorder, as I would later do when I met with the *ngangas* as an observer.

Saturday afternoon. Pierre became violent. We were sitting there, painfully searching for words, when he suddenly leapt to his feet, struck me a blow in the face with his fist, which knocked my glasses off, grabbed an ashtray full of cigarette butts and threw it through a window, smashing the pane, then mounted a chair and began to disrobe. The male analyst tried to intervene, but he did not succeed in preventing Pierre's exhibition. He dressed himself again, before our stupefied eyes, took his place one more, and everything was back in order—save that a cold breeze now wafted about us, reminding us of the incident for the rest of the session. Of course, the pane could have been boarded up with something, but no, the analysts wished us to suffer the consequences of our words and actions.

Then I lashed out at Pierre with something for which he would later say heartfelt thanks. "You had your little scene all ready before you even came in here this morning. I'd have rather had something more extemporaneous!" The words popped into my head suddenly as if of their own accord. They were exactly in line with what Pierre thought of himself—that he was an artificial personality.

Sunday morning. Our session was long, slow. Pierre reproached Marthe for the studied sloppiness of her mourning clothes. And he added, "The important thing for you, Marthe, is to save your skin." Save her skin? How could this have been what Marthe needed to hear? Had she just decided on the life or death of the child she was expecting? She did not tell us. She only explained that she wore her grandmother's mourning clothes because she had been the only person who had ever understood her. And she thanked Pierre all through the rest of the analysis.

The importance of any of our statements could be judged from the quality of the silence it provoked. Very few important statements would be made, but those that were important echoed long, like ripples from a paddle pulled a little harder in the calm waters.

Jocelyne, the most reserved of the four of us, reaped no harvest of advice. We simply told her we did not believe her resentment at being a "little bourgeois Jewess." We helped her realize that the real motive for her being here was not her uneasiness with her ethnic origin or social class. This was really just a pretext for her to do group analysis, we said, for, we thought, she hoped to become an analyst herself one day. Unlike me, she had come as a professional. She already knew all the group techniques. It seemed to me that, of the four of us, she gained the least from our encounter.

Sunday afternoon. Pierre and Marthe attacked me. Jocelyne kept silent. Pierre and Marthe brought up everything, from obedience to the pope to priestly celibacy. I remarked that their language was more filled with religious expressions than was mine. I grew weary of all the target practice and finally offered to leave the group. I saw no advantage to me, I told them, in staying to be their whipping boy. I found myself in the uncomfortable position of the village sorcerer, become the scapegoat, the target of all criticism.

Marthe then said something really scathing to me, something that cut to the quick. "You priests are really a big deal," she said. "You never listen. You have nothing to learn." "Touché," I replied. It was true that, of the four of us, I was the least patient with the long, empty silences, when we really had nothing to say to one another. I could not bear them. I would fill them with words, for whatever they were worth. Or again, several times my three companions had accused me of misinterpreting something they had said. But I recall nothing else to justify Marthe's reaction. And yet she had taken offense. I allowed the silence to orchestrate what I was going to say— then, after a long, long pause, instead of bristling and retorting, I let go, defeated. "Look," I said, "I need you to tell me to stay."

My reaction calmed them down. They needed me, too, just as villagers need their sorcerer in some confused way. The evening concluded in an amiable euphoria, and perfect harmony, each of us having received our allotment of material for reflection over the days to come. Afterward the student came up from his corner and shook my hand warmly. I imagined he had grasped the effect of what Marthe had said to me. I paid my three hundred francs, and I certainly did not feel I had not had my money's worth. The analysts informed us that the fee also entitled us to a private session. But I had no desire for one. I wanted to interpret by myself what had been said to me.

It is startling to be told by someone, out of the blue, a truth that you admit to yourself in secret. Children pronounce such judgments, lightning bolts of accuracy that offend, but we are satisfied just to smile about them.

"You priests have nothing to learn!" And I had thought I was doing everything necessary not to deserve such a reproach. Marthe had made to me the reproach of Jesus to the scribes and Pharisees, and the old complaint often repeated in Africa about whites, especially missionaries. The arrow Marthe had let fly had not only pierced my sacerdotal shell. It had struck deeper still, down within my primordial, family being, down where I thought that the lovely first assurance of my childhood—that truth was mine—had been alive and well. The memory of this searing little sentence figured, without any doubt, in my decision to remain in the school of the *ngangas*, in order to maintain myself in an attitude that was resolutely receptive.

But the most unexpected thing—when all was said and done, the most revelatory point as far as I was concerned—was the request that I had made myself: "I need you to tell me to stay." The Curé of Ars is said to have remarked, "I measure the meaningfulness of anything I say by how much it hurts me." Yes, to stay—to remain with this apparently hostile trio, this living echo of an anticlerical society where the priest is rare, out of place, undesirable, prohibited—was something that was needful to me. For indeed it was needful to me that nothing be foreign to me, no milieu shut off, no part of the world forbidden. What was it? Mission? Faith? Vocation? I hesitate to use these traditional Christian terms, not because they seem inaccurate—they express the experience of over a thousand years—but because they are too limpid, too clear. Really, I had to wonder what vast depths, what region of the high seas, could be the source of these mighty waves that never ceased to drive me toward other shores.

Then too, how was I to explain to myself how all my experiences in Douala country, surely more impressive in other respects, could have failed to make me forget that short little Parisian interlude? I had only one explanation. In Paris I had been personally involved. In Douala I was an observer, a student, silent and reserved— sitting along the wall, outside the battle zone. What else could I do in the *nganga* domain? I could go sit in the midst of the possessed and pursued, the bewitched, and undergo treatment myself. Only, I did not see the need at the moment. Or I could have my eyes opened, to be "with" the ones who heal in the night.

Mysterious the sway of the masters of the night! Of what unsubjugated region of myself had they taken possession? Did they occupy the realm where dreams are born and bred? Had they seized the spot where the most contrary desires mingle—the one to kill and the one to love, the one to make suffer and the one to adore, the phantasms born of water and fire, blood and death, in a perpetual maelstrom like the one I had seen with my own eyes in the course of the night séances at the hands of the *ngangas*. There must be a hidden relationship, I thought, a secret pact, between the *ngangas* and myself. Nothing else could have explained the fascination I felt when I was among them. Since childhood I had always wanted to reach other cultural worlds—to get as far away as I could from my own roots. And now that I had done so, I had the feeling of having arrived in a familiar land.

> Where can I go from your spirit?
> from your presence where can I flee?
>   If I go up to the heavens, you are there:
> if I sink to the nether world, you are present there.
>   If I take the wings of the dawn,
> if I settle at the farthest limits of the sea,
>   Even there your hand shall guide me,
> you and your right hand hold me fast.
>
> Psalm 139:8–10 [NAB]

Chapter 16

Death of the Seer

Loe saw his death coming. He took such risks, he said, in the course of the nights of battle, flying to the rescue of the bewitched, that sooner or later he would be carried off himself. On several occasions he had fallen to the ground, rigid as wood, and nothing could have convinced an onlooker that he was playacting. He now fixed his life expectancy at eight months. I could not take this prophecy of misfortune literally. Neither could Elimbi, his eldest son.[95] It was true that Loe was not wrong about much. But one never knew whether a *nganga*'s statements were not, after all, therapeutic maneuvers.

This was a man in his fifties, and tough as a cat. When he began to waste away, stopped treating others, and put himself in the hospital, we began to be uneasy. His first physician found signs of tuberculosis. Loe rejected the diagnosis. They wrangled about it, and Loe decided to try his luck elsewhere. This time the possibility of a liver abscess was discovered. These divergent diagnoses disturbed Loe very much, and he decided he preferred to go back to traditional medicine. "I know I'll have to go stay in the hospital some day," he told me. "But I have some other things to take care of first."

And then the merry-go-round of *nganga*s started. I shall describe only the oldest of these men, because of his special reputation and influence. Yonas was his name. To look at him—blind, emaciated—it was difficult to imagine his great power. But all up and down the coast his prowess was celebrated, even in song: "Bring us your problem," the followers at solemn treatment séances would sing, "we'll go get Yonas"—*Wanea biso pai, di m'ala nongo Yonas*. With him, Loe knew he was playing his last trump. Years before, the blind old man had performed upon Loe the essential rite of the opening of the eyes. Yonas was Loe's master.

Elimbi told me about the meeting of Yonas and the other *nganga*s. "The blind old man came to our house. You would have thought he saw everything. He asked the other *nganga*s there, 'You came to treat Papa Loe—do you know exactly what's wrong with him?' Nobody said anything. So

212

Yonas said, 'Fine. I'm the one who'll work today. Go home. Consult your men [the ancestors who supply the inspiration for the healing], ask them what's wrong with Loe, and come back Saturday to treat him. I won't be here, but I'll be here in *ndimsi*.'''

"Did they come back?" I asked.

"No, because Loe told them, 'The ones who don't come back with a good medicine will be wiped out.' They were afraid!"

"What did Yonas say?"

"That Papa had caught his malady when he went to treat a patient, and that he wouldn't survive it. But he spoke in an ironical way. He was going to work on it, but Papa couldn't get completely well. He'd just get some relief for a while. Then I knew Papa was going to die. But you know, sometimes science can tell you you're going to die, and you don't die. That's why papa put up such a fight to keep alive. But he really knew he didn't have a chance."

And then Yonas returned no more. The family began to wonder why the *nganga*s were giving up so easily. Many had left saying, "If our medicines line up with the sickness he has, he'll get well."

A month went by. Back from a trip, I went to Loe's quarter with a feeling of apprehension. I noticed the little heap of earth beside the *dibandi* at once. Practically in the center of the helter-skelter of the different little buildings that stood there on Loe's property. When his wives, all dressed in widow's blue, his daughters, and his nieces saw me arrive, they assembled at the doorstep, as custom prescribed when a friend of the deceased came to visit. They welcomed me, and preceded me to the grave site with cries and lamentations. Until that moment, these dismal laments had seemed to me artificial and overdone, but now I felt thankful to those women for having taken it upon themselves to express the emotion I felt, that I might keep silent. Curiously, the last scene of *The Seventh Seal* came back to me—the film in which Bergman sketches the world of possession and sorcery. When death comes at last, the woman says, simply, "tuss"—meaning "silence." And I said to myself, "Be quiet, forget yourself, pray." From my inmost depths, as simply as I could, I asked God to receive this good man into his presence.

Elimbi, who had stayed by my side all the while I stood before the grave, had a question to ask me. "Papa spoke to you very often. Didn't he tell you anything?"

"No."

"Not the slightest thing?"

"No," I replied. "I was like a child for your father. I was a friend and a child, as far as his science was concerned."

"Because he didn't tell us anything either. Three days before he died he didn't say a single word any more—nothing!"

Loe's silence had disturbed his family. The last wishes of someone about to die were to be gathered, observed, kept sacred. This was the strictest of rules. Loe's muteness had left serious questions of succession unresolved. Had it been due to his difficult character, or was it simply physical incapacity.

Everything I knew inclined me to think that Loe had saved what he had to say until he could say it in more solemn fashion, and with a better chance of being obeyed, by the expedient of a phenomenon he knew better than anyone else: the *bejongo* trance.

Nine days after his death, two women fell into a trance: his third wife—Elimbi's mother—and a former patient who had often been seen attending Loe's major treatments. Papa Loe, a number of witnesses agreed, had dictated his last will through these women's mouths. His family received their words with gratitude. Thanks to them, the principal sources of conflict had disappeared. When various persons would recount for me, emotionally, what had happened, I accepted their accounts as given in good faith and truthful, for I had witnessed such trances myself.

As a general rule, circumstances would prevent me from carrying out a complete investigation of a like report. The families would be too upset and excited by the phenomenon. Only on rare occasions had I been able to do a thorough examination of it. The *bejongo* trance, which summons the intervention of the ancestors, is a social mechanism in the service of group unity, a safety valve. Its effectiveness rests on the solidity of genealogical ties, and on the conviction that the ancestors still have dealings with the families that they have visibly left. The possessed woman will have personal reasons for having the ancestors intervene. She will not find any means of having her rights recognized through ordinary channels, and will resent this, anxiously and mightily. The trance affords her her only opportunity to express herself. At that moment, she will no longer be aware of what she is saying, it is for the ancestors who will be speaking through her. The group will have to render her justice, and comply with the instructions from beyond the grave.[96]

Loe had had four last things to say:

1) "I have died over a matter of land." This was a comforting revelation. He had not been killed by any of his relatives. Suspicions, resting on the various diagnoses of so many physicians and *nganga*s, had run rampant ever since Loe had begun to be treated, and had spared no one. And yet this was but a half-revelation.

Everyone knew that Loe had been risking death for a long time, defending property rights in a zone of the city where they had been hotly disputed. Loe had fallen victim to the last skirmishes of a long-standing battle. Many years before, German colonists had pushed the Douala back from the banks of the river in order to be able to build a port and warehouses. The Douala, in turn, had seized quarters farther away from the river, and it was said that the Bassa who had tried to interfere were met with all manner of resistance, including sorcery and poison.[97] Loe was everlastingly running into conflict with these Bassa neighbors of his, and he would talk to me about it from time to time.

The poison theory, then, was not to be excluded as a possible cause of Loe's demise. I asked a Cameroonian physician, who had done his medical studies in Europe, whether an abscess of the liver—the last diagnosis at the hospital—debunked the poison hypothesis. He replied that hepatitis could indeed be of toxic origin. He said he knew of a plant that caused a viral hepatitis that was slow to show its presence. But it would have been necessary to attend the patient regularly in order to be able positively to arrive at this conclusion.

2) "All my children are to share my estate equally." Here Loe's third wife, the one reporting the father's last will, betrayed her special interest. Loe had never legally recognized their son, Elimbi. And yet he considered him his firstborn and heir, for neither of his first two wives had given him a son. An old quarrel had driven Elimbi's mother to take the boy with her when she left his father. To punish this infidelity, Loe had never taken official steps to recognize their child, which he would have had to do if Elimbi was to have been his heir. This declaration from beyond the grave had saved the situation in the nick of time.

3) "It's no use looking for money. There isn't any." The widows could breathe easily. Now no one would dare to try to force them to reveal the places where they had perhaps hidden the family savings. The decedent's declaration would obviate endless digging and searching.

4) "Nkongo is in charge of the *dibandi*." This last declaration of the decedent's will was far from least important, to my way of thinking. It seemed to me to be a difficult thing to carry out. Nkongo had come to stay with Loe, thirteen years before, as a patient. He had attached himself to his *nganga*, never leaving him after that, and rendering inestimable services, with assiduity, good humor, and practicality. He was Loe's only disciple. The entire weight of the master's legacy would fall on his shoulders.

"It's a big responsibility to take care of Father's *dibandi*," he said to me. "The *dibandi* is like a treasure. If it weren't for the *dibandi*, Father wouldn't have all his goods, his lands, his houses, everything. Now he's left it to me, and I'm not even a member of the family! It's true I know all the treatment theories—exactly like Father. I know how the *dibandi* is set up, from one end to the other. We've been to the forest together and we've found all the barks that are there. There's only one thing I don't have—the double sight."

I asked Elimbi for his viewpoint on Nkongo's promotion. "Papa wants Nkongo as his successor," he said. "But Nkongo doesn't see. The only one who can settle this thing is the master who opened Papa's eyes—the blind old *nganga* who tried to heal him. The man is very good, the best of the good ones. He should perform what we call *tole* on Nkongo—put drops under his eyelids so he can open his other eyes."

Double Sight

Those who enjoy double sight, and those who are reduced to the mere use of their simple mortal eyes, are worlds apart. I had once had to pay the price of ignorance in this matter, while Loe was still alive, on the occasion of a divination session. He had invited me to come into the *dibandi* and study with him the case of a woman who had come to consult him. It was an unusual invitation. "You do the visit [the examination] the European way," he had said, "and then I'll do it the African way."

I accepted. I questioned the woman on the reasons why she had come. She quickly learned I was a priest, and spoke of her conjugal disputes. Her husband, a railway employee, had assured her that she would be his only wife—then, after the marriage had been consummated, she learned that he already had a wife and five children. Then she herself did not become pregnant. And so all the husband's money and attention went to the first wife. The patient fell ill as a result. I thought I ought to tell her that, after all, she had not entered into any definitive contract with this man, because he had deceived her in an essential matter, and that she could consider herself free.

"That wouldn't change a thing," she replied. "Men are all scamps."

Loe went at his part of the "examination" altogether differently. He avoided using any acquired knowledge. He "saw." Without asking her any questions, he described her physical troubles—and he was right on target, to judge from all the nodding and shaking of the patient's head. He talked about her family, and about a certain uncle, who could have been the cause of her misery. Finally he asked her: "Am I lying?"

"No, what you tell me is true," she replied.

Now Loe demanded a meeting with her husband. "We're going to have to persuade him to be present the night of the treatment."

I could see the *nganga*'s tactics at work. Antagonists were driven to avowals, and if possible to reconciliation, because this would be the sole guarantee of a complete cure. But this time Loe's stipulation was too difficult, and we never saw the woman again. Doubtless she had found a less demanding *nganga*. I was struck that Loe, unlike me, had asked her but a single question—"Am I lying?" He had just gone ahead as one who saw.

The vast importance ascribed to vision can be explained only in reference to Bantu anthropology. I shall sketch only a few particulars here, the ones that will be essential for an understanding of what will follow.

Everyone has four eyes (*miso manei*). As a rule persons close their two visible eyes at the hour of death, and open the other two in the kingdom of the ancestors. But it happens that certain persons (*brwusu*) are born with all four eyes open. This anomaly, at once feared and desired, is discovered when a child catches a glimpse of someone passing by, and then it is learned that that person has died. In such a case, parents generally hasten to have the pair of eyes that see the invisible "put out" (*tuba*), by a special treatment, for a child does not have the strength to bear such revelations without harm. Those who "put out" eyes also have the power to open them.

Thus those human beings who have both pairs of eyes at once, those of the living and those of the dead, serve as intermediaries between the two worlds. They can see the underside of society. And so they have the task of intervening when sorcery rears its ugly head. It is from among these individuals that *nganga*s are recruited. "You know," Elimbi said to me, "the spirit is what makes a human being, and that's what sees double."

Nkongo, then, had no choice but to obey Loe and take the *dibandi* in charge, without having his eyes opened. Yet he hesitated, and he might have procrastinated indefinitely, had it not been for certain new portents that forced him to make the commitment.

"Papa Loe's made a little boy talk, too," Nkongo told me.

"What boy?" I asked.

"A child about eleven or twelve years old. He doesn't even live here. He lives back there a way. He's the brother of the wife of one of Father's relatives. He repeated what Father told him to say."

"Did you hear this child? What did he say?"

"I was there. So was Elimbi, and everybody. First he said, 'Nkongo is in charge of the *dibandi*.' Papa Loe's big brother said no. 'This is impossible,' he said. 'Nkongo isn't even a member of the family. This medicine is a family matter. Are you going to leave this to a stranger, and get yourselves a batch of prohibitions into the bargain?' "

According to Nkongo, Loe had also prescribed a number of other things, by this same medium, concerning respect for trees on the property and the danger of riding a motorbike. He had announced that one of his daughters was expecting. And he had said a number of other things, including two instructions for Nkongo that finally forced him to make a move.

Nkongo was ordered to organize a major night séance, a *dikute*, for the purpose of restoring to the *dibandi* its lost power. More precisely, he was to call Loe's *jengu* wife back to the place she had deserted when Loe had died, for without her, the *dibandi* was an empty hut. (Loe had always declared that he held his powers from his mystical *jengu* spouse. This liaison made him an *esunkan*, the highest rank in the *nganga* hierarchy.) And at midnight, Father would speak. The child who had transmitted the wishes of the deceased had outlined the ceremony to be followed in its minutest details, and I can testify that this plan was scrupulously respected.

The second command provoked a moment of panic. "The child also said that Father had left some money hidden in the ceiling, and that I was supposed to go and find it to give to his widows for their support. And he said nobody was supposed to know just when I would go looking. Otherwise I wouldn't find this money. Then Papa Loe's big brother and Elimbi got mad, and said 'This is not possible!' Then the child said that when I went to look for this money, all I had to do was take along a witness."

"But the first time, Loe said there wasn't any money to look for!" I said.

"And now all of a sudden the child says there's some hidden in the ceiling!"

"That's true, and we simply don't understand. We don't know how to put the two things together."

"Have you tried to find the money?"

"We tried, but everybody made us look for it right away. There were four of us, and we looked in the ceiling, but we didn't find anything. I don't know if it's true or not. Father said we were supposed to look in secret. That's why they didn't see anything. Unless there's another reason. . . ."

"What do you think about it?" I asked.

"It bothers me," Nkongo replied. "Things like that do happen. I know they can happen. There's proof. For instance, the night before the little boy spoke, Loe's second wife asked me for some black cloths that Father had kept in his *dibandi*, so that she could do some sewing on them. And then the boy said, 'Father allows Nkongo to give his wife the black cloths.' And yet nobody knew what I'd done, and it was night when I finally put those cloths back."

The first *bejongo* trances I had witnessed had seemed to me to answer to the secret expectations of the group, and reinforce its cohesion. But this time the boy's demonstration looked suspect. I did not imagine the boy was playing games any more than the women had been, but his exaggerated performance was beginning to take the structures of custom down a peg or two.

The most straightforward outcome of this series of episodes was the announcement of the great ceremony that Nkongo had to conduct according to the instructions given. It would take place the following Saturday. I helped Nkongo gather a little money for the occasion, and I had decided to watch him very closely: he was "blind" (he did not have double sight), but he had to conduct himself as a seer.

Rendezvous with Death

As a general rule the atmosphere of a night ceremony is generated progressively. One must await the approach of midnight for the drums to beat their fullest, and for the pitch of fervor conducive to trances.

That night though, I arrived early and was surprised to find the crowd already bubbling with excitement. It was raining, and they had all crammed themselves into the largest of the huts, at the end of the courtyard—the elder brother's house. I noticed a number of persons present whom I had never seen at Loe's—men of tradition, doubtless come from the neighborhoods along the river. Their absolute impassivity contrasted sharply with the frenzied trances seizing one wife or relative of the deceased after another. Two *nganga*s in showy red costumes saw to good order. Neighbors peered in at the doors and windows, drawn by the high drama of this ceremony. Would Loe speak again? I had never seen the presence of a dead person rendered so palpable. You will struggle in vain against such demonstrations, foreign as they are to your sensibilities. They are contagious. You are won over.

Before the rain was over, the assembly transferred to the courtyard, in front of the *dibandi* where Loe had practiced for twenty-five years. His grave was a little hillock to one side. No innovation had been introduced since his death—the space was still a square, marked off by planks resting on cinder blocks, and serving as benches, and, as one side of the square, the facade of the *dibandi*. In the center, the sacred bush arose, with a trunk as thick as an arm and branches to the housetops. The staging could not have been lower key. There was a general assault on the benches, but on account of the unusual size of the crowd, five or six rows of persons had to stand.

Alone in the *dibandi* for the first time, and hence out of view, Nkongo docilely executed the rites. "In the *dibandi*," he later told me, "I did as Father used to. I whistled and rang the bells [to summon the ancestors]. And I talked to them, inside myself: 'I know that you [the ancestors] are here. I can't see you, of course, but you know me. I know Father is here, too. He may be dead, but he's here. You know me—I'm Father's son. And I'm giving you orders as Father used to do. When he was with me he commanded me to talk to you. So I'm talking to you right now. So here I am now, just about ready to go out. You're here, and you see everything, and hear everything. I know absolutely nothing. You're here. I ask you, I beg you, to protect me against my enemies who may be in the courtyard. I'm like a blind person now.' After I said that, I broke an egg and spread it all around."

Nkongo came out of the *dibandi* into our midst, and tried to intone a few chants, when the others gave him a chance. He wore a red and white robe, and danced along the benches crammed with visitors; he did not approach the center. There was an indefinable exaltation and wantonness in his gestures. Why was he wearing that kerchief on his head? With its red border falling along his neck, it gave his light, mulatto face a look of childishness. He was too timid to dance where the master had danced. Gradually I noticed that that place had been taken by Eboa, a nephew of Loe, who had spent his childhood here, and who flaunted a high and mighty offhandedness. I had never seen him before.

Now Eboa called for silence, and held a laconic conversation with both *nganga*s, all in grunts and mime. Finally he started giving Nkongo orders. I thought he must surely be attempting to take Loe's succession upon himself. But no, Elimbi would later explain to me, even though "Eboa could do the work, because he's the one who knows the most, of the whole family—more than Nkongo," still, Elimbi assured me, "he probably wouldn't accept this work. He's with Criminal Investigation. He wouldn't want to waste his time. He'd never make the sacrifice." And indeed, Eboa did not become Loe's successor, and I never saw him again.

Perceiving the discomfort of Nkongo's situation, an old man I did not know stepped in to intervene. "This child does not see," he cried to the nephew, the detective. "Lay no trap for him! And the one who has four eyes—well, let him make no use of them! When you dance—even tiny movements of your feet or your hands—I can explain what it means. . . . I know you're fond of *ekumti* [occult battles]. You don't come around here just for fun; you've got to go tickling your brother, right?" Tickling meant starting a fight. Before a ritual combat, adversaries provoked one another by jabbing with their fingers.

"I don't know, I don't have four eyes," someone in the crowd called out. "I just came to dance. I'm not looking to kill, you don't have to kill me first. I was Father's best companion during the treatments. If I was a killer, you think I'd admit it?" And there was a general brouhaha.

"Understand me well!" the old man replied. "This child before you is our adopted son [a child of the day—*mun'asu nya mwese*]. He is not of our family. Nobody better try having fun by setting a trap for him! Father Loe hasn't shown himself yet, but when he comes out, nobody'll feel like testing this young man any longer! If you try now, Father'll see to it that you get wedged [*kudumane*]. This child is here by Father's will, and we accept him. This is why I have risen [to speak]. I am a man of peace. 'Who sows war, reaps war!' Somebody may be better than I, but he won't be better than Nkongo!"

The old man's little speech was right to the mark, and was followed by applause. There were a few more dances, then three young men of the family took hold of Nkongo and led him to the center of the square around which the others were seated or standing. They they took up *mwandando* branches—the "cane of the dead," whose ritual importance for peace and good government throughout the land I had often remarked—and began to switch him. I followed this rite with attention, because so many cultures employ it as the sign of the passing of power from one person to another, or of accession to an office.[98] And my neighbor, the man who had often before helped me understand the obscure, but essential, gestures of Loe's courtyard, whispered: "This is the enthronement."

Was Nkongo being made a *nganga* before my very eyes? Afterward he told me he had not known the rite could have such importance and such effect. "The late Father had ordered me to prepare three *mwandandos*, to be whipped with, through the *bejongo* of the little boy. If I was going to want to do the work Father ordered, this was the only way to give me the courage and spiritual strength for it."

It was the little boy, then, who was said to have laid down the prescriptions for this extremely rare ceremony. Who could have inspired him?

It was nearly midnight, the hour when Loe was manifest himself. Suddenly there was some commotion on my left. Loe's first wife rose to her feet, in a trance. Her spectacular seizure incited a chain reaction. Twelve persons very quickly fell into trances—Loe's wives, his grown daughters, two former patients (including Kwedi), and—a rare occurrence—two men. Eboa and Nkongo, the *nganga*s, circled the writhing bodies as calmly and cooly as if they had been judges at a country fair. Clearly, they had no wish to become entangled in this encounter with the ancestors.

It would have been fascinating to know the meaning of this trance for each of those who had entered into it. For example, what did this moment represent for Loe's eldest daughter? While her father was alive, she had lived apart from the family, a lost daughter. The day he was buried, she was actually driven away. Tonight here she was, readmitted. Some of those around sought to interrupt this out-of-place demonstration; others wished it to be allowed to take its course.

Strange and wild was the spectacle. Molded into a long, black spindle, the young woman was seized by some force that now would bend her backward, now whip her forward, like a pliant reed. She clutched the white trunk of the bush that grew in the middle of the courtyard, the one they called the "outdoor *dibandi*," and shook all over, together with the bush, until it looked as if she could go on shaking forever.

Conditions were right for the sudden event. But nothing happened. The possessed were mute.

"You don't force them," Nkongo later explained to me. "You never force them."

"At midnight I counted twelve trances," I said. "But no one spoke!"

"Father was there, though. Starting at eleven-thirty I could feel his presence. I was Father's valet, you know. When he was alive, if he came by, for instance, and I didn't see him, I could smell him. From eleven-thirty on, I could feel inside me that he was there. That was when things went into high gear."

"But no one spoke."

"My wives fell over, but they didn't speak. That is, Father didn't speak. Father saw he couldn't speak, that Saturday, because the news had spread all over. A whole crowd came to hear him. And his enemies were there, too, plenty of them. Enemies we know—Bassa folk, those who say the land belongs to them."

The scheduled program stayed right on time. Now it was time to go to the only two places where one might find Hélène Yambe, Father's mystical *jengu* wife, who had deserted the *dibandi* the moment he died.

We started our procession, then, toward the little rivulet we had visited so often in the course of Loe's treatments—the backwater of the Mbanya, celebrated sacred stream of the Douala people. There Nkongo danced and sang. Then he led us through the quarter (where nary a one was sleeping that night!) to a great, deserted intersection, all the emptier-looking for its purposeless streetlamp, hard by the Grand Stadium of Douala. Loe had constructed his first *dibandi* here, when it was still part of the wild. There we were, then, a hundred anachronisms, milling strangely about in this place of tar and concrete. Once in a while a taxi would whip around the corner, barely brake in time to keep from hitting us, and continue on its way.

Nkongo told me later what he had been doing all this while. "Down at the riverbank I talked with the water, according to the orders I had: to find the *jengu* river-woman. It was to make her come back. I told the water I was nothing but a messenger from Father. If his wife Hélène was there, she was supposed to come with us. And if the water knew it was keeping Hélène somewhere, it had better give her to us! I waited a little bit, then we went to the intersection.''

"Did you have the feeling that Hélène Yambe came back to the *dibandi* with us?" I asked.

"Hélène came back. She's in the *dibandi*.''

"How can you be certain?"

"I'm certain. . . . After he died, Father told me I had to go have my eyes opened. Usually if you only have two eyes, you don't see. There are things that happen that are invisible. But when I was living with father, I could feel, for instance, when somebody from outside was there. I could feel it. My body knew there was a strange body there. He didn't tell me, I didn't hear anything, I didn't see anything, but I felt it inside me. My blood noticed there was a strange body.''

What might we call this physical faculty of perceiving an invisible presence? It is the *nganga*s who have it in the highest degree, but it is strongly developed in the uninitiated, too, and I can include myself in their number. It is not a sixth sense, alongside the other five, nor is it the sum of the other five (as Nkongo once put it), but it is a property of the body taken in its totality.

I was greatly impressed one day when an old *nganga* of the Kribi region confided something to me. We were sitting on the sand, watching the equatorial sun in its rapid setting, when he said to me, in an altogether natural tone: "You see, I've been a *nganga* for forty years. I've been with the ancestors and water spirits so often that I know exactly when they're around. It's usually at this time of day that my body tells me.''

The rites dragged on through the last part of the night. The songs were from the traditional repertory now, and became elliptical and allusive— referring to the dead, to the *mïengu*, and to sorcery.[99] But hearts were no longer in it. Most of the rubbernecks had gone home, disappointed in the mute, departed *nganga*. The little family group was alone. Rice and fish were spilled onto the floor for the ancestors, and served on plates for us. A woman in a trance quickly circled the men, and solemnly led Nkongo to the *dibandi*. Eboa calmed her, and everything wound down to an end. The rain began again at dawn, and that was enough to send us all home.

A few days later, Nkongo was sent by the company he worked for to Ngaoundéré, a city in the north. All by himself, he was to solder all the guard rails around the big floodlights in the stadium and the new railroad station. It was his first assignment on his own, and he returned from it happy and content. It had been a useful diversion, far from Douala, the *dibandi*, and their attendant problems.

We got together, and he described his position clearly: "I want to work for a company. I want a new life. But this *nganga* business keeps chasing me! If I have a vision, in a dream, that will give me back some strength. I'll be forced to accept. But I'm not going looking for the vision myself."

Nkongo's wait-and-see policy seemed wise to me, and I took care not to intimate any other. He had already spoken to me in this same sense. "If the departed father really declares that it's still I who must keep his work going, and if I refuse, sooner or later he'll show me that I have to be a *nganga*. At first, he himself didn't want to be a *nganga*. He wanted to be a carpenter. But he had certain gifts. It was his destiny to be a *nganga*, and that's the work he finally did."

I wondered if Nkongo would ever have that decisive dream. For the moment he lacked a real desire to be a *nganga*. And I thought that without such motivation, he would never dream that dream. It was more than a matter of an attraction to modern business life. I knew a young man, called Ngea, who had given up a dance band he directed, from which he had had quite a decent living, to retire to the bush and practice traditional medicine. Nkongo was afraid. He lacked his master's "punch," and perhaps would never acquire the taste for battle that was one of the prime indicators of the *nganga* calling. "I realize," he told me, "that if I get double sight I could catch my death. In fact I'm sure that if my mother knew all this, she'd tell me to quit."

Nkongo's hesitations, which I followed closely day after day, produced a great effect on me. I was now convinced once and for all that double sight was the entryway to the *nganga*'s enclosed garden. Perhaps I could have penetrated a little way into the secret world of the initiated in Nkongo's shadow. But I concealed my disappointment from him. There could be no question of my influencing him, in any manner whatsoever, to set him off on a path he would never totally accept.

There was only one solution and it had been inextricably intertwined with the logic of my research for five years now. That solution was to try the experience myself—to leap over the wall. But who would be willing to open my eyes? Perhaps one person only: Din.

Chapter 17

The Eyes of My Goat

I was personally acquainted with some thirty *nganga*s, all up and down the coast. Why should I have had to approach Din to open my eyes? True, he was the first *nganga* I had actually seen at work. And he was the only one who had behaved toward me as a master toward a disciple—and that from our very first meeting. On February 5, 1971, he had himself taken the initiative of inviting me to Engome's night séance. I still remembered how packed with meaning his gestures had been. He was at once the witness and the occasion of my repeated astonishment—and from time to time he would turn to me with that certain smile of his, as if he were saying, "See? Understand?" He had placed me at his side from the very start of the night, by having me come to his *dibandi*. The reader will recall that it was there that I had seen him, for the first time, lying on his back with his eyes closed, perfectly motionless, plunged into that quasi-cataleptic state in which he had access to invisible realities—to the world of *ndimsi*.

From that day forward, our friendship gradually grew. Still, as I have recounted, our first steps were difficult. I could only stammer a bit of Douala at the time, and he was not really very good at it himself, having come from the island of Malimba, a hundred kilometers away. There was a certain mistrustfulness between us. He must have wondered what this European priest's ulterior motives were. For my own part, I was taken aback by his affability and attention. Was he merely out for all the money he could get? Was he just playacting? But then we met again and again. Our relationship changed, as I have described. He "made me dream," he "armored" me against sorcery. And then one day, as if it had been a whimsical notion that just popped into his head, he declared that he would open my eyes one day.

Finally, by way of thanking me for having stood by him during the court proceedings, he had named his last child for me, just after being released from jail and just before fleeing to his island.

And now, a few weeks after Loe's death, just when I was wrestling with this problem of double sight, Din reappeared. Coincidentally, just about this same time, Chief Betote Akwa, the leading figure of all the Douala, who knew about my work, told me one day simply, "They'll open your eyes." Finally, a Frenchman I knew, and whose keen mind and considerable experience I admired, spoke to me at length of the visions he had had as a result of the ingestion of psychedelic substances. All these things converged upon my sensibilities, and aroused my enthusiasm. I decided to visit Din, to ask him whether he was still disposed to give me "the sight."

And Din gave this answer: "I want to know if you ask the sight in order to heal, or if it's just to keep it for your own use. If you want to heal others, when you're in Europe, the way of the whites, you'll have to be able to see to increase the strength of your sick patients. But if you just want it for yourself, say so."

Before responding, I made a rapid inquiry as to whether one can have one's eyes opened without becoming a *nganga*. The answer was in the affirmative: the rite sufficed unto itself, and did not oblige the beneficiary to make a future commitment. Indeed, there existed an ancillary social function performed by those who merely stood watch—kept their eyes open to see what was going on in the "night," in the invisible world. They were like sentinels, and had no other function than to watch and warn.[100] And the practice of traditional medicine seemed out of the question for me. Everything I had gathered thus far indicated that the first condition for success in this area was a deep congruity between the healer and the patient at all levels. How would I be capable of managing the symbols that penetrated my patients through and through if I were not penetrated by them myself? I had healed Dieudonné because he had joined me in my own world. Could I ever play that game of accusing persons of sorcery?

Initiation to double sight—that and no more—seemed to me to be a reasonable objective, recognized by tradition, and perhaps the only one that would be accessible to me without playacting.

Now I could reply. "My desire is not to become a *nganga*, but if you are willing to open my eyes, I would be grateful to you. My purpose is to know (*bia*) and to understand (*songtane*) the way you do. It does not seem to me that this would be possible without 'seeing' (*jene*)."

"I understand," said Din. You don't want to see in order to heal. The Pygmies taught me how to open the eyes of others, but there are terrible prohibitions (*le mbenda jita*). No *nganga*, if you go to one, will open your eyes. He'll tell you stories till you're blue in the face—all dreams.[101] But I promise you I'll do it for you."

A bit later in our conversation, Din continued: "The problem is to get started. I didn't bring all my things here. I haven't any *njum bwele*, I haven't any *ngopange*. Seriously, if I had those two barks we could start right away."

"I'll get some, no matter what."

I had no idea how much trouble I would have procuring those two barks. What I took for an inconvenience or misfortune was actually a step in the initiation process. A *nganga*'s disciple must learn the price of bark!

First I went to Etame Dika, the oldest person in Bonabéri, for help in procuring the *njum bwele*—the plant whose adult stalks kill all plants around it.[102] This is why it is found in the center of a clearing, and it is this property that is perhaps at the basis of its reputation: its bark is used to keep sorcerers at a distance. Din claimed to have had a meager amount of it in his enclosure when he had lived with Ekwala.

Etame Dika was at pains to let me know what I was asking. "When you've got *njum bwele*," he said, "no other medicine is a match for its strength. If you go to look for it, you have to be strong yourself—tough, in good condition, to be able to remove this strength from the earth (*nginya wase*). You have to stand naked before the tree. Before you take a piece, you have to pray. This is the way it was in the time of our ancestors, too. Rare are those who possess any *njum bwele* today. Myself, I've never seen any in the wild."

Several *ngangas* whom I approached took refuge behind a prohibition in order not to have to supply me any *njum bwele*. The prohibition was a serious one, I was told. It made the donor sterile. One of them, Tokoto, spared me no details. "I'm sorry," he said, "but I can't touch any *njum bwele* today. I was with my wife last night. It could make her sterile. I have to wait."

I made the rounds of every *nganga* I knew in Douala, and returned to Din crestfallen. Well, things were not so bad, after all. He did keep a piece of *njum bwele* on his island. To his view, the problem would be the other bark, the *ngopange*, which not many *ngangas* knew about along the coast. It was a most special tree, and it was the Pygmies who had taught him its power in the old days. But there was an old man who knew where to find it on the outskirts of Douala. So a few days later off we went, all three of us, to find it.

It was a journey of detours and dead ends. *Nganga* apprentices have great difficulty in believing that a miserable little piece of bark is worth its weight in gold only if they have taken great risks to get hold of it. It is not surprising that candidates for discipleship are rare in our time.

In Search of the *Ngopange*

> Violence among the peoples of the earth,
>   violence everywhere!
> Then a tree, ancient of days and crisp and dry,
>   spoke wise words yet once again. . . .
> And another tree, of mighty reach and order,
>   sprung full timely from deepest earth,
>   from great Indies, all underground,
> With its lodeleaf on its boughs,
>   bore burden of fresh new fruit.
>
> Saint-John Perse, *Vents ("Winds")*, 4–7

According to the old man, the tree was to be found nearly forty-five kilometers up the Wouri, the river flowing down to the port of Douala and used by the Germans in early colonial times to gain access to the interior of the country. And so, one morning, Din, the old man, and I took the regularly scheduled little motor dinghy up river, to pass the night in the village of Bwene, on the river bank, and then to go out to the tree at first light. We were going to have to traverse a country marvelous to behold, and all aflood, the great kingdom of caiman sorcery—Kwedi's land.

First we had to find a stable place in the boat in all the bustle. Everyone seemed to wonder who we were. A priest? Why is he going to a Protestant village? And that one with him—he doesn't look like a catechist. But soon the familiar purr of the motor over the glassy surface of the water and the jovial atmosphere made our presence forgotten. When we got to Bwene we disembarked.

I saw nothing of the inundated village, but I did vaguely make out the outline of a range of houses behind the cocoa trees. The dwelling where we were to pass the night was just a few steps from the mooring, right along the river, but these few steps were difficult going. The water in flood season was so high that it came all the way up to the threshold of the front door of this rectangular building (one story, like all homes in the south). Its cinder-block walls had been newly coated with cement, and the roof was layered with shiny sheets of aluminum. By rural standards the ones who lived here were prosperous.

The door opened, and there stood a stocky young fellow in rubber boots. He was intrigued with us at first, and stared a good long while after we had made our entrance. But his wife was a relative of our old guide, and the moment he introduced us as friends of his, we were completely welcome. The young proprietor eagerly led the three of us into the main room, which took up nearly half the house, and invited us to be seated at a heavy, square table.

Now neighbors came paddling along, tied up at the door, and came in to say hello to the strangers and look them over. A medical technician, who seemed a bit addled to me, remained behind a while after the others had stepped back down into the boat. He made me uneasy. He talked too much. He said he was the only Catholic in this Protestant region, and declared himself a passionate devotee of Gregorian chant. Finally all seemed in good order.

Then all of a sudden I felt (rather than heard) a muffled din, coming from the direction of the village—and I noticed that my companions were suddenly on their guard. The master of the house took a standing position at the entryway as if he might have a job to do. His wife quickly took their three-year-old child and went to the kitchen. Din showed signs of irritation, and the old man who had brought us here, with his forehead on the table, seemed in consternation. Then, at this very moment—by coincidence, although doubtless I was the only person in the house to consider it such—the house shook. The newspapers reported this brief earthquake three days later. My companions looked at one another in utter helplessness.

Night had fallen now. I heard a nearby voice, and the splash of a paddle. It was the village crier, making the rounds of all the houses, with: "Good villagers, sleep on the ground tonight!" He was warning them to be vigilant in view of certain things that might come to pass. And suddenly I understood. Closed up in this house, practically in a clandestine gathering, we were in an excellent position to be accused of sorcery.

I had been in this absurd situation twice now. I had still not learned my lesson! A European traveling to a village on the outskirts of Douala, accompanied by a stranger, and for an unrevealed purpose, could very well be a trafficker in human beings. He was buying Africans. He was having a sorcerer kill them, so that he could force them to work for him on his invisible plantations. This is sorcery, *ekong*, and it arouses unforeseeable emotional reactions as I had learned to my rue in the escapade of the roadblock. So here were were, thirty kilometers from Douala, far from major highways, in a flooded area, and we were caught. If I now went to see the local chief, what would I tell him? The truth? That we were here to look for a bark endowed with occult powers?

Happily, we were saved by the smooth functioning of traditional societal mechanisms. At about eight o'clock we heard some pirogues paddle up. The master of the house, once more planted on his threshold, informed us that the chief and other notables were arriving. Ten men silently entered the dwelling. Then there was more silence. Finally the oldest among them spoke up, declaring that Bwene had never received such illustrious visitors—how was it, then, that the chief had not been accorded the opportunity to greet them? I answered that I was not in the habit of disturbing the chief when I spent just one night in a village. I told our visitors who I was and presented identification. I also gave the names of some of our former students from this region—adding that they would be surprised to know that I was not allowed to sleep over in their village.

Now came the protests. Of course we could stay here the night. But just one night. Din intervened, and with great aplomb. "What is this joke? We're taken for sorcerers, when we're just the opposite—a priest and a *nganga*! We're here just to find good hunting country!" (What did he mean, "hunting country"? Was he being ironical?) The chief asked my blessing for a peaceful night, and the delegation withdrew.

The chief's action produced an effect perhaps intended from the beginning. It calmed the populace. After his departure, the muffled uproar died away in the distance, and our little hut was plunged once more in silence. And yet, stretched out by Din's side on the one great bed of the house, which our host had left to us, I was unable to close my eyes the whole night long. The reasons for this were twofold. First, the mosquito netting over us hung down onto the mattress in such a way that insects could easily make their way in, but could not easily make their way out. But more especially, I could not keep my mind off the potential consequences of this latest predicament. The real danger was that someone in the village might die tonight. Then we would be held responsible, and the notables would not necessarily have the authority necessary to prevent reprisals. Din seemed sleepless too. Did he have the same apprehensions?

At five o'clock the next morning, our host, together with a friend of his who had a good reputation as an oarsman, Din, our old guide, and I—five of us—stepped into a little pirogue. From five to nine we sloshed ahead in a driving rain—that heavy, warm, implacable rain of the tropics, against which there is no defense. We had to row up river, then into a little tributary, then through the forest itself, which had become an immense lake. Our host, though, had been seized with a sudden, high fever, and we had had to leave him at one of the last houses we passed before entering the forest. I attributed the fever to emotion and anxiety. He had had to obey two contradictory imperatives, one of hospitality, the other of security. The news had come that if anything happened to anyone in the village, his son, his only son, would die.

Relieved of one of its passengers, our pirogue now advanced among the tree trunks, over a surface devoid of any landmark. I felt doubly out of my element in this forest fallen prey to the waters. I have never traversed it, even in the dry season, without a twinge of anxiety. Life was so exuberant here. You could become lost, die on the spot, and be reabsorbed into nature's everlasting work of regeneration, without anyone's knowing about your disappearance. Ordinarily this forest exuded the intoxicating odor of fermentation that, in the woods of more temperate climes, rises to the nostrils only after a heavy rain. Today, however, all flooded as it was, it had become strange and oppressive. Deprived of its wonted scent, it seemed cut off from the earth by a shroud of deadening water.

By nine o'clock I was sure we were lost. I laid down an ultimatum. If we did not reach the tree within another hour, we would turn back. Din and the old man said nothing. Half an hour later, as if our route had been calculated to the last meter, we came up along a low island in the waters. The old guide leapt out of the boat and pointed to an enormous trunk. It had not a single limb, but shot straight for the sky, and was lost in the branches of the trees around it. It was the *ngopange*.

With a broad gesture, Din held the three of us at a distance, and he approached the giant alone. He completely disrobed. Standing naked before the *ngopange*, he recollected himself a moment, then circled the tree, spitting perfumed condiments against its bark—*bongolo* and *njansang*—in token of pacific intentions. He placed a bottle of wine and some tobacco at its foot. Then, as if he were addressing a person *(moto)*, he begged the tree to grant him his desires.

"Here's what I said," Din explained to me later. " 'It is I—I have come to beg a favor [*musima*—often mistranslated "luck" or "fortune"] of you. I am killing no one. I am only doing my work. But if anyone approaches me [metamorphosed] as an animal, to kill me, may it be that one who dies. Open my eyes once more! Upon a time, it was you who opened them, you, *ngopange*!' " [103]

Then he went at the tree with his machete, and we others were finally allowed to approach as well. Rarely have I assisted at such a sober, yet triumphal, liturgy. And rarely have I so deeply penetrated the truth of what is called (not very accurately) animism. There is a striking similarity between a tree and a naked human being. Each is sovereign in its members, for the one is fitted out with arms, and the other with branches. Their relationship is undeniable. There in the presence of Din and the *ngopange*, the intuitive veneration I had had for trees in my childhood came rushing back to me. It was not the monkey that was the ancestor of the human being. It was the tree.

Din summoned me to come right up to the tree and gather the slabs of bark he was slashing with great slices of his machete. I put the slabs into a hempen bag—big hunks of living bark, with gray skin and red flesh. My hair, my hands, my shirt suddenly became soaked in a violent scent, the odor of a vat of new wine, strong and intoxicating.

When the bag was full, all dripping with sap from pieces of bark that were over an inch thick, we left the place, without glancing backward. [104] The rain had stopped. The journey back was royal recompense for the trip of the early morning. Now the swimming forest seemed a park, such as romantic poets dream of. Gilded birds swooped low over the waters, to be doubled by their reflections, as if they had been sweeping down over a mirror. Alighting on arches of giant grass, they watched us pass. Our little boat was all but immersed in the waters embracing it. Borne along by the current, safe as the birds perched on the dead trunks as we floated past, we rowed no longer. Our pain had been rewarded. We could glide with the stream now. We were victorious, and we savored the moment.

We resumed contact with humanity at the first village, where our host, still with a fever, came back on board. As we covered the last miles we heard tom-toms, relaying the news of our return to the dwellers of the river bank. I could feel that Din was uneasy. He kept squinting into the little coves and crannies of the bank. We delivered the patient and his friend to their homes, then headed for Douala without further delay. I did not rest easy until I met our old guide two days later. Nothing had happened in the village since we had left.

Master and Disciple

Now I could appreciate in all serenity how close this trip had brought Din and me together. We had taken the same risks, we had surmounted the same difficulties together. At the trial, Din was the only defendant. I had the easier part. Here, master and disciple were on the same level. I realized that the main obstacle to my initiation—the real reason for Din's initial diffidence—had just been removed. He had gained the conviction that, if he opened my eyes, perhaps I would not use it to kill him. (It was an astounding revelation for me, and I would grasp the logic of it only much later, at the end of our road together.) Here are some of Din's reflections in the course of our meetings:

"Now, try to understand. I am telling you what I think because you love me. If you tell someone the truth—if you show someone *ndimsi*—the one you show it to will kill you. The opening of the eyes is the key to the forces of the earth. I am risking your killing me. But I'm not sure you'd want to. You could have done it at the trial. All you'd have had to do was to refuse to be a witness.

"There are those who say, 'the whites are going to make you lose your strength. If you open the eyes of a white, he'll kill you.' But the white won't kill me. He wants me to open his eyes so he can see. That doesn't mean he wanted something else. They say it's not good to show these things to whites, because they'll get hold of this force. But I won't refuse. This way I'm going to be working all the way to Europe [in *ndimsi*]!"

Now that he had driven from his mind the danger of death that I seemed to represent for him, Din declared himself prepared to enter into a contract with me. A contract is a convention obligating each of the contracting parties. Din was offering me double sight. What was my part of the contract? According to the most common opinion, the only acceptable compensation in such a case was the gift of a person. Caïn Dibunje Tukuru, who was right at the heart of tradition, assured me that this was indeed the case.

"There are some *nganga*s who require you to kill someone if you want your eyes opened," he said. "Then that person belongs to them. It's not only *nganga*s who act this way, but it is they who can teach others. This kills many persons in our country, and these practices have been forbidden. They put an herb juice in your eyes, to open them, and you become a killer too."

Din himself had told me, maliciously, about his colleague Loe when the latter was still alive: "You know, Loe used to be a carpenter. Well, he went and had his eyes opened, and he killed some of his own people for it, because that has advantages!"

The term *ewusu* comports all the ambivalence of the personage who bears its name. It is a word with strong emotional connotations. *Nganga*s love to flaunt it, and clients whisper it of them secretly. But *ewusu* also designates the born sorcerer, the cannibal sorcerer, the worst of all, the perverse one, the one who does evil for evil's sake, the born adversary of the *nganga*. The reason for this paradox must be sought elsewhere, beyond the categories of sorcerer and antisorcerer, at the very roots of the notion of power. *Ewusu*s are born with a power engrafted in their very person, be it for the community's weal or woe. Because it is a matter of individual privilege, and not of a power granted by the group, it arouses hostility, generally in nascent form—that is, suspicion.[105]

I was unable to believe that Din expected me to offer him a human life. I decided to let him take the initiative and prescribe my part of the contract himself. And then one day, in the course of one of the rituals in which he was having me join him, as he sat talking to me, to his ancestors, and to his *miengu*, there before his display of barks, he finally decided to broach the crucial question.[106]

He spoke to his barks and herbs: "I'm going to ask him what he's going to give me in exchange for my instruction—what great deed *(eyembilan endene)* he'll do for me. To open someone's eyes, custom says you ask for 'an animal without hair on its body'—a human being. When you've killed that person—then, and only then, they put something in your eyes, and you start seeing at night, you start knowing everything. But I refuse to do that. I do not agree to this transaction *(mba na titi ten)*. That's not the way I've learned to do things. Now, it's you, your trees and herbs, who opened my eyes. But instead—he could bring a goat."

Din repeated this declaration from time to time over the next few days. It was official then, and I could go on with the initiation in good conscience. But it did not resolve the question of a stipend. Besides the ritual compensation—here happily limited to the offering of a goat—I was to offer the *nganga* a gift. Nor did Din delay in reminding me. He refused to "tax" me—demand a sum of money from me, which, he said, would have to be considerable, something in proportion to the service rendered. You didn't "tax" a priest. He would be satisfied with a gift that I would have to choose myself. I offered him 5,000 CFA francs (about $20) on the spot. But Din explained to me at once how ridiculous my offer was. "Think about it!" he said with a great guffaw. "I get 5,000 francs for treating somebody's piles!" And he recited a proverb for me: "When you go see the *nganga*, always carry something under your arm"—that is, a gift. So I decided to take a little more time, and really see what I was able to suggest.

But before sealing the contract, I still had doubts to admit to Din. After all, he had admitted everything to me; surely I must requite in kind. He had been open with me about the risk he was taking in opening my eyes. Surely in all honesty I had to reveal to him how little I believed! I wrote out my confession before I read it to him. I wanted my words in Douala to be just right. This is what I wrote and then read to him:

> Din, I want to speak frankly with you, lest there be the shadow of a lie between us. It was you who offered to open my eyes, four years ago. I had not asked it—I did not believe I should see better afterward than before. And I have not changed my mind. But today, I think this would bring me wisdom. Why? Because after the ceremony we shall be so bound together that you shall teach me much about life.

I watched Din's reaction closely and anxiously. Would he stop everything now? But he made no answer at all. To my stupefaction, he did not even make any allusion to my declaration. And yet he had surely listened to it with the greatest attention. How was I to interpret such indifference?

I repeated what I had read, paraphrasing. Still no reaction! Not a nod. Not even the little smile of the initiated. Without saying a word, he simply continued preparing the ritual of that day. I was at a loss to know how to interpret his silence.

A series of mishaps now interrupted our project, just when it seemed to be coming to its conclusion. Each of the two of us fell ill, and we went off in different directions, he to Metet, some 350 kilometers from Douala, for a hernia operation, and I to Paris for diagnosis and treatment of a mysterious sore throat. On my return, I learned that his health was now worse than before. The operation had been successful, but he had gone back to his island and fallen ill once again. One day I received a little note he had dictated, asking me to come to his assistance.

I underestimated the earnestness of the appeal, and merely sent him some money so that he could come to Douala for treatment. To this suggestion I added a request: not to forget the *njum bwele*. His reply, written in French by someone on the scene there, was a dreadful shock:

I thought you loved me for the love of God. I didn't know it was for the medicine I would show you. . . . I explain to you that I'm in my last agony and you don't come to see me! And you tell me to bring everything necessary. I did not feel good from that letter you wrote me. We *nganga*s are numerous. Because I am sick, you can go to another. My respects. Din.

These lines, biting and pathetic, in a crisp, proper French that lent them even more solemnity, cut me to the quick. Everything seemed finished between us. How could I win his pardon? I decided to seize the first opportunity to join him on his island. Meanwhile I tried to convince myself that he had perhaps exaggerated his condition, and that his letter was not really that of someone on their deathbed.

Then suddenly, the next day, I had a new surprise. Din was now in a hospital in Douala, conveyed there by members of his family. His physician, whom I alerted as to his patient's status in the community, diagnosed tuberculosis and cirrhosis of the liver, and declined to commit himself as to the chances of recovery. I visited Din daily, and there was no more talk of double sight.

But when I was alone, I thought about Din's silence following the confession I had made to him. On the very threshold of my initiation, I had the feeling of knowing no more than I had the first day. What did this "sight" consist in? To be sure, there was no question of interviewing Din on the subject, in the present state of affairs, but at least I could seek to formulate some hypotheses of my own, in order to try to see things a little more clearly.

First Hypothesis: Double sight is simply nothing at all. In this case, the initiation of candidates for double sight would consist in revealing to them that there is actually nothing to see—that the celebrated realities, in which they are of course correct to believe, are, after all, really only invisible. They exist, but no one perceives them. This could doubtless be a traumatizing discovery. There must be a gradual initiation, to help candidates bear the disillusionment, and prevent them from superficially concluding to the unreality of the other world. The difference between an ordinary person and the initiated, then, would be very great. The former believes that the ancestors still live, and has the conviction that seers actually encounter them. The initiated believe just as much in the ancestors' survival—but they know that no one sees them. This would explain Din's silence. In doubting the vision, I was getting dangerously ahead of the pedagogical process. His absolute silence, impossible to interpret, had been calculated to keep the cards facedown.

I had seen the initiated in action on the occasion of a little village drama on the coast, near Kribi. It was Christmas afternoon. All the villagers had assisted at my midnight Mass, then at my morning Mass, and had begun their scheduled dancing on the broad sand boulevard. Suddenly there was a sort of violent commotion. Women rushed headlong for their houses with their children, and the village was abandoned to the men. A Canadian tourist there for the dancing was startled out of his wits, and prudently returned to the beach. The explanation was quite simple. A sacrilege had been committed: A woman who had had too much to drink had wandered into a building where some young men were assisting the mask-wearer of the secret male society called *Munjeli*, to vest. At nightfall, the ancestors, furious, began striding through the village. The women and children cowering in their homes heard the roar of a tornado as the ancestors passed. From my window, I could see the initiated producing a loud, throbbing noise with a rhombus—a hollowed-out twist of creeper trunk, swung by hand in great arcs. If the women knew what it really was, they took great care not to let their children know—that what was out there in the dark was not really a swarm of ghosts, but a troup of angry men.

Second Hypothesis: Double sight is stimulated by hallucinogenic herbs. On the coast, "the sight" is bestowed by placing in the eyes two drops of a vegetable brew. My informants were unanimous on this point. I wondered, then, whether the barks and herbs from which the liquid was made might have hallucinogenic properties. The *ngopange*, for instance—might it not have some psychedelic virtue? This would explain Din's zeal to obtain the bark. The initiation would then have an affinity with ecstatic experiences the world over, stimulated by Mexican peyotl or Turkish opium. Nor did I need to find my examples on other continents. Right here on the coast of Cameroon, for example, there was the *eboga* tree. Its root contains a powerful stimulant. German colonialists had used it to drug their forced labor when the Douala-Yaoundé railway was under construction. The *eboga* is the ritual plant of initiation in Guinea and Gabon; it is so celebrated there that it has given its name to a religion.[107]

I have been encouraged in this hypothesis by Din's statements on the occult powers of alcohol. I had long believed that he would invent a pretext to justify his frequent state of inebriation, for which he was presently paying the price in the hospital. Now I began to suspect he had need of alcohol to maintain the exaltation and intensity that were indispensable for the conduct of a long night séance. I remembered what he had said: "I have to make you pass the test of wine, because I love you. When the moment comes, you'll have to drink. You'll drink, and the ones who work with you, the *miengu*, the dwarfs [the ancestors of the Pygmies], they'll drink too. When you drink, you lose all track of time. That's very important. During a night séance, I make everybody drink, so I can see clearly what work I have to do. I even make the sorcerers drink, the ones who've bewitched my patient. When they're drunk, they soften up, and are willing to make a deal. For example, they say, 'We want a goat and 6,000 francs.' I give them what they ask for, and the patient gets well."

Perhaps Din was getting ready to put an elixir in my eyes that would have the same properties as *eboga* or alcohol, and would widen my vision.

Third Hypothesis: Double sight is the revelation of the imaginary. By "imaginary" I mean the dreams and phantasms so often and so unjustly relegated to the scientific refuse heap, all the seemingly foolish and useless images that were finally rehabilitated by Freud. After all, they represent the mighty currents of drives and desires that unconsciously orientate human relationships. Once they have been snatched from the night, they become a treasure trove of information, one all too rarely made use of. Initiation, then, would here consist in revealing to candidates the seriousness of the workings of the imagination, and in helping them to retain and select dreams and images by providing a code for their interpretation.[108]

In this hypothesis, one could easily understand the value attached to a bark, the great trouble undergone to obtain it, and the ceremony over it before it is placed under one's pillow. The presence of this bark, with its prestigious reputation, and its echoes in the cultural depths of the sleeper, will infallibly produce important dreams. The initiation would be complete the day the candidate takes this world of the imagination for a true vision of reality, in all its precision.

If this hypothesis were to be correct, I would be a difficult disciple for my master. My unconscious, despite all my good will, did not respond to the same signals as his. It was not altogether sensitive to the same symbolic structure, for it did not belong to the same cultural universe.

Of the three hypotheses, which one was correct? I decided to try to get the answer clear in my mind, in spite of Din's illness and resentment. Besides, I had some decisions to make. I had just been informed by my superiors that

I was to leave Cameroon at the beginning of September and go to Abidjan, the capital of Ivory Coast.*

It would have been of no use to attempt to hide from myself a sense of relief at the idea of escaping the world of the *ngangas*. But I also felt a deep sorrow at having to leave this land I loved so well.

This sudden news clouded my personal skies, to be sure, just as in the skies over Douala country, clouds within my own being crisscrossed one another helplessly, without intermingling, all at the mercy of the anarchic winds. But the same news also obliged me to work very quickly. I was on the point of harvesting the fruit of five years of research, and I had no right to abandon my goal so shortly before its attainment.

The opportunity that presented itself was precisely the one that had been Din's sarcastic advice—to go see another *nganga*. This year, as every year, during the long school vacation, I was to spend several weeks in Kribi, the other coastal port, where I did not lack for friends in the milieu of traditional medicine. Now I decided to apply to them. I had made this decision not without a certain uneasiness. I appreciated the priority Din accorded experience over knowledge, and his respect for the importance of a length of time. I recognized the mark of an authentic initiation here. My time in Kribi would be brief, and I should have to find an all-purpose *nganga* who could satisfy my curiosity. I recognized that I would run the risk of falling into a certain spirit of "doing ethnology." And I had promised myself I would avoid that. But I could see nothing else to do in the circumstance.

And so I made a number of attempts to find a cooperative Kribi *nganga*. The first ones to whom I applied all found excuses to refuse. But then I went to see Madola. Madola spoke French, and in previous years he had always admitted me to his treatment sessions, as often as I wished. I had never met a *nganga* as obliging as Madola. He had received his initiation in Guinea, in a framework of the Bwiti religion, which makes use of the psychedelic plant *eboga*.

"*Eboga* is a very delicate thing," Madola explained to me. "When you've eaten enough, you get drunk and you vomit. When you've finished vomiting, you die. You're like a corpse. It sends you such a long way, all the way to—well, I might as well say it, all the way to heaven. You see things that can't be seen in life. If your father and mother are dead, you find them up there. They teach you to practice medicine. They tell you, 'Here's the way to treat this disease, you do this and that!' You sleep four or five days, and it's the bishop [He used the English word meaning, here, the great Bwiti hierarchy] who brings you back."

*The Jesuits have set up an "Institut Africain pour le Développement Economique et Social" here—INADES. Per se there was nothing unusual in this change of assignment. The Abidjan community belonged to the same jurisdiction in the internal organization of the order as did Douala. Those familiar with the Jesuits know that they are expected to be ready to betake themselves to any region of the world, as their founder, Ignatius Loyola, had demanded— "even to the regions of the Turks," Ignatius had added, without malice (supreme courage and availability, in his day). There was nothing heroic about my going to Abidjan.

Evidently there could be no question of having myself initiated in this manner. But Madola had likewise learned the art of opening eyes with drops, as is practiced on the coast of Cameroon, and he proposed that I try it.

At the far end of the Catholic mission grounds in Kribi was the old convent. It was vacant now, and one morning at six o'clock I met Madola there. We set up a little spot on the second floor where no one could see in. Then Madola spent a long time bathing my face with a large leaf soaked in water, and began speaking to his ancestors. He invited me to invoke mine, which I promptly did. Now he placed several drops of a bitter concentrate, which stung a bit, on the crown of my head, in my nose, and finally, in my eyes, with little funnels made of leaves.[109] Then he directed me to look straight at the sun for a quarter of an hour. It was seven-thirty now, and the sun, just over the tree tops, was already fearfully bright. Madola had advised me the evening before of the necessity of exposing my eyes to the sun's rays, and when I hesitated, he added:"Either you trust our herbs or you don't trust them." I decided to "trust" them, then, but I reserved the right to halt the experiment if it was not working out.

At first it was like watching a land sparkling with fire, and I thought I could feel my eyes being hammered like a brass gong. Madola cooled my face from time to time. By the end of the quarter hour there was a sort of miracle: the sun blinded me no longer. I had a feeling of deliverance, and something like a touch of pride at being able to stare at the fiery star in all tranquility.[110]

The experience over, we sat quietly side by side. Madola had warned me: "You'll be afraid. Afraid of seeing the evil spirits. When you see them, you'll start shaking!" I "saw stars," all right, but I saw nothing disturbing.

That night I had horrible nightmares—the price of my insensitivity that morning. The next day we did the same thing all over again. The day after that, the sun had disappeared behind rain clouds. Would the third day of contemplation have to be postponed? To my surprise, Madola explained that the sun was not so important—the initiation was a matter of three days, and the eyedrops were the decisive factor.

"You mean looking at the sun isn't to open my eyes?" I asked.

"No," replied the *nganga*. The sun removes impurities from the eyes. It's the drops that open them."

Before we parted I presented Madola with a modest gift, promised him to say nothing about this along the Kribi coast, and betook myself to Mama Enge, an old *nganga*, to be treated for the beginnings of conjunctivitis, with the help of a secret balm she used.

I was still convinced that Madola had not been playing games with me— that he had performed the appropriate gestures over me, and used the right herbs and barks. But I had the feeling that he had only followed a recipe. Without the proper existential context, the recipe alone could have no meaning and power for initiation.[111] I returned to Douala still interested, but just as perplexed as before.

"This Power, to Remember Me By"

A pleasant surprise was in store for me when I arrived. I found Din improved, and sitting up in his hospital bed. He took the initiative in speaking to me—in a sort of code, lest our conversation be too intriguing for the other patients in the ward—of the next steps in my initiation. He had sent his son Bata to his island, with the mission of fetching the *njum bwele* and the necessary "objects." I must now await his discharge from the hospital and Bata's return. The physician, aware of what manner of personage his patient was, had followed the course of his illness with attention, and had restored the *nganga* to health. I did not yet dare to tell Din of my impending departure for Abdijan. Nor did I say a single word about the questionable experiment in Kribi—like someone concealing an act of infidelity.

And so, upon his discharge from the hospital, Din invited me to come see him at the home of a discreet, trustworthy relative of his. The latter lived in one of the lower quarters of Douala, far from Deïdo, and Din could "work on me" here without stares or suspicions. I found the house only with great difficulty, amid a tumble of dwellings all with the same rusty iron roofs. There was no road for getting there. You had to zigzag your way along walls, around piles of garbage, past outhouses, and over homemade sewers. The house Din had indicated was dangerously located on a hillside over a putrid stream, and it was the middle of the rainy season. I went into the house. Din invited me to greet the several persons who were chatting in the tidy little parlor, although I would not be having any contact with them. Then he led me to a back room—four earthen walls, covered over with a grey coat of cement, and pierced by a single window looking out on a bare wall. There was a big bed, where one might sit on the edge, and an equipment case, where Din had his material all arranged. Adjoining was a toilet, with a bucket for a washbasin. That was all. The quarter was one of the most densely populated of the city. Yet I had the feeling of having been removed from the world. We sat down, and Din began to speak.

"I've already told you that I feel a great friendship for you," he said. "But I was resentful. You sent me a letter directing me to rejoin you when I was sick. You didn't consider me a friend. You didn't understand that I loved you in the name of God. I was all but dead. You know that it is true.

"Still, I've decided to do what I promised you. But there are laws *(mbenda)*. Someone who wishes to have their eyes opened, and has no money, cannot have this desire satisfied. It can cost over 100,000 francs. We don't like to do this work on just anybody, because the one whose eyes we open is the first to fight against us. I told you I won't tax you, but I'm waiting for a deed [a sign, a gesture]. Look at my situation yourself!"

A few years before, this statement would have awakened my mistrust. Today it seemed altogether natural. I knew that *nganga*s deserved their stipends—that they were not tips—I knew that I would be getting my money's worth. Din was paying me a great compliment by leaving the judgment of the gift to me. I gave him a 70-meter-long fishing net. The islanders of Malimba would be able to cast it into the sea, nightly, from October to December, and gain an income from it. It was a handsome gift, and I could tell that Din was pleased with it.

I took advantage of the occasion to tell him of my coming departure. I would be leaving Cameroon for Ivory Coast, I said, with a good chance that I could come back to see him every year. For a moment he was absorbed in disappointment, and was silent. Then he said simply, "I'd like to leave you this power *(mianga)*, to remember me by."

August 5. Din had donned his red robe. Bata and I were seated on the edge of the bed, in the back room, safe from the gaze of the indiscreet. "Even my wife mustn't know," said Din. Bata had just completed his second year in a trade school in town, where he studied electricity. He was tall and svelte like his father, and had the same brown eyes. (But his silky face was no more like his father's than the pelt of a young antelope is like a drumhead.) His father wished to teach him the *nganga*'s trade, and Bata was very interested. He had not had the experience of a Nkongo, for he had not lived with his father on the island, but he had the enthusiasm of a neophyte. "I'm going to give my son wisdom. He'll learn long at my side. For seven years. If his manner of life suits me, I'll keep him. Otherwise I won't give him this gift. Why so long? Because he can't pay. But he can work."

On a chair before us, in battle formation, all the equipment lay displayed, from the cowrie shells and the mirror, to the miniature saber I had brought Din from Paris. I saw no chains or hooks: I was not guilty of sorcery. Carefully arranged on the floor were five barks and three herbs. Din winked at me as he pointed out the *ngopange*. I recognized the blossom and leaf of the *ngonda balemba*, too, the "sorcerer's spice" that he would give me as viaticum every time I went on a trip. Everything was here, then, to guarantee the success of the experiment—the ancestors, the "objects" (the *mianga*), and ourselves.

Now Din addressed the ancestors. "I wish him to see," he prayed. "I ask that he see, as I myself see. May nothing be hidden from him. May he see. Any country at all—Europe *(mbenge)*, or other regions. May he see. I am afraid neither for him nor for myself. They say he's going to kill me. Well, then let him kill me! But he has helped me, a number of times. No, he won't kill me. First, he'll be forbidden *(mbenda)* to kill me. And I wait for death from God. May he see, for better or for worse. May he see. May he be able to continue his work in good conditions. I ask all this in the name of God *(Loba)*, who gave me the strength to see."

Din made a sign to Bata who left the room and returned leading a goat. My goat would have a very important role in the coming rites, and I had gone to purchase it, that very morning, in Din's company. Din had wished to select it himself, for it sometimes happened that animals that already were "persons"—were dishonestly sold a second time—an exchange that I decided I should have to learn more about. Din had had a bit of fun at my expense at the market. Because this goat was to replace me, it ought to look like me, so he chose one with a round belly! "Besides, she's heavy with kid," he added—"she'll kid before she dies, and we'll be that much ahead." The goat there before me in the room, with her distant, indefinable look, obviously had all the desired characteristics.

Din handed me the little horn with the powder of five barks marinating in the juice of three herbs. I placed one drop on top of the head, and in each eye, of my goat. Bata, translating everything his father said, whispered to me, "Say something in your dialect." I said simply, "I wish to see, as Din sees." I had to straddle the animal nine times, to transmit to it all the evil I bore within me. This goat, in recognition of its sad heritage, would be giving me both its eyes, so that I might see. This is all I understood at the moment, and I promised myself I would question Din about my scapegoat more at length at another time.

Nine times too—that decisive number—I must straddle the ritual objects lying in the little horn, then open both hands, in a respectful gesture of acceptance, to receive anew the precious horn. On nine consecutive evenings, I was to place a few drops in the corner of each of my eyes before going to sleep, as well as on the top of my head, and report my first dreams to my master.

"This will open your eyes interiorly *(o teten)*. This will open your memory, and will show you the future. This will wash your brain. Little by little, not all at once. Even when you've stopped putting the drops in, your eyes will remain open—and you'll *see*, in broad daylight. You're like a pupil just beginning—you're starting in first grade and going to the highest."

When the ritual was over, I questioned Din about my goat's fate, turning my questions every which way to get at the logic and mechanism of the identification.

"You've gone across this goat and my objects nine times," Din replied. "That means any bad luck that can be loaded on you goes into the goat *(mbey's nyolo)*."

"What's going to happen to her?"

"She won't be eaten. She's reserved for *ndimsi*. Nobody'll be able to touch her. She'll die all by herself. She'll be buried like a person. She'll go where the *manga* are." (The *manga* are the goats the *miengu* keep.)[112]

"Are you going to keep her?" I asked.

"Yes," Din answered, until she dies. I don't think it'll be long before she kids. These medicines here'll kill her." Din meant the drops.

"Are you sure you're not going to kill her yourself?"

"Absolutely not. The drops'll be enough."

"When will she die, exactly? In a year?"

"I don't know. That depends on how powerful the drops are. She'll get them every night. They're strong. You'll see for yourself how it goes with her."

"But when you treat a patient, aren't you the one who kills the goat?"

"Yes," Din said, "to save the patient, I kill the goat. We cut off her head and feet and bury them with 6,000 francs. Everyone there eats the rest. But you've noticed I don't touch this food. I don't want to risk killing a patient."

"Is the goat me?"

"The goat *is* all your bad luck.[113] She *is* whatever's bad in you."

"Did the Pygmies have a ceremony like this to open your eyes?" I asked.

"Yes, exactly like this one. But they used a *mbudi* antelope [something like a water buffalo] instead of a goat."

I was not trying Din's patience without an ulterior motive. There was nothing surprising about his using a goat. *Nganga*s depend on a goat for every major night treatment. But I had remarked certain anomalies, which could not have been due to Din's creative imagination, for these rituals follow precise rules, and function in terms of a coherent whole. I questioned the master in order to know where he placed me in his universe. His responses enlightened me considerably.

As a general rule, a goat takes the place of a person who is sentenced to death by sorcerers. This is why the *nganga* sacrifices it, in the course of the night, before the eyes of the family, in whose midst is inevitably to be found at least the sorcerers' accomplice, if not the sorcerers themselves. For "your sorcerer is always one of your own." In my case there was no reason to sacrifice the goat, or have anyone eat it, because there was no one who had bewitched me. I was not a victim of sorcery. On the other hand, it must die, little by little, because I was taking its eyes, and because it was receiving all the misfortunes destined for me.

At the risk of vexing Din, I returned to the subject of what was going to happen to myself. If the goat died before my eyes were opened, would my life be in danger? "Absolutely not," Din responded unhesitatingly. One purpose of my question was to ascertain whether Din considered the goat to be a guardian spirit-animal.[114] His response in the negative did not surprise me.

A guardian spirit-animal, one capable of metamorphosis, is generally wild, undomesticated—a panther, a snake, or an elephant. A goat is the most domesticated of all beasts, so much "a part of the family" that it can symbolize the family. When an inheritance is distributed, the parts of a goat serve to designate the portion to be allotted to each member of the family. When a goat is served in the course of a festival meal, morsels are distributed to those present in accordance with each one's place in the family hierarchy. In Douala society the goat—so homely, so familiar—and edible—can be substituted for a person altogether naturally. But in explaining my identification with my goat, Din was being faithful to traditional

Bantu anthropology. He did not make a radical identification, as he would have in the case of a guardian spirit-animal. That is, he did not say, "The goat is you." He said, "The goat is all your misfortunes." My goat then, was a member of that mournful, submissive herd of scapegoats.

Initiation

From this point on, I shall limit myself to the highlights of my initiation, simply transcribing extracts of the notes I took daily. These extracts will record both the main lines of the initiation, and certain details that seem to me to be of particular significance. For I now found myself in the place of a student coming to the Libermann School for the first time. You answer when your name is called, write down whatever is dictated, and rise on signal. You do not yet have the necessary distance to be critical and objective. As a matter of fact, Din compared my situation to that of a pupil in a school more than once during the course of these rites.

The rite takes place either in Din's own dwelling, where he is keeping my goat and "working on" her, or in my own room, where I follow his instructions. My room, as I have said, was in our little house in Deïdo, where I lived with three of my colleagues from the Libermann School. Each of the three had accompanied me to a healing session, but none enters into the action in any way. I scarcely spoke to them concerning my initiation while it was actually in progress, although I did so at a later date. From time to time one or another of them would caution prudence, but none ever suggested I abstain from the experience. I appreciated their discretion at a period when I was reduced to silence simply because I did not know what to say.

August 6. Din asked me to tell him about the two dreams I had last night, which I did.[115]

He commented: "This sort of dream performs work *(yi ndoti y ben ebolo)*. When you put your heart into something, God answers. So you've started to dream. You'll see lots of things, good and bad. You won't tell anyone about them. You'll keep quiet. Still, if you see that one of your friends is going to be arrested [set upon by sorcerers], go ahead and tell him or her to look out."

I understood that Din was opening my eyes, as agreed, simply that I might see, not so I could interfere—except to warn a friend.

August 7. Din got up last night to "work on" my goat. He put two drops in its eyes, the same drops I had administered.

This afternoon, a double rite:

1) We went to the river for water, to a place where the *miengu* ancestors are supposed to hide. Then back to the quarter. Din put the five barks and three herbs in the pan of water. I wore a white loincloth (white is the *miengu* color. Bata washed me with the water and wished me good fortune (grace, *musima*). He passed a red hen back and forth over my head (classic blessing rite).

2) Bata and his father got the *dindo* ready, with a rooster, various herbs, and weeds. (I knew its meaning very well—fortifying, "armoring." When this dish is made up for a sorcery victim, the *nganga* takes none of it, for the reasons I have given above. Din excused himself here too, but only because he was on a salt-free diet by doctor's orders.)[116]

August 8. I reported a peaceful dream to Din; he made no comment. The ablutions were as the day before.

I asked him, "Did the Pygmies wash you too?"

"Yes, but for you we're bringing the *miengu* water here. I had to spend six days in the river."

I remarked to Din that my eyes were full of mucus. He decided to replace the eye drops with drops on the top of my head; so he made nine little pricks there, and forbade me to wash my hair.

August 11. My goat is on its last legs, gasping for breath. Din's wife remarked to him in my presence, "You don't like people very much, do you?"—an allusion to the Spartan treatment to which he was subjecting the goat. (Din hadn't told her why.) I suddenly felt the desire to take a picture of "my goat." But I turned away from the idea as from a "bad thought."

I told Din about some more dreams. They were much more clearly conflictual than the earlier ones.[117] Din said, "Tonight before you go to sleep, put drops in your eyes and say 'I want to know who's fighting me.' "

We went through the ablutions a third and fourth time. Bata was bathing my face. Din was away, so Bata asked me, "The things you see—is it like in the movies?"

I thought a moment, then replied: "Your father's teaching me to take certain dreams very seriously. Dreams can show important things. Usually we don't pay any attention to them."

August 13. I told Din about my two nightmares the night before: a classroom uprising, and a flooded city. He had no comment. I never paid so much attention to my dreams. Din's personality, rites he's performing on me, the *nganga* conflict atmosphere—all this has to have something to do with my nightmares. They're all I remember when I wake up. Other dream images, in a kind of limbo, don't seem important.

Din has decided this will be the last night I put drops in my eyes.

Din says we should wait till August 16 to meet. August 15, the feast of the Assumption, was a religious holiday and a day of rest for him, too. He saw no incompatibility between his rites and those of the church.

August 16. Din gave me a little package of herbs to put under my pillow at night. Then in the morning I'm supposed to swallow them before eating anything else.

I asked, "What are these herbs called?"

"I'll tell you when the time comes. You have time. I don't work on you every day now, because you're in an advanced class. Don't worry; nothing bothers us."

August 18. Din asked me, as usual: "Did you sleep?" He doesn't usually talk about "dreaming," *ndoti*. He talks about "seeing." I told him my last night's dreams; they dwelt on conflicts among individuals.

August 19. Din had warned me he was going to ask me some questions. ("For the first time!" I said, and we both laughed.) So today he did, but I noticed he wasn't trying to learn anything; the questions were pedagogical.

Din asked me, "Do trees and plants eat?"

"Yes."

"Do the herbs that'll be opening your eyes eat?"

"Yes."

"Who's going to feed them?"

"Er—well, me," I said, and I gave Din a coin. In return he showed me one of the herbs he was using to open my eyes and told me its name.

August 21. I told Din my nightmare: auto accident (near miss). But Din is no longer at all interested in details of my dreams. He listens distractedly. He just makes sure I have a certain type of vision, with adversaries and allies.

Now I can list and recognize all five barks and three herbs that open the eyes.[118]

August 22. Din, his wife, Eric-de-Rosny (their son), and Bata came to dinner. (Din would say "Elic-de-Losny": there is no *r* in his language.) It was a great event for them and for me. I was not sure my master would accept, until the last minute. It was vacation time—only one Jesuit was there besides me. The cook, who had guessed I was having my eyes opened, served us at table. I played my recording of the first treatment, nearly five years ago now. Din smiled slyly.

August 23. Din gave me another package of herbs to put under my pillow and swallow first thing in the morning.

The goat is still alive. I feel a certain emotion when I look at her.

August 24. Another nightmare, at daybreak: a cigarette lighter, with the gas escaping. I can't stop it; I'm being asphyxiated. I woke up. I swallowed the little ball of herbs. All of a sudden a great moment came. My eyes were opened. I saw persons killing one another. It was a visual sensation.

Everything Din had long been telling me unwound like a thread from a spool. "The sight" is mainly the revelation of violence among human beings. You have to have great strength of character to look brute reality in the face. Without initiation, with pedagogy, this vision would make one mentally ill, or hurl one into the circle of violence. Society is organized so as to conceal from its members the violence that can break out among them at any moment. Dreams speak of it very clearly. It would be a dangerous revelation for society; that's why the *nganga* is a dangerous personage.[119]

I listened to the morning news on the radio differently this morning, deafened by the conflicts in the world.

August 26. Din has a high fever. I told him about my dream. No comment. Then I told him of the great event.

He said, "I tell you the truth, don't I? Just the way it is. If I tell you this, or that, believe me."

I asked him, "If I want to open somebody else's eyes, can I do it by going at it the same way as you?"

"Yes."[120]

August 28. Din was still feverish. His daughter was worried, and told me, "I don't understand. We've tried everything. He's getting sick again!" I thought I heard a tone of reproach in her voice. "Don't understand" means "understand only too well." That is, somebody has it in for her papa. Does she suspect me?

August 30. Din's fever was down, but he still had nervous spasms. Now Bata tells me: "I don't understand." I try to reassure him. But am I in any position to do so?

I saw Din for the last time before leaving Douala. He reminded me that my goat would not be put to death. She'd die in her own time, and he'd have a funeral for her as if she'd been a person.

"You're going? Watch out for your body. Pray God your trip will be all right, and you can come back, and find me alive when we see each other again. But nothing bad will happen to you. And if trouble has to come, you'll see it ahead of time."

The new fishing net was behind the door. I turned around for one last look. In the back of the room, practically lost in thick black fur, dull, enigmatic, were the eyes of "my goat." Those eyes were all but closed now. Between the animal Din called a person, and me, there was still a sacred relationship. I turned to go, filled with a sense of reverence.

Chapter 18

Afterthoughts

To tell the truth, in the beginning I had had no intention of writing about what I learned from the *ngangas*. Not that I had scruples about revealing any secrets—Din knew I would be writing about all I had seen and recorded on tape, and he had never made the slightest objection. He was not shocked or offended at the publication of my first book. He had asked me only not to refer to my apprenticeship when I happened to be moving in his sphere of influence. But I had received no other requests for secrecy. For my part, however, I had decided not to publish the complete list of herbs and barks Din had used, lest they be employed in a parody of initiation.

From the day things really began to happen (August 6, 1975), I was bound to daily rituals. I sought to follow them blindly, and—perhaps for the first time—not to take any critical distance, but simply to jot down the few notes I have transcribed above and not much more, just enough to get me through this maze of experience. This simple activity, which took all my time, had absorbed all my attention, as well. Now I was about to leave Douala, after so many years there, and change my whole professional orientation. Yet I was not even concerned. Had I been bewitched?

I preferred rather to compare myself, more prosaically, to a passionate devotee of chess, who would become totally wrapped up in the particular game going on at the moment. For example, I had never heard tragic news on the radio the way I listened to it now, as it was reported in the announcer's monotone. It stood out in a special, new way now, and seemed to acquire a realism and truth that leapt right out and seized me, as if I had just received the gift of hearing. At the same time, by way of a kind of intellectual echo, I seemed to understand the meaning of my initiation.

Din had not tried to make a visionary out of me. It was nothing as poetic or prophetic as that. He had only opened my eyes to the hidden world of violence. As a matter of fact, when I say "violence," I am still yielding to my passion for abstraction. I know several words for "violence" in Din's language, and I doubt whether I even heard them all in the context of my initiation. Din was satisfied with simply opening my bodily eyes, along with my interior eyes, to the spectacle of persons' being jealous, hating one another and killing one another. The moment finally came when he no longer had any need to condition me. Now I saw for myself. In the days that followed, after the initiation, far as I was from Douala, I continued to see any little conflict most graphically, right in front of me. One of my new colleagues, in Abidjan, noticed it. The experience had made me a little like a touch-me-not, those little flowers that fold up at the slightest warning. Din had placed me on "standing alert."

One thing still puzzled me, however. I had been promised a vision of apocalyptic proportions. And yet, intense as my felt reaction had been, it had not had its expected breadth. I recalled what one of my students had told me when I asked him whether I should have my eyes opened. "I'd be too afraid, myself. I don't have the nerve to face the *nganga*s. I'm too simple. But if a priest, like you, had his eyes opened, there'd be nothing anybody could do to him."

It took the active intervention of some of my readers to make me decide to go on with a description of my experience. They had been following me in my journey, from afar or close at hand, and had called me short on certain points, posing precise questions. "What do you mean exactly by 'visual sensation'?" "Did you see persons killing each other as in a motion picture, in greater or lesser detail, scenes you had never seen, or were they things that had already been recorded in your memory?" "Did you have an original 'hallucination,' or did you simply have a *revelation of something you had looked at countless times and never really seen?*"

I put this last phrase in italics because it describes my actual experience quite well. No, I was not the subject of any form of hallucination, apparition, ecstasy, or visual delirium. Perhaps it is because my psychological defenses are so strong that I have always kept my lucidity even along the lengthy path leading to the *nganga* world, where so many others have succumbed. I have never yielded to the phantasmagoric. But my claim is that in the very early morning of August 24, 1971, I clearly saw. I saw violence, cold and clear. For perhaps the length of a second, I saw a thousand pictures of world conflict, superimposed on my field of vision as if by a cinematographic effect.

Nkongo, too had been tireless in his descriptions of the universe of the initiated as a terrifying battlefield, where he would never dare to go. And I could still hear Madola, my Kribi *nganga*, standing at my side on the second floor of the abandoned convent and telling me, when the sun experiment was over, "Now, don't be afraid." As for Din, had he not long hesitated to open my eyes for fear I would kill him?

I wrote one of my colleagues in Douala about how surprised I was at my relative insensitivity. He sent me a helpful reply:

What Nkongo and Din mean by "sight" is certainly not what we mean. For them, "sight" is mainly a functional matter. They have to succeed in a difficult task. Just to survive, they need to know what evil-intentioned beings lurk about them and their patients. For Din, "sight" is first and foremost a power. For you, not being involved in the same therapeutic battles, this "sight" is bound to be something intellectual: "violence exists." This is basically knowledge—"wisdom." This essential difference was virtually present from the beginning, in the two differing social situations: Din lives by his work as a *nganga*, and you are caught up in your work of research.

Indeed what was at stake in initiation obviously was less meaningful for me than for a *nganga* postulant. The effects of my initiation were unavoidably dulled in me, because I was not concerned in the same fashion. I did not understand the meaning of my initiation, or why I had failed to grasp it previously, until August 24, a few days before my departure for Abidjan. All of a sudden it came to me. *Initiation into the function of a* nganga *consists in opening candidates' eyes to the acts of violence being committed around them.*

Din had been drumming this into me for years. It was something that was perfectly evident to everyone who dealt with the subject, whether they were "sighted" or not. And I had been looking elsewhere. It had never occurred to me that I would need an initiation in order to dare to look violence straight in the eye. I had been kept from this insight by a flaw inherent in all cultures: the incredible difficulty we have in entering into the notions and attitudes of others.

Pity the poor stranger! Strangers have to compensate for their blindness, for their inability to feel and react on their hosts' wavelength, by taking an intellectual approach. They have to reconstruct something that others have simply inherited. I had never understood, until the moment of Din's final intervention, why such long patience was necessary—all the toils and privileges of initiation— in order to have access to the spectacle of violence. I was like a dull, stubborn schoolboy. Why have an initiation when violence is so evident a daily basis to the most ordinary mortal? I did not know that one great building block in the *nganga* cultural edifice was still beyond my view.

A thousand observations, and some reading, had shown me that, in a traditional society, everything conspires to conceal violence. Society hides it, seeks to conjure it away. If violence were to come completely out into the open, society might well collapse. How often I have felt this violence, like a smoldering fire. For example, I have seen it in the Deïdo quarter, among the men, sitting peacefully, the children playing ball, the women slowly making their way homeward—when suddenly one car crumples into another. No one is hurt, but everyone dashes headlong to the scene, glued to the spot around the drivers, cramming themselves into the space of a few square feet, as if released from some straitjacket of order, and ready to fight. Faced with such dangers, society is very adept at creating institutions, customs, habits instilled in childhood—to hide from its members the power and potential of violence. Among all the systematic deterrents, perhaps the most tested and most refined is sorcery.

It took me a while to accept this paradox. Sorcery, which passes for the unleasher of the worst frenzies, is the abettor of the established order and domestic tranquility! Nor was I alone in the discovery. Where sorcery reigns, public mores seem more pacific, children calmer, and armed brawls, suicides, and murders less frequent. This is not by accident. Sorcery furnishes its own antidotes: the antisorcerers—the diviners, exorcists, *ngangas* and *khamsis*. The secret of their success lies in their contacts with the invisible, the knowledge possessed by the initiated. If the paroxysm of violence is not accessible to ordinary eyes, if the real conflicts take place and the real accounts are settled on the battlefield of the invisible, then it is useless to be locked in battle before the eyes of all, and public order is the gainer. I can still see the two men I dined with one evening, seated on the same bench and greedily sharing the same bottle. I knew, as did all the other banqueters, a mortal enmity existed between them. One of them was the presumed murderer, by sorcery, of the other's son. But to see them together at the same table, no outsider would ever have guessed it.

The upshot is that violence has its edge dulled, that it is camouflaged and thrust aside—save to the eyes of the initiated, whose function it is to look it straight in the eye and to act upon it, for the safeguarding of society.

But at what price? *Ngangas* have a perception of the conflicts crushing their patients—a perception that is incomparably clearer than anyone else's, and astonishingly precise, thanks to their artful exploitation of the imaginary. In this particular society, where the censorship of violence is so well organized, dreams and phantasms in the night are the universal safety valve for the release of antisocial aggressiveness. "Dreams perform work," Din said. "Dreams are true," another *nganga* said to me. The effect of their action, taking place within the imagination, is tenfold, because they bear on precise objectives: the denunciation of sorcerers. "I sleep—"Loe told me, "I sleep, and I see as in a dream the mistakes others make. Sometimes it comes from God like a light. And if this light appears a second time, ah, then I'm happy. I see how I have to heal, how I have to fight in *ndimsi*."

The real fear the candidate for initiation feels—the fear I did not experience—comes from elsewhere. I finally understood it, thanks to my own initiation. Without it I would not have believed in the flashing visions they claimed they had, and so would have passed over the essential thing as well. The great fear of the future that candidates feel has its roots in their anomalous, nightmarish social situation. It is a lonely position to be in! In lifting the cloak of violence, they are swimming against the stream of social inclinations, and those of their own upbringing as well. Officially, candidates are to become antisorcerers. But they will be continually suspected of having become just the opposite, because the antisorcerer, too, must perceive violence and manipulate it. The prospect of so singular a societal position has a traumatizing effect that a Westerner has difficulty appreciating. The need for a progressive initiation can be seen, then.

Great care will have to be taken in selecting candidates for the vision. The time necessary to evaluate their mental and emotional equilibrium will be long—seven years, according to Din—before they can be permitted to perform so dangerous a function.

Northern societies doubtless have as much reason to fear violence as do any other. Their governments have all sorts of guardrails for protecting themselves from it. But willy-nilly, naked violence, impossible to contain, infiltrates public life. Class struggle, strikes, mass demonstrations—all win acquiescence and acceptance. Theories circulate to the effect that there is such a thing as good violence—that crises are not only inevitable, but necessary for social development, and hence legitimate. These ideas penetrate us like the air we breathe. They immunize us, they prevent us from reacting as the apprentice *nganga* reacts. Modern society, in authorizing manifestations of violence, deprives itself of the secret offices of the imaginary.

For my own part, I am certain that my relatively cool reaction to Din's treatment was owing first of all to my acceptance of the Christian faith. Christianity has a different outlook on violence from the one presented by sorcery. Jesus Christ's decision to take upon himself all the violence of the world, and become its sole victim, its voluntary scapegoat, has, in the gospel, a decisive liberating effect, not all of whose consequences have been evaluated and appreciated.

Unlike the system of sorcery, which manages to sidetrack the threat of evil provisionally, for the sake of the unity of the extended family, Christianity claims to suppress it radically. The deed has been accomplished, as far as Jesus Christ himself is concerned, but it remains the task of each one's individual liberty to authenticate it in their life. Any doctrinal structure this revolutionary will inevitably influence the attitude of its followers toward violence. But when their faith becomes tepid, their aversion to violence diminishes. In fact, I wonder whether modern Western society, so long marked by Christianity, will not simply have to allow itself to see all its violence burst out into the open one fine day.

Today I realize that my initiation at the hands of Din was not actually my first. In the framework of my own religious life, I had already passed through a form of initiation known as the "Spiritual Exercises," under the supervision of a director.[121] On more than one occasion, a Jesuit devotes a month to this programed spiritual journey toward a conversion of outlook. He learns techniques of contemplation, nor is he spared the vision of violence. But, after the first few days, the life of Jesus quickly becomes a model for contemplation and imitation. The exercitant is penetrated with the certitude that Christ has vanquished death. Thus, in a way, I had already had my eyes opened to violence, even before Din began to treat me. Neither he nor I could realize, at the moment, that we were embarking on a retouching project. We were superimposing a second layer on what was already there.

This raises the question of the legitimacy of my initiation. This question has been proposed to me in the following terms:

> When a European is initiated into a vision or sight, that will not thereupon be made use of for acting upon society and transforming it, is this not simply having a *nganga* "go through the motions," in the name of friendship?

Technically speaking, double sight as such is accession to an official function in the hierarchy to which the initiate belongs. For example, some persons in traditional Douala society perform the role of sentinel, without having to take part in the combats of *ndimsi*. On my request, as we have seen, Din was willing to accord me this simple vision. Thus my initiation was a homogeneous part of a greater whole, one ordained for the unity of families and the healing of its members. The description of Kwedi's healing can afford a glimpse of the expertise needed to perform such an act of healing.

For Din, my initiation was an episode in his encounter with the West. I trust it was a special, meaningful one, not artificial. Din was surely a lone eagle. And yet he had lived on the edges of the Occident ever since he had been born. Toward the end of the last century, members of his family had built the first school on the island of Malimba, as well as a number of chapels. Din was born in 1915, the very year British gunboats pursued the Germans up and down the Sanaga River. And now, in his work as a *nganga*, that most indigenous of occupations, he was discovering Europe in his clientele. Were not his most difficult patients students, caught, according to him, in the nets of European magic? He saw his own son, his possible successor in the practice of the traditional exorcisms, approaching tradition with the affected disinterest of a whole new generation of urban youth. But Din let Europe in without really offering any resistance. I discovered, in Din, an unlimited capacity for acceptance. It was a property of his culture, porous as cinder.

As for myself, I consider my initiation an incomparable experience—doubtless one of the mightiest, and certainly the most ambivalent, of my life. I shall never be a perfect initiate, in the African sense, but neither can my initiation simply be compared to any of the various journeys undertaken by persons of my own culture, as in psychoanalysis. The recognition and assimilation of a number of forgotten childhood memories does not constitute analysis, and Din never attempted to make me face myself in depth as an analyst would have done. The violence he revealed to me was always that of others, not my own, and in this he was consistent with the logic employed by traditional societies in writing one's own ills to the account of others.

Whatever be the nature of the experience I have had, I am happy with its outcome. There could never have been any substitute for it. I have gained vision, I have gained "the sight." That is, I have gained the capacity to look at the things of life in the manner of the people of Douala country, with the extreme delicacy of their perception of group conflicts.

Was it not this outcome—modest in appearance, but crucial, vital—that I had sought some twenty years, ever since my arrival in Africa? Like a long-distance runner, at rest after maximum exertion, I now find myself more at ease in the jumble of everyday relationships.

To be sure, it would be absurd to pretend I had eliminated all distance between Din and myself, or between my other Cameroonian friends and myself. The problem of true relationships arises anew every day. But this problem is now reduced to normal dimensions for me, reduced to the dimensions of any relationship problem between one human being and another. As the most critical of my friends wrote, concluding a letter: "After all the internal conflicts you've put Din through, and the graciousness with which he gradually surrendered, how can we not feel that we are assisting at the birth of a love between human beings across the chasm of their cultural differences?"

Return

After being eight months away, I was given the opportunity, in April 1976, to return to Douala for a few days, and I seized it with both joy and apprehension.

As my plane began to circle the mangrove touching down on the runway, I held my breath. I had hung over this swampy delta a good score of times, but today the inextricable tangle of waterways, the omnipresence of water, gave the landscape the physiognomy of an invaded territory where the human being had no place. My eyes fell on a few pirogues, scattered over the surface of the water—tiny twigs on a huge green carpet. Perhaps I even knew the names of the persons in them. I glanced at my fellow passengers, one after another, and smiled within myself. Not one of them could have imagined how much closer I felt to those fishermen than to them, though the ratio of the physical distances was precisely the inverse.

I went there with a predetermined objective. I would devote this short sojourn to making my departure from Douala official. I felt a little uncomfortable about all the persons who had gradually made me one of their own. How many of them wondered whether I had perhaps been doing a little game-playing: learning their language, schooling myself in their customs, appropriating some of their secrets—and then simply disappearing?

In some cases I had already formalized my departure—for example, in the village that had first held me prisoner for suspected sorcery, and then later adopted me. Its chief, Caïn Dibunje Tukuru, considered me one of his own family, and had even given me his name. It was painful to have to leave him. But I had told him the news, and he had gathered his notables and had me summoned. He invited me to announce the news. I told the august gathering that my religious superiors were sending me to Abidjan. Slowly the elders sipped the whisky I had brought, then pronounced their decision: "We are sending you to Abidjan." Finally the chief had me present the palms of my hands. Then he moistened them with saliva, looked straight into my eyes, and recommended me to his ancestors.

But there were other friends whom it had been more painful to leave. I thought more and more uneasily of Loe's family, whom I had abandoned so brusquely, practically turning tail and running. And especially I thought of Din, my initiator who had been lying on his sickbed dying when I had last said goodbye to him. I had thought of him every day these eight months since.

My first visit, then, would be to Din. I was in such a hurry to see him—and yet, to my own puzzlement, I kept putting off the moment, fearing the worst. For eight months I had had no news of him. And so I arrived at his house ready for whatever I might have to hear. The surprise would have been rather to see his long, lanky silhouette once more, and hear his nasal, taunting voice calling me. There was an old woman alone in the front room. In my haste I violated all convention and asked her, before even greeting her, if Din were home. She answered in a neutral tone, without lifting her head, that Din had long since died. The news struck me almost without wounding me, so thoroughly had I done my secret preparation. But I was stabbed in a section of my heart that I had left unprotected when the old woman added, after a moment of silence, that Din had died just two days after my departure.

Bata, the old woman informed me, was taking a driving lesson at the nearby drivers' school. I went there and without any preliminaries, as if we had never parted, he recounted to me the circumstances of his father's death. Din's state had worsened in the hours following my departure, and no one had been able to persuade him to return to the hospital. He died very suddenly, and apparently without suffering. His corpse rested on the island of Malimba. That was where his youngest wife and their son, little Eric-de-Rosny, lived today. They had taken everything with them, the treasury of barks, the instruments of power, the net, and the goat.

Immediately after the burial, Bata added, he himself had returned to Douala. It had not been work that called him here, for he was unemployed. But at the end of the ceremony an old man had dropped a remark that had made Bata decide to leave the island: "Now that Din is no more, the road is open."

Without any transition, Bata informed me that part of the family judged me responsible for his father's death. We were standing at the door of a room where an instructor was lecturing a group on the basics of the traffic code. I did not flinch, but the environment —these students learning to drive, the ordinary sounds of a street—lent this latest news a singular realism, a "realism of broad daylight."

Bata had spoken in a conversational tone, without any apparent animosity. And he added—perhaps this explained his calm—that the immediate family's suspicions were directed more toward Ekwala, his old host, who had once reported Din to the police. According to Bata, Ekwala had actually boasted of having caused his death. "But we don't know the European *ndimsi*," Bata added evasively.

I held my tongue, knowing from experience that denials served no purpose. I preferred to nourish within myself the hypothesis that Din, stricken with incurable cirrhosis, had allowed himself to die after having transmitted his power to me. Bata and I agreed to meet at his home the next day, when there would be a chance of seeing the family.

The "European *ndimsi*"! Bata's phrase contained a terrible logic. It haunted me the whole afternoon, to the point where I lost my desire to visit the other families. Everyone in Douala country knew that a *nganga's* apprentice could become a sorcerer's apprentice. The temptation is great to kill the teacher, by *ndimsi* means just discovered, and take over the master's power. Then the master can be forced to toil as a common slave—but what a powerful one! Everyone knew, too, the role played by Europeans in the devastating slave traffic of times gone by. Din had died just after having opened my eyes. What a coincidence!

This was not the first time I had found myself caught up in the logic of the Douala system of interpreting interpersonal conflicts. But until now I had always been able to stay in control of my emotions. Today, I was suspected of murder by a family I loved, and it was the murder of their father! You can use all the "good sense" you wish, you can "armor yourself" against a like accusation, and relativize its real force—but something breaks down within you.

All night I recalled Din's prophetic words: "They tell me not to open the eyes of a white; he'll kill me." Had I taken his doubts seriously enough? Now I understood better how heavily he must have been burdened with hesitation, and interior combat. "They say he'll kill me. Well then, let him kill me! But he's helped me, several times. . . . No, he won't kill me! In the first place, he won't be permitted to kill me." From the very beginning of our meetings, five years earlier, in designating me as his assistant, he had already made a statement that was unintelligible to me then, but I had recorded it, and duly entered it in my notes: "I won't open his eyes, otherwise he'll take advantage of it to kill me!" Why had I been so casual about this?

In giving me double sight, Din knew he was risking his life. I saw his face, up close before me, Din sniggering and dancing, sure of his power, Din lifting his warrior mask to smile at me, Din gray as death, lying on his bed, while his double hastened to the field of battle, Din suffering, Din tracked like a wild animal from his cell to the police headquarters waiting room and back again, Din exhausted to death the day I left him for the last time. Little good it did me to tell myself that the immediate family "preferred to accuse Ekwala." I could not get away from the face of Din and fall asleep.

But no, it was impossible that I should have killed my master! However his death might be interpreted, in Western or traditional fashion, or unless a psychosomatic thesis or *ekong* sorcery were invoked, it flew in the face of the facts to say that I had killed him. I raised a protest within me against the injustice that victimized me, along with all the numberless persons suspected of sorcery in the villages or in the city, who were driven into a corner and obliged to hang their heads and keep silence. "At first you react," the *khamsi* had told me, "then you keep still, because that's all you can do." In my mind's eye, I saw the old village *nganga* again, all barricaded up, my so-called accomplice. I saw Clara, the alleged killer of her own children, and so many shut-up faces of accused persons I had stolen glimpses of in the course of so many encounters.

In Douala colloquial, where cynical comparisons are rife, the innocent victim is called the *nyama boso beta*, the "meat just inside the pantry door." This is the flesh that is always eaten first, out of convenience. But mine would not be. No, I had not killed Din, and I would give the family to know this the next day, when they gathered to hear me.

To the family I went, then, and found Bata, his mother, and his sister— the young woman whom Din had sometimes called in during rites that involved me, to assist her father in some of the last steps. She was a waitress in a restaurant, on maternity leave for the moment, and she had given birth to her first baby, naming him for her departed father. I recognized as well the faces I had so often glimpsed in the parlor when I came to visit Din. Each time I had entered here, I had seen them, placid, benevolent, always in the same places, as if they had turned to statues. Uncles, aunts, and cousins? I had never been very sure of the exact relationship. Din was gone, but they stayed. It was eleven o'clock in the morning, and so the several men who had to go to jobs were not present at the meeting. Bata invited me to be seated on the shaky chair that had always been pushed toward me when his father was alive.

I started to talk. I told them about my life in Abidjan. Fortunately my Douala vocabulary came back to me easily—doubtless the circumstances stimulated my memory. Abidjan is a city as big as Yaoundé and Douala put together. Almost half the residents there come from neighboring countries—Upper Volta, Mali, Niger, Nigeria, Guinea, Ghana, and Benin. The proportion of these foreigners is comparable to that of the Bamiléké in Douala. . . . They flood into Abidjan in the hope of finding employment. . . . Still, there's less unemployment there than in Douala. . . . Certain quarters are more modern and luxurious than the ones here, it's true, but there are worse slums there, too. . . . I work in an agency called INADES,[122] with priests who are confreres of the ones who teach in the Libermann

School, and with some specialists in economics, history, and sociology. . . .
We're trying to help make life more human, trying to help develop the
economy of the country without crushing the rural population or the foreign immigrants, trying to introduce youth to a modern life that respects
custom, trying to acquaint them with the gospel without violating the African soul.

I said all this as if I had been on fire. The family heard me out, but from a
great distance. They were more concerned with following what was going
on between themselves and me, between the lines. A baby began to cry.
They gave it back to its mother. They gave me a glass of beer. A fly fell into
it. They emptied it and filled the glass again. Other little incidents interrupted my words, but this was not the reason for the veil of indifference
that seemed to be stretched between the family members and what I was
telling them.

Their interrogation was mute, but I knew what each one of them was
asking me. All the while I spoke, I was begging them from the bottom of my
heart to believe that I had not killed Din. Then all of a sudden it was as if I
distinctly "saw" something. I saw that they had understood me and that
they trusted me—and this vision was perhaps the most concrete result of my
initiation.

There is a communications wavelength that anyone too attached to precision cannot use. Before getting to know the Douala people, the most effective language I knew was the one that most closely matches words to reality.
But my visits to Din and other *nganga*s had hastened my discovery of
another type of communication, one not altogether unlike contemplative
prayer. In Africa I saw it utilized by the whole population, in all circumstances. And it was at the most unexpected moments that I best perceived
this mute communication.

How often I had been irritated by the verbiage of African speakers who
manipulated formulas and concepts with an air of self-satisfaction and lack
of involvement that seemed really ridiculous. But little by little, I became
sensitized to messages that some of these persons were transmitting behind
the pomposity of their rhetoric. From the looks on their faces, you think
that the audience must be sitting there thinking, "This speaker is just gar-
gling words at us." What they are actually doing, however, is listening very
carefully to what the speaker is saying to them *in another way*.

Prudence dissuaded me from going to Malimba to find Din's child, who
had my name, or his young mother. It was not that I had no desire to see
them again. Far from it. But I was making it a duty to find Bata a job. I
knew a team of religious men who lived a monastic life in the heart of the
city: the Little Brothers of Jesus, disciples of Charles de Foucauld. The only
distinctive feature about their humble dwelling was that they had a chapel
that pushed a little farther out toward the street. When they were not pray-
ing, they were working. One of them was in charge of a mobile team of
unemployed young men of various talents who lived in the quarter, and who

were each learning a trade on various construction sites. They adopted Bata, who had already had two years of training as an electrician in a trade school. Here he had the opportunity to put his modest knowledge to work— a very difficult first step for an apprentice like himself, given the current conditions in the labor market.

"When I Think of You, I Eat You"

Once I had acquitted myself of this task, my heart felt freer for another visit, one just as important in my eyes as my visit to Din's family. I wanted to go and see Loe's family. (To be sure, I had no intention of limiting myself to the world of the *ngangas*. I was looking forward to restoring ties with other old friends and I found the days too short to go and greet them all.)

Loe had been dead over a year. On my way to his house I prepared myself to find signs of an agony almost as terrible as that of an individual: the agony of a group. I recalled the irascible character of Loe's older brother, now the head of the family. I recalled the ambiguous situation of Elimbi, Loe's eldest son but cut off from his family by a legal technicality. I recalled the contempt surrounding one of his daughters, who was considered a runaway.

Loe's return from beyond the grave, in Elimbi's mother's trance, had not been enough, perhaps, to give this family the cohesion it needed to survive as a family. At least this was my thought, as they all rushed out to greet me, from all the little houses scattered about what had been Loe's property.

Everybody talked at once, amid the hugs and kisses. They asked me questions, then gave me no time to answer! We just stayed standing, all together, in the middle of the courtyard. I felt the warm rush of welcome passing between each of them and myself, but I certainly did not feel it among themselves. All this noise was covering up a deep silence. I suddenly had the impression that I somehow represented their Father Loe, back among them for part of a day.

Finally the elder brother took me into his house. A part of the family followed. I was asked to recount my new life in Abidjan. From my own side I was afraid to ask any questions. I did assure myself that Elimbi was still at his job, and that everyone's children were still going to school. Then as I was getting ready to go, Nkongo, Loe's old disciple, arrived. I invited him to go back with me, intending to ask him the questions that were burning on my lips.

Once in the car, I kept silent for a moment before asking my questions. I had to catch my breath. I felt like one of those tree trunks adrift in the Wouri, swept loose from the piers. Little boys try to climb up on them, but in vain—they are too slippery, and they spin in the water. This family was clinging to me as if they had been drowning. And I was content to float on by, without being able to come to their aid in any real way.

Nkongo confirmed these first impressions of mine. Nothing was right any longer in this family, once upon a time inspired by such a great man of custom. The elder brother was selling the land by plots without the consent of the rest of the family, and keeping the money, Nkongo told me. He took care only of his own children, leaving to their fate the widows who had been left in his charge. Elimbi was still living a shuttle life, now with his father's family, now with his mother's. He had never been legally recognized, and could exercise no authority in his father's family. Loe's youngest wife had taken her child and fled, doubtless to her native village. The daughters reared, as best they could, children whose fathers had disappeared. Nkongo was helplessly witnessing the dissolution of a family with but a single thread to cling to: the certitude that the one buried in the courtyard was still living among them.

Nkongo asked me to drive him to the cement factory, where I had found him work before I left, across the bridge spanning the Wouri. I had never paid much attention to it. I had preferred to contemplate the islands up the river, watching the pirogues of the fishermen disappear behind them.

Through Nkongo's eyes, then, I observed it attentively for the first time. It seemed to have been set on the ground like a silver cube, with cylinders of all sizes—long, or pot-bellied, or fluted—mounted all around. Trucks came here day and night for cement. At first, Nkongo had been put to weighing the trucks on the scales. Now he worked in the clerks' office, checking the indicators that assured a proper mix. He spoke of his promotion in terms of initiation.

I watched as Loe's disciple receded into the distance, with his slow, confident pace. I could not help thinking that Nkongo at the factory was like Nkongo in the *dibandi*—before that amazing scaffolding of powerful barks, charged with energy, which his master had accumulated. His tranquil assurance was the same. He was utterly confident, in either place.

Nkongo had let Loe's *dibandi* run down. I had noticed that when I entered the courtyard. But his neglect did not mean that Nkongo doubted the power of the barks, or the presence of the ancestors, or the intervention of the water spirits. It was only that the factory took the better part of his time, and the *dibandi* and its sacred guests got short shrift.

We had strolled about a bit, and Nkongo had spoken to me of his projects. He was saving part of his salary to build a little house to move into with his bride-to-be. At the factory he sought to win the confidence of his superiors, and so improve his situation. He had joined the union, in the hope of obtaining a more flexible work rhythm for himself and his fellow workers. He sounded like a young laborer of Boulogne-Billancourt. Nkongo was becoming an independent individual. All unawares, he was taking his distance from traditional society, and adopting a lifestyle where you must count only on yourself if you hope to succeed. The change in Nkongo was not really the product of a reflective choice, however, but of a series of small decisions that were pulling him into the great current of modernity.

Din and Loe had disappeared without leaving heirs who could take over their function. My recent brief visits had revealed to me in a striking manner the huge chasm formed by this break in the line of succession. Family and faithful were having to reorganize their existence without benefit of the physical presence of these masters of the night, who had so long been accustomed to gather them together and reconcile them. I had known other successful *nganga*s in the vicinity, but none had had such a place in my life. Suddenly I felt, in my own turn, and poignantly, how much I missed Din and Loe.

There was only one more person to see. From her—unconsciously as yet—I sought a sign: some solid reliable token that my secret ties with the rulers of the night had not been severed. I went to see the mountain *khamsi*.

I set out at dawn, traversing the Deïdo quarter, and slowly covering the more than a mile of bridge that crossed the Wouri. The port was waking like a beehive on my left; on my right the banks and the islands seemed to drowse after the night's secret activities. The bridge was the only connecting route between Douala, the economic capital, and the rich Bamiléké country. Dreamers call it a symbolic link between the modern world and tradition. In reality, this seemingly inoffensive bridge favors modernism and hastens the death of customs. The residents understood this very well when they demanded that the Batignolles Company cast certain offerings to the bottom of the deep, to appease the *niengu* before pouring the last arch. The engineers guffawed, then complied, understanding nothing.

This morning I did not even look to see whether Mount Cameroon appeared on the horizon, or was lost in mist. I drove distractedly, with my eyes all but closed, trying to collect the memories that blew back to me in gusts. Loe, his young wife, his elder brother, and Nkongo had formed a single group in this car that fateful night we all crossed the bridge to answer the old *nganga*'s call, and fall into a trap. Now I had crossed it a hundred times, on my way to the same village, where I was called Dibunje, after the reconciliation. With Din, I had passed beneath it in a launch, in quest of the glorious bark *ngopange*. The whistling of the breeze over the water, the strong smell of silt, and the slapping of the waves against the arches, all jostled my memory.

Then came the long trip up the mountain. As usual, it took me several hours to reach the Batié Pass. About noon, I turned off the asphalt road that ran along the ridge, and headed down the little dirt trail that led to the *khamsi*'s hut. Even before I arrived, I could make out the file of visitors crouching in the shadow of the hut, waiting their turn for a session with the diviner. The *khamsi* was seated near the door where she always sat. Before her was a patient, whom she was scrutinizing. The tableau had not changed. The personages seemed permanently painted in black on the ocher wall, and the house stood cut away against the green and dark brown of the mountain, all bright in this midday.

As I drew near, the *khamsi* detached her gaze from her patient and raised her head. I saw a broad smile gradually form on the round surface of her face. "How glad I am to see you!" I said, and I asked the child at her side kindly to translate this sentence. In her turn the *khamsi* pronounced several words to me, which the child translated into French. I asked the young interpreter to repeat it, to be sure I had understood the meaning, so much had her words both surprised and delighted me. Perhaps it was just a formula of politeness. But for me it was one of the most powerful statements that have ever been addressed to me. "The *khamsi* says," the child repeated, careful to pronounce every syllable very clearly, "that every time she thinks of you, she eats you."

Appendix 1

Glossary of the Most Important Douala Words Used in This Book

Phonetic Equivalents, Douala/English

Douala	English
a	ä (cart)
e	ā (bake) or ë (let)
i	ī (life)
o	ō (flow) or ô (ought)
u	ōō(loot)

G is always pronounced hard, as in "get."

Bato (sing. **moto**) Human beings *Bato ba mianga* (lit. medicine persons), *ngangas; bato ba lemba, bato b'ekong, bato b'ewusu,* sorcerers. See *mianga, lemba, ekong, ewusu.*

Bedimo (sing. **edimo**) Ancestors, the dead.

Bejongo (sing. in disuse) Trances, in which the ancestors speak through the entranced subject.

Bobe (pl. **miobe**) Evil, malice.

Dibandi (pl. **mabandi**) The sanctuary where *ngangas* amass their *mianga* and instruments of power; the special place where they invoke the ancestors and the spirits in the practice of traditional medicine. From the verb *banda,* protect, conjure, exorcise.

Diboa (pl. **maboa**) Disease, sickness, malady, in the broad sense.

Dibokuboku Any of a particular group of aquatic nympheaceous plants. *Dibokuboku la wonja* (lit. *d.* of free persons), the leaf of this plant, round and as large as a

261

plate; frequently used as a symbol of unity to be restored or preserved; reputed to calm heart palpitations; the *khamsi*'s *mbömbu. Dibokuboku la bakom* (lit. *d.* of slaves), a plant related to the former, but physically smaller and of lesser importance; likewise used in the *nganga*'s *esa;* used to calm heart palpitations; its leaf is green on one side and brown on the other; the *khamsi*'s *pankhwi jüm.*

Dindo (pl. **mindo**) Sacred meal celebrated at the close of a treatment, consisting of the meat of the animal sacrificed, medicinal herbs, and a plantain called *miele ma sese.*

Eboga *Tabernanthe iboga,* any of a group of apocynaceous bushes whose roots contain hallucinogenic alkaloids. The name is a Fang word , and the plant is prized especially by the adepts of Bwiti-Fang, a new religion in Gabon, which has not taken hold in Cameroon, but which inspires certain rites of healing performed in the region lying on the Cameroon-Gabon border.

Edidi, a person's double during life; *edimo,* the double after death.

Edimo (pl. **bedimo**) A deceased person, an ancestor.

Ekong (pl. **bekong**) The sorcery of traffic in human beings. *Ekong* practitioners *(bato b'ekong)* form an association whose principal activity consists in putting to death, by methods invisible to ordinary eyes (for example, by means of the *nyungu*), designated victims, who are thereupon deemed to travel to invisible plantations (for example, on Mount Kupe) to work for their new masters. When Africans or Europeans in Africa suddenly become rich, it is commonly attributed to *ekong.*

Ekumti (pl. **bekumti**) Invisible *ndimsi* battles.

Esa (pl. **besa**) A ceremony performed for the purpose of banishing misfortune, consisting in a quest for the cause of the ill, protestations of innocence, ablutions with the *dibokuboku* leaf, reconciliation, and elimination of the cause. The rite is practiced at all social levels: in the family, at the hands of a *nganga,* and in circumstances where all the Douala take part.

Esunkan A *jengu nganga.*

Evu Sorcery, in the Ewondo language of Yaoundé. Cf. the Douala *ewusu. Evu* is connected with a myth of the origin of power and disorder upon the earth. The myth, which gives the sorcery its meaning, is unknown to the Douala of today, but is still recounted in the central and eastern regions of Cameroon.

Ewusu (pl. **bewusu**) Cannibalistic sorcery. The *ewusu* followers form small groups for the purpose of devouring victims furnished by each member in turn. The practice, invisible to ordinary eyes, has as its only purpose to do harm to persons and thereby augment the power of the group members. One is born an *ewusu.* Formerly the word was neutral in its connotation, but today it is frankly pejorative.

Eyembilan (pl. **byembilan**) An example, sign, or gesture.

Janjo (pl. **manjo**) An insignia of authority, made of raffia fronds, and resembling a feather-duster.

Jene la ndoti A meaningful vision beheld in a dream, to be distinguished from an ordinary dream *(ndoti),* and representing important events, which must be interpreted by a diviner. From the verb *ene,* see.

Jengu (pl. **miengu**) Water genie, water spirit, water ancestor. An ancient representation shows a little black creature with a great amount of hair, very large, protruding eyes, and turned-up toes. The modern representation is of a white woman with long hair (the *mamy wata*). The *jengu* bestows wealth on men and fertility on women.

A secret Jengu Society formerly played a very important role in Douala society, moderating and counterbalancing the power of the chiefs. It disappeared with the German colonization.

The *jengu* is accorded the same honor as the ancestors themselves. Certain prominent persons are deemed to have a *jengu* spouse.

The public cult of the *miengu* has disappeared in our day, but it perdures in a context of illness and healing, by means of invocations, possessions, and trances.

Kwa A certain tree, whose bark is poisonous. In former times it was used in an ordeal of guilt and innocence. If the accused could drink the water in which the bark had been steeped, regurgitate it, and survive, they were deemed innocent. The practice is in disuse today.

Lemba (pl. **balemba**) Sorcery. Only by birth can someone be a "person of *ewusu,*" but one may become a "person of lemba" *(mota lemba).* The *mota lemba* is a person who acquires harmful objects or products *(mianga ma bobe),* and uses them in an invisible manner to harm other persons.

Loba Traditionally, heaven, or the God of heaven; to be distinguished from the God of earth. *Loba* is the word preferred by Christians for translating "God" in the biblical sense.

Londa To be full; to "armor." The *balondedi* are those who are "charged with power."

Male (sing. in disuse) Contracts of alliance.

Maya ma bobe (lit. blood of evil) Bad blood; sign of a serious disease; misfortune deliberately caused.

Mbenda (pl. **mambenda**) Prohibition; rule, law.

Mbenge The West; Europe; the outside world. Shipping to Douala from abroad generally arrives from a westerly direction.

Mbeu'a nyolo (lit. loss of the body) A grave illness. The common Cameroonian translation into French as *malchance,* "misfortune," is correct only with the understood reservation that the "misfortune" referred to is deliberately provoked.

Mbodi (pl. **mbodi**) Goat.

Mianga (sing. **bwanga**) Objects charged with power; medicines. *Mianga* can be helpful or harmful. *Nganga*'s are *bato ba mianga* (lit. medicine persons).

Miengu See *jengu.*

Miso manei (lit. eyes four) Double sight. An ordinary person is born with four eyes, of which two are closed during life, to open only when the other two close in death. Seers have all four eyes open in life: two see the visible world, two the invisible. *Tele la miso* (lit. to open the eyes), the seer's initiation ceremony.

Moto (pl. **bato**) Human being.

Mudi (pl. **midi**) The vital principle.

Musima (pl. **misima**) Grace; good fortune, success, a cure that has been granted; (by extension) good luck received.

Mwandando (pl. **myandando**) *Costus afer,* any of a group of zingiberaceous plants used in numerous rituals: at the consecration of a chief, the annual Douala festival (the Ngongo), treatments, and the like. The *mwandando* is a sign of peace. In olden times it was planted at the entrance to a village, where food was placed for the ancestors; hence a synonym, *mukoke mwa bedimo,* ancestors' sugar cane. The plant resembles sugar cane.

  Mwandando is also used medicinally, in the treatment of various diseases, as for meningitis in children.

  Mwandando is the *khamsi*'s *nkwengkang.*

Mwititi Darkness; the world shut off from ordinary eyes.

Ndimsi (pl. in disuse) World of hidden realities, where destiny is decided. Those who can penetrate this reality—persons endowed with "double sight"—have the power to act on health, sickness, and the future, for the good or ill of ordinary mortals. Certain seers refrain from the exercise of this power, being content merely to observe what transpires in *ndimsi.* From the verb *dima,* to become dark.

Ndoti (pl. **ndoti**) Ordinary dream. To be distinguished from the *jene la ndoti,* or dream of vision.

Ngad'a mudumbu (pl. **ngadi**) (lit. bullet from the mouth) A casting of lots; a sorcerers' weapon.

Ngambi (pl. **ngambi**) A diviner, an oracle.

Ngandó (pl. **ngandó**) Caiman, a crocodilian; caiman sorcery.

Ngando (pl. **mangando**) Feast, festival; mixture of the most powerful barks, a particularly celebrated "armoring" against sorcerers.

Nganga (pl. **nganga**) Practitioner of traditional medicine.

Nginya (pl. **nginya**) Power. *Nginya gobina,* political power (the second word being pidgin English for "governor"); *nginya ebasi,* religious power (*ebasi* = the Christian religion); *nginya wase,* earthly, cosmic, or occult power (*wase* = the earth); *nginya ekombo,* power of the people *(ekombo* = land, tribe).

Ngoso (pl. **ngoso**) Parrot; Douala musical repertoire.

Njan (pl. **njan** or **minjan**) Foreigner adopted by the Douala.

Njom (pl. **njom**) Cause, origin, reason. The word is a most emphatic one, and is applied to *Loba* (God) when one feels engulfed in overwhelming circumstances.

Njum bwele The most celebrated tree of Douala tradition. Its bark enables the user to hold sorcerers at a distance. It is used in a number of rites, including that of initiation.
   Other traditional trees honored for their power and cited in this book: the *buma (le Grand Fromager* of Deïdo); the *bongongi* (the great tree of Bonabéri); the *eselebako;* the *ngopange;* the *ekon;* Loe's *selebenge;* Madola's *bovenga.*

Nsote A bay tree having particularly sweet seeds. The *nsote* signifies peace and unity. The Bamiléké name is *dethum.*

Nyambe The traditional name for the God of the earth, the Ancestor of ancestors. Christians have adopted *Loba,* God of the sky, to translate "God" in the biblical sense, instead of *Nyambe;* the word still occurs, however, even among Christians, in the following formula of welcome: *"Nje tuse?"* Response: *"Nyambe."* ("What gives life?"—"God.")

Nyolo (pl. **manyolo**) Body.

Nyungu (pl. **nyungu**) An invisible snake, at the service of sorcerers; the rainbow.

Appendix 2

Dreams

I conducted a survey of various *nganga* friends of mine in the city of Douala concerning the world of sleep, and thus was able to gather the traditional teaching on dreams and visions in rather nontechnical language, as one might explain something to school children. These experts were at different levels of professional familiarity with the subject, but their responses converge.

The Ordinary Dream and the Dream of Vision

All the *ngangas* surveyed made an elemental distinction between the (French) *rêve* and the *songe,* or the mere dream and the dream of vision. The Douala language marks the difference by using *ndoti,* "dream," for the mere dream ("Anybody can dream, babies dream")—and *jene la ndoti,* which I translate *songe,* and which means literally, "dream vision," the dream that reveals reality. The difference between the two is of the greatest importance: the former has no significance at all, whereas the latter has tremendous meaning.

"Ordinary dreams are sometimes true and sometimes false," Tokoto told me. "You can't very well tell the difference. But dream visions are always true: persons want to know what they want to know, and they find out. Here's an example. When I had my first wife, seven years ago, I wanted to get myself to have a dream, and find out whether we'd just live a plain, normal life, or whether there'd be something dramatic, something bad. Well, I dreamed someone was speaking behind her back to disturb her. And sure enough, we're separating. [This was true.] And she'd sworn to me it could never happen. But she's been unfaithful. I took her to court and won. She appealed, but I told her, 'Remember what I predicted seven years ago!' "

The *songe,* the vision dream, goes beyond a simple warning. It is the communication of a fait accompli, as it were, even though it regards the future. The anxiety of someone awakening after an unusual nightmare, then, is easy to understand. If it has been a real *songe,* a *jene la ndoti,* then that person can be sure that what they have seen will actually come to pass. The vision dream partakes of prophecy: it unveils truth.

Normally dreamers themselves realize that their dream has been a *songe,* a vision dream. There is no need to have a diviner say so. Everyone has had their apprenticeship in the elementary code of nightmares, as drawn up by the cultural universe into which they have been born. There remains the problem of interpretation—the movement from the confused certainty that some danger threatens, to a clear knowledge of circumstances and persons. Here the *nganga*-diviners become indispensable. (Today, the two functions are most often joined in one person.) Two similar vision dreams can have different meanings, even opposite meanings.

For example, what does it mean to see water in a dream? Din explained: "Somebody dreams about being carried off to the water. This can be, for instance, *ekong* sorcerers acting. Or it can be that the police will come and arrest the person the next day.[123] But suppose someone dreams he or she is surrounded by water. That's not bad. This time the water keeps the evil spirits from coming to this person during the night. Somebody else might dream it's fire, being surrounded by fire at night—evildoers can't get near." A diviner's work is first and foremost the exercise of the art of discernment.

Provoking, Interpreting, and Overcoming Dreams

The *nganga*-diviners have means of provoking dreams. Every *nganga*-diviner has a particular secret *mianga* recipe. Tokoto told me: "When I want to have a look at something that's not going right, I put the root of this herb under my pillow before I go to sleep. You know you're going to do that, but you don't tell anybody else. You just lift up your pillow a little bit, slip it in, and go to sleep. And then, while you're in bed, you don't have real sleep this time, you have a different kind of sight of everything that's going on."

Mianga—so often lightly referred to as "medicines," or "remedies"—are a global designation for all the means of power that a *nganga* is called upon to manage, and whose force for good or ill infinitely surpasses the dimensions of their modest package. They are always objects; they are never personalized. They can be composed of plants and barks, or made of leather, bone, or iron. Their shabby appearance is actually an advantage: it recalls that their true strength is not of the order of things visible.

The interpreted *songe,* provoked or not, reveals a precise and certain event. If it announces a baneful event, those responsible must be exposed. And indeed it is impossible for the Douala to conceive of any action, especially a hurtful one, whose source is not in the intention of some person or persons. It is the delicate mission of the diviner-healers discreetly to reveal to the family the name of the one who has woven the plots.

Once the discernment process has been completed, the time has come to intervene. Without neglecting organic medicine, the *nganga* officially carries on the combat on the level of dreams. If the *nganga* manages to expel the troubled dreams of vision, and restores the normal course of sleep, the client has been cured.

"The doctor works to cut out *(ke)* the vision dreams, Din explained. "He works to finish *(bole)* them. Suppose the patient can only dream he's being followed, for instance, or that he's being tied up and beaten, or that he's getting married at night. This illness comes from enemies. They're the ones who're after him like that. If the doctor manages to stop all this, it's over." Thus in any overall treatment, treatment of the dream itself has priority. Hence a major treatment is inaugurated by a sort of antinightmare ceremony, where a dramatic structure is created that represents the opposite of the nightmare: the good graces of the departed are invoked and guaranteed, the patient passes the night in the midst of a benevolent community, the sorcerers are driven away by fire, water is used in special, purifying ablutions, the sufferer is replaced by an animal, which is then sacrificed.

"You tell the *nganga* what dreams come back often. Then he tries to finish your dreams. Then he treats your sickness," Din explained.

Double Sight

Both victim and *nganga* accord an important place to the *songe,* the visionary dream. For ordinary mortals, the dream of vision is a very special moment when they have fleeting access to the mysterious reality whose key is in the hands of the diviner-*nganga.* Hence the great importance sufferers attribute to unusual dreams, so that they go to consult an oracle about their meaning. The oracle, day and night, sees with perfect clarity what an ordinary mortal sees only in bits and pieces during sleep. The dream is clear and true in itself, but it is like a flashbulb: it leaves its environment in shadow. But diviner-*nganga*s have eyes for this reality—they have *miso manei,* four eyes, the double sight. They see in darkness *(mwititi)* as in broad daylight, and they intervene in the battles *(ekumti)* of the invisible world *(ndimsi).* "The dream [the *songe*] is the alphabet of the understanding of *ndimsi,*" was Din's way of putting it.

The gift of vision, the gift of double sight, may be bestowed on someone in a dream, it may be received at birth, or it may be received in the course of an initiation called "school." This ability to pierce the dark is so integrated with the personhood of the chosen one as to be quasi-natural.

"There are slots [i.e., categories] of dreams," Loe told me. "There's the dream provoked by sorcery. I can take that away from you and cure you. But there is also the dream-by-nature. Take that away and it'll kill you—now you don't see anything any more, you've had your eyes put out."

The last of the three paths to vision, that of initiation, is accompanied by its proper rites, of which the last step is the administration of a liquid in the eyes, drop by drop. "Then you notice your body's changed," said Tokoto. "There are times when you're in some place and you say, 'No!' and your body says, 'No! I have to get out of here! The police are coming!' You get out of there, and sure enough, the police come."

The thread of logic linking the ordinary dream, the visionary dream, and reality, became evident to me. But it is a logic that is valid only in a vaster cultural context, wherein all that exists is shot through with the cohesiveness of that context, and wherein one recognizes that the greater part of reality, the most determinative part of reality, escapes ordinary eyes—as is borne out by countless night séances.

Appendix 3

The One Who Came Back from the Dead

Appendix to Chapter 5, "*Ekong* Sorcery"

"Can persons come back when they've been sold?" I once asked Loe.

"It's very rare," he replied. "I just don't understand these stories. They do come back. My brother was one. He'd been sold to the Hausa [Muslims from the north]. It's always Hausa, or Europeans who buy them. My brother died. He was buried, and forgotten for years. But his body didn't stay in the cemetery. They awakened him, as if he'd been asleep. When he came back, they'd changed his looks. He was black when he'd left, and now he was brown. He'd had carbuncles on his bottom, and when he came back he didn't have them any more. But it's very rare."

I asked Din the same question: "Do the dead return?"

"No, they lead another life over there, they can't come back any more."

"But I'm told they can!"

"Well, those particular ones have been released."

Through the good offices of friends, I met one of these revenants. He had a booth at the Deïdo market, a place teeming with Hausa. He dressed and acted like a Hausa, but his face was unmistakably Douala—round, and a bit ruddy. He swore that the Douala he spoke was his native tongue, and claimed to be related to a well-known family of Bonabéri—another quarter, across the bridge. He admitted that his first name was Muslim, but insisted that his family name was Douala. Of course, it was scarcely usual for a child from Bonabéri to be converted to Islam, and be reared, and marry, among the Hausa. The market superintendent gave me permission to write up his interpretation of the phenomenon.

"He didn't die naturally," the superintendent said. "It was a result of *ndimsi*. He was buried in the Bonabéri cemetery a good thirty years ago. They mourned him, and yet he hadn't really died. The sorcerers took him away at night and sold him to the Hausa of Lagos [Nigeria]. And then one fine day here he was back, alive. He himself recognizes that this is his native country. 'I'm home,' he says. When the Douala saw him they said, 'That fellow died! What's he doing back here?' And he began to recognize his friends and relatives. But when his relatives wanted to take him home, the Hausa said, 'No, you don't, he's one of us!' The trouble is, the conditions of sale are not known. [Had there been a record of the sale, the family could have the sale price and taken the home.] He doesn't live in Bonabéri, he lives in the Hausa quarter. He dresses like a Hausa. He knows everybody in the market. Ninety

270 THE ONE WHO CAME BACK FROM THE DEAD

percent of those who come to the market don't know he's a Douala. And yet his mother is still living in Bonabéri, and sometimes he goes and sees her on his motorbike. There's *ndimsi* at the market, but each according to its kind: there's the Nigerians', there's Ewondos'. . . ."

The Hausa-Douala merchant himself did not have to be asked twice to come and explain his side of the story, in the Douala language. This was understandable, of course—he was eager to intercept any interpretation that might be to his discredit. "I don't want to say anything that'll get me in trouble tomorrow. I'm not afraid of you, because you're a priest, and if you want me back tomorrow, I'll come back tomorrow," he averred.

"I'm telling you, others are making up stories about me," he said. "I can't tell you whether somebody can die and come back, but there are lots of troubles in the world. The Koran tells me you can't have any other faith: 'Thou shalt not believe in anyone besides Me, the one true God.' I'm with the Muslims, that's all. I haven't changed. I won't change. The Koran doesn't let you go around telling things all wrong, and saying things that aren't so. 'Thou shalt not repeat the tales thou hearest.' The Douala, when they've had something to drink, tell you anything. If you want a drink, take some vinegar and Perrier, and put that in the liquor. That kills the strength of the liquor for you. Do you ever see a white get drunk and fall down in the courtyard?

"What happened to me when I was a small child—there isn't much I can tell you and sign my name to it. I started working for the Muslims when I was seven or eight. I was out of the country, in Lagos, where the traffic had sent me, and I traveled with an old Muslim. I've been to Caduna, Onitsha, Enugu, and Yahe [Nigerian cities], right over the border from Cameroon. Then Mamfé, Kumba, and Douala [Cameroon cities]. I don't know how many years I spent out of the country. Over ten years. I left at age seven, according to what my father told me, and I was already paying taxes when I came back. When I got back nobody said anything to me. I didn't know a thing. I stayed in New-Bell [another Douala quarter], and started up a little business, in the way of the Hausa—you know, selling cloth and little jewelry things.

"That's when they started saying, 'Oh, look at that fellow!' They'd decided I was a certain Douala child they remembered. 'Here's your father, here's your mother, here's your brother, here's your friend!' I was surprised. 'How can I be a Douala?' I said. I asked myself how this could be, that I'm being taken for a Douala. And they told me, 'We don't know how the world is made, but don't refuse us.' That's why I decided to agree with them. But I told them I couldn't change my religion. And they said, 'Fine, you can keep your religion.' "

I recounted these two versions of the story to Douala friends, and they were not surprised. This man was not the only one to have had this happen to him. Another had a stall in another market. Years ago, I was told, in the days of pirogue-racing, when less vigilance was exercised over children, the Hausa engaged in kidnaping. Then the vagaries of trade and travel had restored missing persons to their homeland. These versions coexist, but the one proposed most often, in the popular milieux where I moved, was the first. The presence of such an exceptional phenomenon—persons back from the dead—reinforces belief in *ekong*. It occasions anxiety, for it confirms the fate of the majority of sorcery victims (they do not return). But it reassures, as well: it is proof of the survival of near relatives who have died as a result of sorcery.

Appendix 4

Two Ceremonies Compared

Synopsis of a Douala and a Bamiléké Ceremony Performed for the Purpose of Finding Employment for the Subject

Some Common Aspects

Loe, the Douala *nganga,* treats his son Elimbi.

Pauline Nkwedum, the Bamendjou *khamsi,* treats her son Jean Fotsing.

Functions of the officiants: Loe is an *esunkan,* a prestigious *jengu nganga.* Nkwedum is a *khamsi,* a diviner.

Identical objective: To gain employment for the eldest son of the officiant.

Meaning, or sign value, of the ceremony: In both cases, the lifting of the curse preventing the subject from finding work—in other words, the securing of family harmony, the regaining of family equilibrium.

Rituals: The rituals are similar in their broad lines. First there is an appeal to God and the ancestor, then purification by water, then confession of innocence, then a prayer or an expression of desires, and finally an expression of encouragement to the subject to seek employment.

Regarding sorcery: The conception is identical in both cases.

Sacred plants: Four of the most important of them are identical in both cases, under different names:

Bamendjou	*Douala*
Mbömbu: various uses for the protection of sacred persons and objects	*Dibokuboku la wonja:* various uses for the protection of clan unity

An aquatic nympheaceous plant

Pankhwijüm: for washing the face	*Dibokuboku la makon:* for washing the face. Loe washed Elimbi's face with the *dibokuboku la wonja,* instead. But on other occasions he did use the *diboku-*

271

boku la makom to wash the subject's face.

Acantheaceous plants

Dethum: friendship, unity
Nkwenkang: peace

Nsote: unity
Mwandando or *mukoke mwa bedimo:* peace

Costus afer (zingiberaceous)

Note: The bonds of the Bamiléké with the Bantu, and thus with the Douala, seem stronger than reputed. Larry Hyman, an American researcher, has arrived at the same conclusion on the basis of linguistic criteria. The parallel ceremonies cited here manifest related structures. Arguments based on linguistic characteristics and ritual system are considered less tenuous than arguments based on other criteria.

Appendix 5

Ekongolo Finds Her *Jengu* Spouse

Appendix to Chapter 13, "Order Lost and Restored"

In the course of a treatment at the hands of a *nganga* of the coast, in Kribi, a woman named Ekongolo fell into a *jengu* trance. I took a photograph, and later brought it to her. Upon seeing the picture, Ekongolo told me of her encounters with Ilina, her mystical *jengu* husband.

"You fall into this sort of thing without noticing it," she began. "If you hadn't shown me the picture as proof, I wouldn't have known it happened. There I am, and he can come into me. My feet start feeling cold. This cold starts creeping up to my head, and finally my eyes turn back into my head. After that I don't know what I'm doing."

"What's his name?" I asked.

"Ilina."

"How do you see him?"

"I see him in dreams. He looks like a white person. . . .

"Usually when I have a dream I jump into the sea. I go down to the very bottom, and lie down, down there, and he comes. Then I come back up. You see, sometimes I go to dangerous places in the sea, where human beings don't go. It's like a chasm. When I get there, I jump in, and go in that way. I sleep there, at the bottom of the water, and I start hearing little sounds—'kwang, kwang,' like that—then I see something like stars, with my eyes. I stay inside there as if I were in another world. Then all of a sudden I come back out. Then I'm surprised, and I say to myself, 'I've been in the water!' And when I come out like that, I'm coming out of my sleep. And I say to myself, 'That was a dream I was in!' That's what I usually see. But see him, with my eyes, right in front of me? No, I don't see him that way."

Appendix 6

The Various Traditional Manners of Preparing and Administering Medicines

(From E. Zipcy, F. Pelissier, and D. Lemordant, "Ethnopharmacologie camerounaise," *Journal d'Agriculture Tropicale et de Botanique Appliquée*, vol. 23 (1976), nos. 1–3.

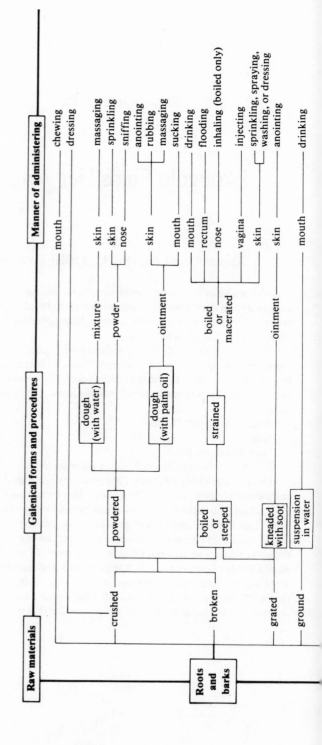

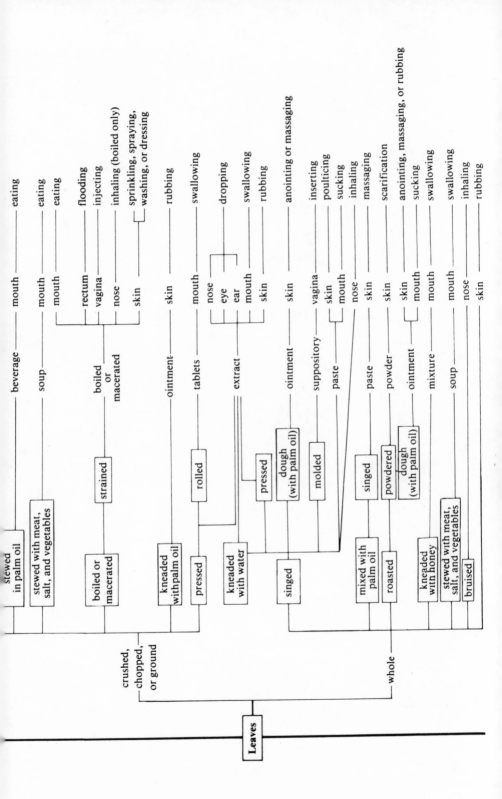

Notes

1. "La lutte contre le choléra: Liturgie de l'*Esa* à Douala," *Abbia*, nos. 29–30 (Yaoundé, 1975).

2. *Ndimsi: Ceux qui soignent dans la nuit* (Yaoundé: CLE, 1974).

3. I am very grateful to the editors of Editions Plon for their attention to the preparation and polishing of the manuscript for the French edition of this book, and to Orbis Books for the translation into English.

4. For the pronunciation of Douala words, see the beginning of Appendix 1.

5. Georges Balandier, *The Sociology of Black Africa* (New York: Praeger, 1970); idem, *Ambiguous Africa: Cultures in Collision* (New York: Meridian, 1969).

6. René Bureau, *Ethnosociologie religieuse des Douala et apparentés* (Yaoundé: Recherches camerounaises, 1962).

7. For the political background to this strike, see J.-F. Bayart, *L'Etat au Cameroun* (Paris: Fondation Nationale des Sciences Politiques, 1979), pp. 129–30.

8. Paul Claudel, *The Tidings Brought to Mary: A Mystery* (Yale University Press, 1916), pp. 30–31.

9. *Etudes* (Paris), May 1970, pp. 737ff.

10. I shall not use the term "sorcerer" in this book with reference to Din or his colleagues. But I shall use it for a category of frankly maleficent persons called in Douala tradition *bato b'ewusu, bato ba lemba,* or *bato b'ekong.* See the Glossary of Douala words, Appendix 1.

11. No term in French or English seems satisfactory to me. The World Health Organization proposes *tradipracticien* ("tradi[tional]practitioner"). *Guérisseur* ("healer"), which seems to be gaining currency in Cameroon in place of *féticheur, marabout, docteur indigéne,* or *professeur,* recalls for French readers a category of personages still practicing in the European countryside, but enjoying a much more restricted reputation and social power. My interlocutors sometimes also use *guérisseur* for *nganga* when they speak to me in French.

12. In this book monetary sums are given in terms of the currency of Cameroon—that is, in terms of Communauté Financière Africaine (African Financial Community) francs. One thousand CFA francs are worth about four dollars; 24,000 CFA francs, then, will be worth approximately a hundred dollars.

13. *Katapula, Eso mawuta, Mulopo mwa machine, Sangwa mianga, Ngoma.*

14. I recorded his words and later had them translated. (Din allowed me to use a tape recorder whenever we were together, including the night séances.) He knew the difficulty I had in understanding him and even sent me after the recorder when he had an important piece of information for me. Not only did Din not speak French, but even his Douala was not the best.

15. Johannes Ittmann, *Volkskundliche und religiöse Begriffe im nordlichen Waldland von Kamerun* (Afrika und Übersee, vol. 26, Berlin, 1953); E. Ardener, *Coastal Bantu of the Cameroons* (London: International African Institute, 1956).

16. I owe these preliminary explanations to a schoolteacher, a member of this family, who was to assist at the ceremony with me. He styled himself a skeptic, but said he wanted to keep an open mind, in view of so many inexplicable things he had witnessed since childhood.

17. Until I better understood colloquial Douala, I used my students as translators. I edited their work only when they departed from the original, or to clarify the French they were writing. I generally permitted them to choose the words and the turns of thought. This gives my translations a style rather like that of my other interviews, those recorded directly in French. It seems to me that this is an appropriate way to deal with a certain de facto linguistic homogeneity created by my interlocutors' bilingual culture.

18. Here "washing" and "misfortune," or "ill luck," have an entirely different connotation from their ordinary Western usage.

19. "*Kwa* designates the *erythrophleum guineense,* the poisonous sasswood tree. The red bark of the roots of the young tree is still used today. In former times persons under suspicion of sorcery were sentenced to drink this beverage. Sometimes they themselves demanded it in order to prove their innocence. The bark was fetched from the forest by the accused, then chopped and made into nine little balls, which the accused had to swallow. They would drink as much of the poisoned beverage as possible and hope to be able to vomit it all up while singing and dancing. If successful, the suspect was absolved of suspicion, and could demand satisfaction of the adversary. But if the suspect began to stagger, without vomiting, it was a proof of guilt, and the suspect was hanged or beaten to death. Because this sort of ordeal is prohibited today, the *kwa* is no longer given to the person, but to a chicken. What happens to the chicken is then observed, and judgment is pronounced: punishment or restitution. (See Ittmann, *Volkskundliche Begriffe,* the article on *kwa.*)

20. Whiskey, rum, and gin, introduced on the coast by the first European traders, became the traditional festive drinks, more highly esteemed than local distillations.

21. See Appendix 3, "The One Who Came Back from the Dead."

22. Monetary values of bygone times, which remain unaltered in *ndimsi.*

23. For caiman sorcery, see chapter 13, "Order Lost and Restored."

24. In support of my hypothesis I adduce the following supplementary arguments. Cameroonians who dream they are being carried off, with hands bound, toward a river or the ocean as a slave, without being able to recognize the face of their abductors, are most anxious to find a *nganga* as soon as possible. Further, the peoples who dwell in the interior say that the *ekong* sorcery that rages among them comes from the coast.

25. And now the children already had a new song about me.

O bi mo, o wo,
O bi mo, o wo,
Nun mukala ndedi, o wo,
Nun mukala ndedi, o wo,
Nu m'ande bato, o wo,
Nu m'ande bato, o wo?

("Do you know him, *o wo*, do you know him, *o wo*, the white who takes pity, *o wo*, the white who takes pity, *o wo*, who buys persons, *o wo*, who buys persons, *o wo*?")

26. See Bayart, *L'Etat au Cameroun*, p. 274. The author mentions this episode, of which he had read in my earlier book *Ndimsi*, as an illustration of his thesis on the struggle for political power on the part of youth against the traditional chiefs. But my book had not mentioned that these scouts were also members of the Cameroonian National Union Youth movement, and that the chief's son, who pacified them, was the local leader in the latter organization. This more overtly political element has never been evident to me, on the part of either of the two groups said to be in competition in this way. At the moment of the events here related, membership in the single national political party was not a popular thing with the Douala. The Scout movement furnished a better vehicle for confrontations.

27. The fig tree, Matthew 21:18.

28. I have already indicated that Loe's only disciple was Nkongo, a former patient who had been healed in his care, but who was absent during these days.

29. This prayer contains a number of key words. "God" is used in the Christian sense (*Loba*, "Jehovah"). Loe is in no way concerned to conceal his membership in a Protestant church. The expression *a Loba njom*, uttered just before the reading of the gospel, means, literally "to God [belongs] the origination, the causality, the reason." It refers to the mystery of the god of heaven (*Loba*), and has been christianized by missionaries. It is employed when a situation is beyond human explanation. The terms *musima* and *bonam* mean "grace" and "blessing," but are usually translated into French as *chance* ("luck") and *bonheur* ("fortune") as opposed to *malchance* ("bad luck"). This vulgarization or secularization of religious vocabulary explains misunderstandings with reference to the content of the French word *malchance*.

30. I was not to be able to record this confused discussion. Happily, my neighbor, the retiree, would be giving me the gist of it.

31. This is the only instance in the story of the use of the word "disease" or "sickness" in a restrictive sense.

32. The explanation is a particularly dense one, a flashing condensation that associates beings, acts, and things in utter disregard and transcendence of physical laws. It was given to me at the end of the rite, and helped me to feel, rather than understand, the meaning of the term "medicine"—a feeble word indeed for *mianga* (singular, *bwanga*). (The *nganga* are sometimes called "medicine persons," *bato ba mianga*.)

33. One of the barks was that of a tree that every *nganga* knows: the *esselebako*. I have accompanied Din to the tree from which he gathered his own provisions of this bark, eighteen kilometers down the road to Razel. The tree is mutilated to a height of six feet. At its foot lie empty bottles from old libations. "You take the bark," Din told me, "you mix it with balsam. You go into the water, and you throw it there. And you see the animal of the water spirits, the *manga* [manatee, sea cow] come out of the water. They call it the 'spirits' goat. You stick it with your spear, you take it to the village, and you start shouting for joy. Maybe I'll show you this work some day."

34. See Appendix 2, "Dreams."

35. According to one of the Douala, here is the way to "make a quill [a fountain pen or a ballpoint pen] for an exam"—*pongo esao ya kekise*. Pour a little water onto a plate. Place a piece of bamboo on the water. Grate a bit of the bark *eselebako* over the floating bamboo. Now place some *bonkeng* (an herb) in the water, place the pen on top of the bamboo, and cover plate and contents with a handkerchief. Wait three days. Return the pen to its owner. A certain Hausa (actually a native of Saudi

Arabia) gave me another recipe. Read a few verses of the Koran and write one of the verses on a piece of unruled paper. Fold the paper and have a cobbler bind it up inside a piece of leather. Wear it around your neck, in your pocket, anywhere at all on your person, the day of the exam. It may be discarded after the exam. This is called *layaarou* in Foulfouldé, the language of the Foulbés. I questioned a student who used the talisman: "You tell me all your classmates carry this object. Did they all pass their exams?"

"No. Some didn't study."

"So?"

"It's for morale."

36. My colleague René Roi remarked: "You weren't exactly brilliant. You were on your guard. You were prudent. Obviously you didn't want to testify as to this particular instance. You just wanted to take the side of the true *nganga*s. You were weighing your words."

37. I read these documents. They list bruises on the patient's body, and a cranial traumatism, but the observations are formulated in such a way that no conclusion can be drawn as to the cause.

38. The attorney's interpretation differs from the one proposed by the *Commentaire du Code Pénal*, an unofficial text, but all police stations have a copy of it for reference. "The law," says the *Commentaire*, "makes 'sorcery' an infraction *sui generis,* and not a case of fraud. This is why this article falls in the section relating to infractions of the public peace. It is considered indispensable to insure the protection of persons and goods against those who arrogate to themselves any imaginary power" (article 251).

39. Between 1972 and 1981, the situation of the *nganga* improved. Today, without being legally recognized in the strict sense, they do have some recognition, provided they are members of a regional association monitored by the administrative authorities of the government.

40. See de Rosny, *Ndimsi.* See also Appendix 2, below, "Dreams."

41. De Rosny, *Ndimsi*, pp. 235–40.

42. See Meinrad Hebga et al., *Croyance et guérison* (Yaoundé: CLE, 1973), "Le jengu de Claire."

43. When the word *dibunje* receives a high-tone accent on the second syllable it means, literally, "little sprout."

44. The everyday parlance of the Douala has a myriad of expressions to describe the infinite variety of nuances in facial coloring. Between the extremes—"weak tea" and "pure ebony"—there was every possible blend of yellows, reds, and browns, all carefully distinguished terminologically—"sheepskin," "bronze," "tobacco," "tan," and so on—not to overlook a tint referred to as "doe belly" (Ventre-de-biche). I avoided this language myself, however, for two reasons. First, one and the same "black" face can itself have several different shades. Secondly, living intimately with this population, I no longer "realized" that they were "colored." In fact it has happened that I have asked an African where we could have met before—only to realize that it was simply that he reminded me of some white acquaintance of mine.

45. Madame Mylla lived in Paris. She sent love chains to the city of Douala and other large French-speaking cities of Africa for 750 CFA francs, good luck keys for the same price, and Chinese medallions that "found employment for anyone out of work" for 1,000 CFA francs (20 French francs).

46. Their names were not recorded. Nor was that of the school attended by the boy. There are between 20,000 and 30,000 high-school students in Douala.

47. I asked him this question because I suspected that he was here translating into French the word his own language used for the spirits of the ancestors and giving it its traditional denotation. I was mistaken.

48. It had been a long time since I had heard of Madame Mylla, referred to by Dieudonné sometimes as "she" and sometimes as "they." (My own conjecture was that of a cynical, mustached businessman.) And so my colleague Pierre-Marie Mesnier, a former teacher at the Libermann School and an old associate of mine in the Kribi research, then my companion and friend in Paris, paid an impromptu visit to Madame Mylla's address, which any number of secondary-school students in Douala had in their possession. Here are his impressions:

"Madame Mylla is a short, rather plump little woman (dyed hair, the 'fine housewife of the North of France' type). Comfortable interior, in the worst taste. She told me she was seventy-three. To me she had seemed no more than sixty-five, because of her spryness—an older woman's coquettish charm?) She received me politely. I expected a somewhat dark interior, a 'crystal ball' atmosphere, and had even expected to have to say I hadn't come for a consultation. I quickly learned she did no consultations here, and lavished her counsels, by correspondence alone, exclusively on an African (French-speaking) public.

"Here are some bits and pieces of what she told me—things I jotted down right after I left. I think they'll tell you more than my simply going on with my description:

" 'I provide moral education for these poor Africans in the colonies. They're like big babies, you know. . . .

" 'I have an authority with them, a kind of domination, that I wouldn't have with whites. I keep them from doing evil things, like stealing, and so forth.

" 'I'm not into costume jewelry [she repeated this a number of times in the course of our conversation]. First I analyze a person's character and tendencies [by handwriting and astrology], then I lock up in a ring the fluid that will help them struggle against their bad inclinations. . . .'

"She added that she had had a 'gift' for helping others ever since she was a child. It was the priest who baptized her—who was also her cousin and an ophthalmologist!—who revealed this to her.

"She placed great emphasis on the absence of magic in what she did—nothing to pass exams with (pens, ballpoints, etc.), no predicting the future, and no magic wallets that keep refilling themselves with cash. I had no impression she was trying to dazzle me—she spoke of her activities as if she had been talking about being a waitress.

"Does she believe all this herself? It's difficult to say. . . . But she certainly has nothing of the schemer about her. She's convinced that, if she were to go to Africa, *multitudes* would come to testify to their gratitude. I have the impression that she must have a fairly simple way of communicating with them, and that this must be the secret of her success."

49. According to Marie-Cécile and Edmond Ortigues (*Oedipe africain* [Paris: Union générale, 1973]) the relationship between a father and son is not to be conceived along European lines. In Africa, the mechanisms of identification and confrontation on the part of a son vis-à-vis his father tend to be directed toward brothers. The father, who represents the lineage of the ancestors, is unassailable.

But, according to the same authors, the behavior of a boy who has gone to school, and whose father has been assimilated into the modern world, as is the case here, will certainly be closer to that of a European adolescent.

50. *Haec prima sit agendorum regula: sic Deo fide, quasi rerum successus omnis a te, nihil a Deo penderet; ita tamen iis operam omnem admovere, quasi tu nihil, Deus omnia sit facturus* (Gaston Fessard, *La dialectique des Exercises Spirituels de S. Ignace de Loyola* [Paris: Aubier, 1956], p. 305; cf. pp. 306–63).

51. A pangolin is a small toothless mammal whose body is covered with large, imbricated, horny scales. The scales are used in divination.

52. All present understood French, but I felt it would be best to have their friend Oyono translate what I had to say into their native tongue. I thought it might sound too blunt in French.

53. For the political context of the rebellion, see J.-F. Bayart, *L'Etat au Cameroun*, "L'embrasement du pays bamiléké," pp. 64ff.

54. Odette Bialley, *Un témoin de la foi—Gabriel Soh, jeune chrétien bamikéké, 1938–1959* (Yaoundé, n.d.), p. 53.

55. Two diacritical marks will be used in this and the next chapter to indicate (a rough approximation of) certain Bamendjou sounds: ü will indicate a French *u* or German *ü* sound; ö will indicate a French *eu* or German *ö* sound. There is a scholarly transcription of the Bamiléké languages, established by V. Futchantse, but it is not necessary for our purposes.

56. *Dethum* is called *nsote* in Douala. On the coast it is a sign of blessing. It contains black seeds, which have the sweet taste of licorice.

57. All conversations, interviews, and monologues were recorded on tape, and translated daily by Patrice Tankam, native of Bamendjou and a student in Yaoundé, currently on vacation. He did not accompany me, but he later told me exactly what had been said, and thus supplemented the commentaries that others gave me piecemeal on the spot.

58. The leaf of the banana, and, especially, of the *pankhwijum* (in Douala, *dibokuboku la makom*).

59. *Khamsi*s just as chiefs and mothers of twins, hold their power from God (*Si*).

60. Jean must move quickly, before the son of his father's killer undergoes a similar treatment and himself says, "I am washed of misfortune." Jean must be treated and utter the declaration first; otherwise his counterpart could find the success in life that could have been Jean's.

61. Twice I have assisted at the "Great Dance [*Taü*] of the panthers": once on the occasion of a feast of reconciliation after the events of the guerrilla war, on February 24, 1974; and again the following year at the end of the traditional austerity period *(ngu nekang)*, on May 18, 1975. Fifty masked notables danced—before a jeering crowd that was nevertheless impressed—in splendid panther skins, as if to say, "Look out, here we are, panthers!"

62. This refers to the common gesture performed by anyone who feels uneasy or anxious about anything: they grasp a handful of earth and lick it. The same gesture is used in taking an oath.

63. This is perhaps the most important ritual leaf on the coast. In Bamendjou, widows wear it on their heads for nine weeks after the death of a husband. Children, who undergo a rite of protection *(tchop-nekang)* once in their lives, must also wear it for nine weeks. (Today the time may be shortened. "What can you do; the children say they have to play soccer!" railed one who performed the rite.)

64. I managed to grasp the highlights, thanks to the model I had studied in Douala. First there is the purification by water, then the transformation into a panther, then the daubing with eggs, and finally the little packet for the journey. All these rites, I could see, served to protect the young man against his adversaries, to be sure, but more especially to reestablish good terms with his father, without which there would be no social equilibrium possible for him in his life. Later I would be given the key to this first day, and the reason why it did not suffice: "Water washes the face; it does not wash away misfortune."

65. When a baby fails to thrive, and wants to eat only sweet bananas, it is said to have "gone to the kingdom of the children." The *khamsi* ascends to that kingdom by night to attempt to persuade the child to return to its parents. This is why she says she does not sleep.

66. Cannibal sorcery is more ancient than the sorcery of traffic in human beings *(ekong)*. It has greater impact in the more traditional rural areas.

67. Here are three examples of these conversations:

(1) The *khamsi*: "Mammy, who's the one accused of *sa* [human traffic sorcery]?"
The Mammy: "Somebody in our house is accused of *sa*."
Khamsi: "Is it your father's son?"
Mammy: "Yes . . . ."
Khamsi: "Well, it's with good reason."

(2) The *khamsi*: "How are you related to somebody in the jurisdiction here?"
A young man: "He's my father."
Khamsi: "Are there four of you?"
Young man: "There were, but there are only three now. One died."

(3) The *khamsi*: "Are you married to a man with a *ja* [little interior courtyard where funeral ceremonies are performed]?"
A young woman: "Yes."
Khamsi: "Who's all the talk been about in your house these days?"
Young woman: "There's just one thing bothering us."
Khamsi: "What's been bothering you recently? Did somebody die?"
Young woman: "It's about a stepbrother of mine. . . ."

68. Jean Fotsing was soon to find employment in a tavern in Mbalmayo, a little town on the outskirts of Yaoundé.

69. See D. Paulme, ed., *Classes et Associations d'âge en Afrique de l'Ouest* (Paris: Plon, 1971), pp. 308ff.

70. See the comparative table of the two ceremonies in Appendix 4.

71. "There is religion when human beings . . . are capable of relating the totality of their existence . . . to its ultimate foundation: the Absolute, which *non facit numerum* with that existence, because it transcends that existence" (Georges Morel).

72. Until one has passed the appropriate tests, one is a *nkantsö,* but not yet a *khamsi.* This was the case with the child who assisted at Jean Fotsing's photo. As for Pauline Nkwedum, "God had long since settled his choice upon her," the aunt told me. And Chief Sokoundjou said, "They stand out because they have a special talent from birth. Often they have two teeth on top that push the first ones out. At three years old they start telling stories about their grandfathers." God's brand, or mark, upon a person from a very early age is not reserved for *khamsi*s, however. Here is what Gabriel Soh's mother said of him after he was executed by the guerrillas: "I was stupefied to hear this eight- or ten-month old child pronounce words in our

language correctly, and to see him walk long before the normal age" (Bialley, *Témoin de la foi*).

73. *Mama mo'jwo:* A very large thing without precise form or shape; a "mass."

74. "Big thing *(mo'jwo)* lying in front of me"—that is, forming a screen, preventing her from taking an interest in anything else.

75. "I keep being told . . .": Literally, "They" or "one *(po)* tell(s) me. . . ." *Po* designates, simultaneously, God *(Si),* the ancestral household divinities, the spirits, and all the intermediaries.

76. "My Creator God" *(Mboo),* regularly translated "angel" by Christian accommodation, today seems to designate God both as creator of, and as exercising providence over, a particular person. The language of the *khamsi* here does not justify entering further into any distinction between *Si,* usually translated "God," and *Mboo.*

77. But I have seen the *khamsi* take heavier men than Jean Fotsing on her shoulder and spin like a top with them on her back.

78. The main parts of this account have appeared in *Recherches de Science Religieuse,* 63:1 (Jan.-Mar., 1975).

79. Two drums with leather heads, a wooden clapper drum, a battery of gongs and bells, and bamboo stick castanets.

80. Evidence of this conviction was furnished me by a member of the Libermann senior class who was undergoing treatment at the hands of another *nganga.* He used exactly the same terms in describing the divination séance. Here is what I recorded on tape: "The *nganga* began by telling me that I hadn't always been in my parents' hands—that is, that it hadn't always been my parents who paid my lodging. I answered that this was true. And he said, 'You've lived in Samba and Ngamba [faraway localities]. At Samba, you weren't in your parents' hands, but at Ngamba you were in your parents hands.' "

"He actually named the towns?" I asked my student.

"He didn't actually name the towns; he said, 'When you finished your primary school you went to live with your parents.' *I understood* that he was talking about Samba first, then Ngamba."

I consider this testimony valuable because circumstances do not usually permit the mechanisms of divination to appear this clearly. The diviner is deemed to say less than he knows.

81. It took me a good long while to discover the barely perceptible signals by which Loe would suddenly stop the music. He would make a little hook with his right foot in the course of a dance step, or else he would hold his toe in a certain way. I was not the only one to have a hard time with it. Sometimes an unfortunate musician would play his instrument a second too long, and become the butt of a little wave of pleasantries that passed through the gathering.

82. Nkongo translated, "Even if you don't want to say what's in the bottom of your belly, in the end I'll force you to reveal it, make no mistake!"

83. Just at this moment I caused a disturbance. I had a flash camera with me, lying unobtrusively alongside my tape recorder, in the hope of being able to take some shots of this treatment, because I wanted to study it with particular care. At the end of the *esa,* I thought the right moment had come, so I made a little sign to Loe that I would take my picture now. When the family members saw what I intended to do, they wrapped themselves up like monks, and the uncle looked as if he might simply walk out. I quickly laid the camera aside. It had been rather easy for me to photograph ceremonies if I was simply an observer, as at Kribi; but as part of

the ceremony, as I was here, all my deeds and gestures were taken to have some meaning. What were they afraid of? Did they think I might aim my flash as a burst of flame at someone? In any case, to my great regret, I have no photograph of this treatment.

84. The *miengu* have retained their therapeutic function all up and down the coast. Before the German colonization, at the end of the nineteenth century, this function extended to all sectors of social life. A secret *jengu* society, reserved to the nobility, moderated the power of chiefs. It had a special language, known only to the initiated. See Ittmann, *Esquisse de la langue de l'association culturelle des nymphes au bord du Mont-Cameroun* (Paris: Société d'Etudes Linguistiques, 1972). See also R. Bureau, "Le jengu, association de culte," in *Recherches et études camerounaises: Ethno-sociologie religieuse des Douala et apparentés* (Yaoundé: IRCAM, 1962), pp. 105-39.

85. R. Bastide: "The trance is a phenomenon of societal pressure, and not a nervous phenomenon." The trance is the quintessence of a culture, and is not to be explained merely by physiological or psychological causes. Nevertheless, let us note the importance of certain more evident factors: the personal history of each of the possessed, the strength of their convictions, the influence of the night, the conditioning of the rhythms, the stage setting, muscular tension, and the use of drugs. These elements, and many others, provoke a hysteriform change in cases of real trance. For a physiological analysis of the phenomenon, see H. Aubin, "Les méchanismes de la transe," *Evolution psychiatrique*, special no., March 1948, pp. 191-215.

86. "It's a bit difficult to explain in words," Nkongo told me. ". . . It's a certain way of dribbling your hands on the drum, and then there's the sound. When you move your hands around, you change the sound. Sometimes they put their heel on the drumhead, then take it off, then put it back."

87. This plant has "only" a symbolic value, not a medical one in the strict sense. It is used in the ritual of the enthronement of a chief, and in the yearly Douala festival of the *ngondo*. In former times it was planted at the entrance of a village, where the ritual food of the dead was also placed—hence its name, "(sugar) cane of the dead." It is also called *mwandando*. In Western scientific nomenclature it is *costus afer*, a zingiberaceous spice. It is a sign of peace, all along the coast, as well as in the western part of the country, among the Bamiléké. The *khamsi* called it *nkwengkang*. It is similar to ordinary sugar cane.

88. Recall that there are two broad categories of sorcery: one of traffic in human beings, and the other of cannibalism. Vampire sorcery (to which the *khamsi* refers), like caiman sorcery, is a variation on cannibalism.

89. The reptile caiman does not devour its victim immediately, but carries the carcass off to a hiding place in the hollow of a steep bank.

90. One must really want to be healed, to be able to submit to a trial like this. Loe's youngest wife had her whole back burned because she turned away. A few days later, hearing her complain about it to me, Loe remarked, half in earnest, half in gibe, "It's her own fault; she was playing sorceress!"

91. One night, I recall, an old fisherman of the Wouri was seated exactly where Kwedi sat tonight, for the same kind of treatment. While Nkongo and his assistants were slaughtering the goat, the old fisherman addressed it in these terms (while he too avoided looking at it): "May my enemies follow you to the place of the dead, my goat, and when they arrive, welcome them with butting horns!"

92. Some of the active substances taken from tropical or subtropical plants: yohimbine, ibogaine, ouabaine, eserine, vinblastine, reserpine.

93. Georges Morel, *Question d'homme: l'autre* (Paris: Aubier Montaigne, 1977), p. 77.

94. *Dieu aujourd'hui* (Paris: Desclée, 1977), p. 215.

95. Elimbi, Loe's eldest son, who had been treated for ill luck, had been absent during Kwedi's treatment.

96. See Gilbert Rouget, *La musique et la transe* (Paris: Gallimard, 1980), pp. 66ff.

97. See René Gouellain, *Douala, ville et histoire* (Paris: Institut d'ethnologie, Musée de l'homme, 1975), pp. 156ff.

98. "The ceremonial taboo of kings is *ostensibly* the highest honor and protection for them, while *actually* it is a punishment for their exaltation, a revenge taken on them by their subjects" (Sigmund Freud, *Totem and Taboo* [Standard Edition of the Complete Psychological Works of Sigmund Freud, James Strachey, ed., London: Hogarth, 1955], vol. 13, p. 151).

99. Here are some examples:

"The tide comes in at its own time; at its own time the *jengu* comes in."

"Boat, I've pulled you; *miengu* boat, I've pulled you; I've pulled all the *miengu*, and I've pulled you" (a song for Hélène Yambe).

"Freely I go to the bottom of the water. The distance is great."

Songs about the dead:

"I wept, and I did not know that the dead were not human beings." Or: "I wept, and I did not know that [Loe] was not a human being." (That is to say, if the dead had any humanity, they would come when they hear me weeping and calling them.)

"Death does not take a tree, but a human being with branches [i.e., members]."

A song about sorcery:

"O my *jengu*, where were you? See how the *ekong* followers have chained you!"

100. "For the Fang of Gabon, one who has *evu* [access to the power of *ndimsi*] is either a *nem* or a *ngolo*. The difference between the *nem* and the *ngolo* is that the former makes use of his or her knowledge for personal advantage, whereas the latter is content merely to see, as it were, and does not exercise the power that flows from seeing" (Bureau, *Péril blanc* [Paris: L'Harmattan, 1978], p. 143).

101. A meaningful use of the word "dream" in its weaker sense *(ndoti)*. "Dreams" properly so-called are *jene la ndoti*.

102. Johannes Ittmann gives a number of scholarly references: *andasonia digitata L., baphia nitida Lodd, entandrophragm utile Daw.* See his *Wörterbuch der Duala-Sprache* (Berlin: Dietrich Keimer, 1976).

103. According to our elderly guide, the word *ngopange* is borrowed from the Pongo Songo, a language similar to Douala, spoken on the banks of the Sanaga, his native territory. It is the name of a rhizophoraceous plant, *anopyxis klaineana,* "a very large tree, commonly found all the way from Sierra Leone to Gabon to the Belgian Congo [Zaire] and Ubangi-Chari. . . . A tree growing to 40 m. in height and 1.2 m. in diameter. Trunk: straight, and perfectly cylindrical, spreading out only at the base. Bark: grayish, smooth or rough, very thick (to 3 cm.), reddish within . . ." (André Aubréville, *La flore forestière de la Côte-d'Ivoire* (Nogent-sur-Marne: Centre technique forestier tropical, 1959), vol. 3.

104. "The ancestors, and the forces contrary to them, coexist. The latter seek to keep you with them in their sphere. If you leave, you are an escaped prisoner. If you turn about, you risk causing the failure of the favorable forces that are thrusting you outside, for you are giving the impression that you wish to remain in the other

world, that of the ancestors. This means the failure of everything that has been done" (from a letter of Dicka Akwa nya Bonambela).

105. This hereditary power is concretized, for the Beti of central and eastern Cameroon, in the *evu,* conceived of as a little crustacean, like a crab, and thought to live in the abdomen of the person who enjoys this power. There is a myth regarding the creation and proliferation of the *evu,* which the Douala seem not to remember. See Louis Mallart, "Ni dos ni ventre," *L'Homme,* vol. 15, no. 2 (April–June 1975), pp. 35–65. The *evu* recalls the Bamiléké *tok.* The Douala word *ewusu* surely derives from it.

106. Din was having me join him for three kinds of rites. There were rites of communication, with words pronounced before his display of objects (barks, for example, and utensils such as the mirror), and addressed to the ancestors. There were rites of purification, consisting in ablutions with water in which herbs and barks have been steeping. Finally, there were rites for provoking dreams, centering on the preparation of a bark to be placed under my pillow.

107. The *tabernanthe iboga.* See Peter T. Furst, ed., *Flesh of the Gods: The Ritual Use of Hallucinogens* (New York: Praeger, 1972), pp. 240–60. See also R. Bureau, "La religion d'Eboga" (University of Abidjan, 1971).

108. "We have had occasion to study, in all detail, more than 50,000 dreams, of persons ill and healthy, especially from the viewpoint of the relationship between these dreams and the total life experience of the dreamer. . . . Those who devote several hours a day to the intense analysis of dreams, their own and those of others, will discover that it is only after a training period of about a year and a half that they will be capable of inserting their own dreams into personal life-experience" (Harold Schultz-Hencke, *Analyse des rêves* [Paris: Payot, 1954], Preface).

109. These juices had been taken from the following plants, as identified in the Yaoundé national herbological manual: for the nose, *trephania sp.* (menispermaceous); for the head, *piper unbellatum* (piperaceous); for the eyes, *bidens bipinnata* (asteraceous). Barks for the nose, head, and eyes: *musamba* (Yasa for "unveil"— this is a divining tree); *pycnanthus angolensis* (myristiraceous); *bovenga* (the great ritual tree—in Ewondo, *oveng); copaifera tessmannii* (caesalpinaceous), together with some hairs of a breed of dog having marks over the eyes as if it had four eyes, considered a sign of being able to see over great distances.

110. Compare this with the ancient Ewondo rite called *melan,* the rite of initiation into the cult of the ancestors: "Candidates seat themselves on the trunk of an umbrella tree lying in the court. They are brought scrapings from the wood of a bush called the *engela.* They chew these scrapings, together with pimiento berries, *while looking fixedly at the sun"* (T. Tsala, *Moeurs et coutumes des Ewondo* [Etudes camerounaises, no. 56, Yaoundé, 1957], p. 70; italics added).

111. There is a great current interest in obtaining lists of medicines from *ngangas,* together with directions for their use. A collection of a thousand medical recipes, *Malema Makom,* of which I possess a considerable portion, is much in demand. But initiation is ignored. The use of these recipes apart from their proper psychocultural context paves the way to painful disappointments and excessively severe judgments on the efficacy of traditional medicine.

112. The *manga*—the goats belonging to the water ancestors, the *miengu*—are manatees. Thus the earthly family continues to live with its domestic animals, after death, in the universe of the waters.

113. Misfortune (in pidgin, *bad luck*—in Douala, *mbeu'a nyolo)* does not mean

sin, but rather whatever *other* persons have "cast upon" me to harm me.

114. See M. Hebga, *Sorcellerie, chimère dangereuse. . .?* (Abidjan: INADES, 1979).

115. According to the notes I took, at two o'clock in the morning, in my first dream, a group of us Jesuit priests are to build a dwelling. The place chosen is a deep hole, with low walls outlining the shape of a house. The others find the place ideal, but I disagree. In the second dream, we are pole fishing on the bank of a canal. We are not in Africa. The others catch nothing, but I catch a great number of small fish. My companions inform me that there are large fish farther down the canal. Then I catch a fish with a little head and enormous fins, but it goes flapping away over the ground and escapes. I manage to contain my fear of being bitten; the fish bites me, but the bite does not harm me.

116. I took what remained of my portion of this dish and carried it home. Our cook, who was aware of my involvement with *ngangas*, recognized the plantain, cooked in a characteristic sauce *(miele ma sese)* with certain chicken parts, and she said, simply, "You're having your eyes opened!"

117. The themes were still the same—dreams of uproars among irrepressible students, dreams of brawls among Africans, dreams of nameless wars.

118. These three herbs turned out to be identifiable as asteraceous plants. The leaves used by Madola in Kribi to open my eyes were likewise asteraceous.

119. Freud and Girard make the same point, each in his own fashion—the former in *Beyond the Pleasure Principle* (New York: Norton, 1975), the latter in *Violence and the Sacred* (Johns Hopkins University Press, 1977).

120. A *nganga* who was unacquainted with Din later recounted to me the manner in which he himself bestows double sight: "It's a ceremony that always takes place around midnight. You have to have a goat along. Some insist on a sorcerer for opening eyes, but those who know about such things sometimes just ask for a goat. The one who's going to do this for you has spent a long time getting the herbs and roots and barks ready. All this stuff has been mixed, and then, in the place you're supposed to meet, this person puts it in your eyes. Afterward, you get some time to rest. When you put your head on the pillow you're supposed to slip the bark of a certain tree under it. You have another way of seeing. Night gets to be like day in front of you. You see what's happening and what's already happened." This account was proof for me that Din had indeed taken me through the ordinary initiation procedures. The only variation had been that Din had performed the nocturnal rites on the goat alone, for it would have been impossible for me to pass the night in his house without attracting attention.

121. The spiritual exercises of Ignatius Loyola. See, e.g., David L. Fleming, ed., *The Spiritual Exercises of Saint Ignatius: A Literal Translation and a Contemporary Reading* (Saint Louis: Institute of Jesuit Sources, 1978); Gaston Fessard, *La dialectique des exercices spirituels de Saint Ignace* (Paris: Aubier Montaigne, 1966).

122. *Institut Africain pour le Développement Economique et Social,* African Institute for Economic and Social Development.

123. The clearest sign of the presence of *ekong* sorcery is for someone to dream of being carried off toward the sea, hands bound. Is this a phantasmal representation of the memory of the slave trade? The appearance of a horse in a dream likewise provokes panic: the German invasion a century ago?

Other Orbis Titles . . .

THE WORLD IN BETWEEN
Christian Healing and the Struggle for Spiritual Survival
by E. Milingo

When Archbishop Emmanuel Milingo resigned in 1982 from the Roman Catholic see of Lusaka, Zambia, which he had occupied since 1969, many people must have wondered what sort of man this could be, whose gifts of healing and exorcising spirits generated a controversy that reached to the Vatican. *The World in Between* tells the story of his healing ministry in response to the spiritual needs of Zambian Christians, who are still deeply embedded in traditional religions. Mona Macmillan, an English Roman Catholic writer, provides an introduction, epilogue, and linking passages describing Milingo's life and recent ordeals.

Emmanuel Milingo is a Special Delegate to the Pontifical Commission on Migration, Refugees, and Tourism.

Item no. 354   *144pp. Paper $5.95*

JESUS AND THE WITCHDOCTOR
An Approach to Healing and Wholeness
by Aylward Shorter

Modern scientific medicine has achieved wonders in healing human ills. But its benefits are unevenly available throughout the world. And inevitably its emphasis on physical healing has overshadowed the healing of other ills, social, psychological, emotional and spiritual. The world continues to be in desperate need of total healing.

Aylward Shorter, anthropologist, theologian and Christian missionary sees two sources for a restoration of human wholeness. One comes from his long experience in black Africa with its still surviving sense of interdependence with the natural world, of local community and its traditions of healing. The other is the person of Jesus Christ, his presence in the sacraments of the Christian church and his revelation of the healing power of God.

Both the black cultures and the church receive their share of criticism in this penetrating study but in both the author sees new hope for healing a flawed and fragmented world.

Item no. 225   *256pp. Paper $10.95*

CHRISTIANITY IN CULTURE
by Charles H. Kraft

"This book will be welcomed by any biblical or theological student with serious interest in cross-cultural perspectives. The author has brought together here almost all possible information on Christianity in culture. Part one is devoted to the clarification of perspective, especially the needs in view and the reality under scrutiny. Part two divides the cultural matrix into the culturally individual and human community, explained through various cultural forms, patterns and processes. Parts three through six deal with the divine action, the way divine revelation affects cultural transformation and its transcultural significance." *Worldmission*

Item no. 075 *463pp. Paper $14.95*

WEST AFRICAN CHRISTIANITY
The Religious Impact
by Lamin Sanneh
This is a broad historical study of the development of Christianity in West Africa. Past historians tended to glorify the white missioners to Africa; many contemporary historians almost vilify them. Sanneh details both the strength and weakness of the European outreach. Selected by the Editors of the *International Bulletin of Missionary Research* as one of the Fifteen Outstanding Books of 1983 for Mission Studies.

Item no. 703 *304pp. Paper $11.95*

CHRISTIANITY WITHOUT FETISHES
An African Critique and Recapture of Christianity
by F. Eboussi Boulaga
From one of the leading theologians in West Africa, a penetrating analysis of the inculturation of Christianity in Africa. Eboussi Boulaga rejects as a fetish manufactured in the West the Christianity imposed upon and adopted by the African churches. He mounts a constructive and comprehensive African alternative. Essential reading for academics, ecumenists, and missioners.

"Once the depth of Eboussi's critique begins to sink in, once one realizes that inculturation has precious little to do with liturgical vestments and musical instruments but rather with very basic worldviews, with basic human values and indeed with the sharing of power, then the significance of this book begins to dawn. This is a threatening book. It cuts to the quick."

Simon E. Smith, S.J., Jesuit Refugee Service, Nairobi

Item no. 432 *256pp. Paper $11.95*

THEOLOGY IN AFRICA
by Kwesi Dickson
Discerning African Christians have long wrestled with the validity of the expression of Christianity in Africa and have observed the need for a culturally authentic church and theology. This landmark study by a Ghanaian theologian represents a significant contribution to the formulation of a distinctively African theology. Combining a fresh approach to biblical scholarship with a comprehensive knowledge of African cultures, Kwesi Dickson reveals the strong continuity between the Old Testament ethos and African life and thought.

"Kwesi Dickson is among the most important of the African theologians writing today. An understanding of his contribution to African theology is indispensable for all those who wish to be part of the international theological discourse."

James H. Cone

Item no. 508 *240pp. Paper $9.95*